Nursing in Primary Care
A Handbook for Students

edited by

Naomi A. Watson

and

Carol Wilkinson

palgrave

First published 2001 by
PALGRAVE
Houndmills, Basingstoke, Hampshire RG21 6XS and
175 Fifth Avenue, New York, N.Y. 10010
Companies and representatives throughout the world

PALGRAVE is the new global academic imprint of
St. Martin's Press LLC Scholarly and Reference Division and
Palgrave Publishers Ltd (formerly Macmillan Press Ltd).

ISBN 0–333–78192–9 paperback

This book is printed on paper suitable for recycling and made from fully managed and sustained forest sources.

A catalogue record for this book is available from the British Library.

Editing and origination by
Aardvark Editorial, Mendham, Suffolk

10 9 8 7 6 5 4 3 2 1
10 09 08 07 06 05 04 03 02 01

Printed and bound in Great Britain by
Creative Print & Design (Wales), Ebbw Vale

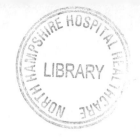

The Late Charles Iddisah
formerly Senior Lecturer, DeMontfort University

I initially met Charles when I was a student nurse in the West Midlands during the early 1980s. He was developing his skills as a tutor with a rather mixed group of precocious adolescents.

We were both equally surprised and amazed to meet again during the final eighteen months of his life. Arriving at the Department of Nursing and Midwifery at DeMontfort University, we immediately recognised each other. He was so pleased that his contribution had made a difference to a now fully fledged Senior Lecturer!

We worked very well as a team, and I was grateful for his guidance, support and mentorship during my introduction to the Managing Care module.

Charles was a warm, kind and patient man. He always had a smile, and whenever invited into his office, one could never escape without a look at his latest acquisition of family photographs, identity badges or library cards.

The staff at DeMontfort experienced a proud moment during 1998, when Charles was applauded for his services to the Territorial Army, to which he was as dedicated as he was to his students and the advancement of the field of nursing.

Charles was an initial contributor to this book. The chapter entitled Death, Dying and Bereavement, completed by Claire Henry, will come to serve as a poignant reminder that he shall not be forgotten.

CAROL WILKINSON

Contents

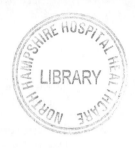

List of figures and tables

Figures

Tables

List of contributors

Jill Barr	Principal Lecturer, DeMontfort University.
Eileen Buchanan	Formerly Senior Lecturer, DeMontfort University.
Jenny Dowling	Assistant Director of Nursing, Leicester.
Paula Heighton	Community General Manager, Leicester.
Claire Henry	Project Manager, Leicester Royal Infirmary.
Sam Maurimootoo	Senior Lecturer and Provost, DeMontfort University.
Danny Pertab	Senior Lecturer, Pathway Leader Dip/HE Nursing (Adult Branch), DeMontfort University.
Lesley Styring	Lecturer/Practitioner, Sheffield Hallam University.
Tom Tait	Senior Lecturer, DeMontfort University.
Donna Young	Principal Lecturer, DeMontfort University.

Preface

This book was written specifically for pre-registration nursing students. The aim is to help them understand the issues which are of relevance to them while they undertake their community practice. This should fill a huge gap in the literature base, which has tended to focus on qualified practitioners. The style of the text is interactive, with varied activities to encourage students to explore concepts for themselves as an aid to independent learning, and to reflect appropriately for portfolio development.

Those practitioners who are supporting students should also find the text useful, especially as a tool to help structure the learning menus of the students they are supervising and assessing in community settings. Equally all students who find themselves caring for patients in the community for the first time will be given a sound introduction to the topic by this text.

The start of the new millennium brought with it a continuation of significant changes, which are having tremendous impact on care delivery in primary care settings. All community nurses are required to contribute significantly to the changing focus of care delivery, not only by delivering high quality care, but also by influencing policy decisions at local and national levels. To do this effectively all students will need to have a sound basic preparation, considering that, once qualified, it is now generally possible to go directly into the community as a first level nurse. The need to provide a service which is as seamless as possible makes it imperative that those who will be working in the acute sectors also have good background knowledge of the issues which face patients, their informal and formal carers and the wider community.

Providing this text for students on community practice should help to supply that necessary background, so that once newly qualified students enter the acute setting, they will have become completely familiar with the concepts of nursing in the primary care sector, and will be able to apply these to their clinical practice. While reference has been made to all members of the primary care team, the text focuses on district nurses, as pre-registration nursing students in the adult branch (for whom the focus of the text was intended) usually spend a major part of their time with this group of nurses. All the activities, however, are equally applicable to most members of the primary health care team, and can be adapted accordingly.

The government's emphasis in documents such as *Making a Difference* (DoH, 1999) and *The NHS Plan* (DoH, 2000) requires clear understanding of the clinical responsibilities required of all nurses and other formal carers. These can only be met if actions are firmly based within the available evidence. This text provides a good starting point for the application of evidence to practice. It is hoped that students and their supervisors will find it a useful tool to help in the generating of new knowledge, to which they must contribute if they are to take the government's policy agenda forward in the new century, and hence make a real contribution to the increased focus on changing practice within primary care.

NAOMI A. WATSON

Acknowledgements

To Carol Wilkinson, who was a tremendous source of support from the initial birth of the idea for this text, through its very difficult patches, to the final submission. Thank you.

To Alan Wood, for help with early computer formatting, which enabled the initial draft of the text to be edited smoothly.

To Jill Barr, in recognition of her editorial contribution in the early stages of the project and her role within the inaugural editorial team.

To Richenda Milton-Thompson, who recognised the potential for a text such as this, and for her invaluable help in making the early drafts take shape. Thank you.

To those members of the team who shared my enthusiasm for the project, and worked consistently to see it through its final stages.

To Balsford Watson, my brother, for providing me with a brief moment of 'respite', when the going got tough, which recharged my batteries to complete the project.

To my daughter Abeni, as an example for you.

NAOMI A. WATSON

The authors and publisher wish to thank the following for permission to use copyright material:

Churchill Livingstone for Table 1.1 adapted from *Community Health Care Nursing* (1998); Lippincott Williams and Wilkins for Table 1.2 adapted from *Introduction to Community Based Nursing*, Hunt and Zurek (1997); EMAP Healthcare for Figure 3.1 adapted from *Nursing Times*, **93**: 52–4 (1997); Roger Hutchinson for Figure 12.2 (1998).

Every effort has been made to trace all the copyright holders but if any have been inadvertently overlooked the publishers will be pleased to make the necessary arrangements at the first opportunity.

List of acronyms

ANS	autonomic nervous system
CFP	common foundation programme
CIS	community information systems
CN	community nurse
CNS	central nervous system
CPD	continuous professional development
CPN	community psychiatric nurse
CRE	Commission for Racial Equality
CSG	Clinical Systems Group
DALY	disability adjusted life year
DN	district nurse
ECG	electrocardiogram
ECR	extra contractual referral
ENB	English National Board
EOC	Equal Opportunities Commission
FIP	financial information planning
GP	general practitioner
GPFH	general practice fundholders
HAZ	health action zone
HE	higher education
HEA	Health Education Authority
HV	health visitor
NHS	National Health Service
NHS and CCA	NHS and Community Care Act
PCG	primary care group
PCT	primary care trust
PHCT	primary health care team
QALY	quality adjusted life year
RAWP	resource allocation working party
RCN	Royal College of Nursing
RRA	Race Relations Act
TLC	tender loving care
UKCC	United Kingdom Central Council for Nursing, Midwifery and Health Visiting
WHO	World Health Organization

Nursing in primary care: an introduction

NAOMI A. WATSON

Learning outcomes

By the end of this chapter you will be able to:

- Identify and define common terminology, which is regularly used.
- Discuss possible variations in meaning, and any significance of usage of the terms.
- Consider the impact of the historical context on the care of sick adults in the community.
- Recognise those factors which contribute to the changing focus of health care, with the emphasis on particular issues for the new millennium.
- Discuss the organisation and delivery of health care in the community and the contribution of district nurses (DNs) within the primary health care team to the process.

Introduction: understanding meanings

The aim of this chapter is to increase awareness and understanding of those factors which may influence the provision of nursing care in primary care settings, with specific emphasis on the care of adults.

Providing care to sick people in the community has been a feature of health services provision for some considerable time. Because of the way this care has emerged over the years, it has had its own brand of controversial issues regarding the way it is organised. The focus, scope and development has not only been the subject of much discussion and legislation, but it has carried with it the use of a number of overlapping terms, which could have a variety of meanings depending on the context in which they are being used. One could argue that some terms have been the subject of 'overuse', and as a result, may have created some confusion regarding meanings, not only for professionals, but also for students and users of the service.

It will be important for your experience as a student in the community that you have a sound understanding of the variety of terms in use, and how these terms are interpreted by members of the primary health care team (PHCT), patients and their carers. As you read the literature, you will no doubt come across the different terms. Being able to identify the context and recognise their meanings is a key factor in helping you to gain a good grasp of the way they have influenced what happens in community practice settings.

Perhaps one of the oldest terms, which may not be referred to very much at present, is 'home nursing'; another commonly used term is 'community care'. Additionally, we have 'community nursing' and 'community health care/community health nursing'. The importance of ensuring that you are clearly aware of the way the terms are being used cannot be over-stressed, especially considering that the meanings may not always accompany their use. Activity 1.1 should help you explore these meanings and the way they may be perceived, before going into your placement:

Student Activity 1.1

♦ Using a jotting sheet, or a sheet from your portfolio, think about the terms used above.

♦ For each of the terms used, write down what you think is its meaning.

♦ Do this exercise as an individual, on your own.

Now you have put your own thoughts on paper, this could form a basis from which to further explore the terms with others.

Your own understanding of the terms in use will be based on a number of factors, which may include your personal experiences or the experiences of friends and family members, as you have understood them. You may also be drawing on knowledge from other modules or past courses you have undertaken. You may not have stopped to think about this before, and could have thought that the terms are quite easy to define. The question is whether perceptions of their meanings are the same, even between staff of the same discipline. The next step is for you to explore this in Activity 1.2.

Student Activity 1.2

♦ Choose a few of your friends, peers and family members and primary care workers (about four or five, where possible).

♦ Try to ensure that they represent a varied group in terms of age, gender, job and social circumstances.

♦ Ask for their views on the meanings of the terms you have defined.

♦ Check for any similarities or differences with your own earlier definitions, and the possible reasons for these.

♦ Make a note of the meanings they identified for you, in your portfolio or in your notes, and see how these compare with definitions from the literature. Make a note of why you think the terms may confuse some people, especially service users.

It is possible that the term 'home nursing', which may still be used by some voluntary organisations such as the Red Cross, is meant to imply care that is being provided by someone perhaps without formal qualifications, not a nurse. Such a person could be a friend, family member or volunteer, depending on the context. The confusion surrounding the term is shown by the English National Board (1992) referring to the need for student nurses to have experience of 'home nursing' as part of their training. So how should this term best be understood? Does it imply that the care being provided is 'below the level of the real thing?' And if this is the case, where do we place the vast numbers of carers, who support their friends, families and neighbours by providing a large measure of care, including some clinical procedures, when nurses are not available?

If the term 'home nursing' implies informal provision of care, by people other than nurses, then the term 'community nursing' suggests a concept of care which is delivered in an organised manner by a group of suitably qualified practitioners. But could the term be perceived to cover just the role of the district nurse (DN)? This may then be understood to mean care which is intermittent, and is not just about general support. Certainly, the concept of 'formal support' by the professionals may be implied, but is it possible that this may be misunderstood? For example, if a team of professionals are providing this service, will they all have similar qualifications, and what will be the perceptions about this provision and those responsible for it, by patients and service users on the receiving end of the care being delivered? You may be aware that skill mixing is now a feature of formal care delivery practices in all settings. The implications of this for patients and carers, and their understanding of the processes, may also influence what is being perceived.

'Community care' is perhaps the term which has been most commonly used. It may be seen as having a much wider meaning, not necessarily relating to sickness, but to other aspects of care delivery which could be applicable to the whole community. It could also involve a perception of a range of statutory, voluntary and private services, which may or may not be easily and/or readily available. This will be further explored later.

You may have been able to use these ideas to consider what you discovered in the above activities, in order to help you to identify the variations and the reasons for them. If you were to do a wider sample of exploration of the terms, you may discover that a range of factors, possibly individual experiences, age, social, cultural and educational background, and even whether or not someone is a nurse, may influence their use, and the way they are understood. Usually, nurses' views are similar, probably because of the way they have been conditioned professionally. This could mean that views may be passed on through this process of socialisation, regardless of their accuracy.

'Community health care' and 'community health nursing' are other widely used terms, and are rapidly replacing older terms. They are certainly identified by the Royal College of Nursing (RCN, 1992) as having clear professional dimensions. These have not, however, been confined to the role of the DN, which should help to raise the awareness of other roles that may be considered from a 'nursing' perspective. In particular, the roles of the health visitor (HV), practice nurse and school nurse may have key influences on the DN's role and on the way the various roles are perceived.

The RCN's definition is as follows:

> Community health nursing is professional nursing directed towards communities or population groups as well as individuals living in the community. It includes assessment of the environmental, social and personal factors, which influence the health status of the targeted population. Its practice incorporates the identification of groups and individuals within the community who require help in maintaining or achieving optimal health. (RCN, 1992, p.6)

When you begin your practice in the community, use the above definition as a measure to see how far the actual practice of the DN and other community nurses is reflected in the statements of the definition. If there are aspects which appear to be missing, try to identify what these are and how they may be incorporated into the day-to-day work of your assessor.

The main aspect of learning here is to remember that the terms commonly used could mean different things to different people depending on a variety of factors. Always be sure to request clarification when you hear them used by your assessor, patients or their carers, so that there will be no confusion about the terms.

Remember that defining 'community,' 'care' and 'health' are important aspects of the learning process, which could also present with problems if not appropriately recognised for possible variations and overlapping views, even in the literature. Turton and Orr (1993) agree that problems of definition exist when looking at the word 'community', but that in a 'nursing specific' understanding it entails describing the location of activities (the geographical area) and then a set of relationships within the environment. These relationships include the social networks which influence the lives of individuals and are important to their experiences. The extent to which these relationships are limited or extended in terms of space is perhaps a worthwhile issue to consider. For example, perceptions of community as a 'place' – the geographical definition may have limitations in terms of the recognition of relationships, which may not have the limitation of space. Social and/or family members that are not local to patients, but with whom they are very much in touch regularly, may be just as important in terms of recognising the contribution to the holistic care of a patient as those who are local to them.

Tadd and Tadd (1997) identify 'community' as a word which is widely used in differing contexts, giving a suggestion of warmth and caring supportiveness, attributes which are meant to be positive and providing advantages, yet many communities experience varied levels of hostility and discrimination, determined by their location and distinct features. Examples of travellers and others, who may face antagonism, are regularly reported in the local and national press. Fostering a 'community' spirit, participating in community activities are terms widely used, which tend to be indicative of the limitation of space in their general understanding. The following areas have been discussed by Turton and Orr (1993) as having specific aspects relevant to location and size:

- Community as social structure, denoting demographic features such as social class and age.

- Community as sentiment, as described by those living within it, or by others about it.

- Community as social activity focusing on available amenities and resources in a particular area.

- Community as locality, mainly denoting physical size and geographical location.

Blackie and Appleby (1998) identify a number of factors (see Table 1.1) which contribute to the creation of group identity and therefore form the basis of a community, arguing that these help members of that group to develop an identity which makes them distinct from others. The consequences could be alienation and social divisions, which may occur both within and outside that community. Blackie and Appleby (1998) also imply that 'community' is not 'community' if it is restricted by space, that is, where people actually reside. This becomes a 'neighbourhood' or locality, usually identifiable as a population unit served by a particular general practitioner.

Whether or not 'community' can be redefined to incorporate the increasing levels of social mobility, which makes distance a key feature in many social relationships, still remains to be tackled by the literature. Tadd and Tadd (1997) agree that the radical changes in the concepts of community are inevitable, given the constant changes in family and social structures, and the increased mobility and technological advances, which minimise drastically the effect of distance.

The word 'care' is also widely used, equally denoting varying perceptions of its meaning. Hennessy and Swain (1997) argue that care and concern are

Table 1.1 Factors contributing to group identity

Culture	Socioeconomic background	Language spoken
Ethnicity	Education	Past experience
Race	Occupation	Unemployment
Religion	Area of residence/region of the country	The law specific to the country where the community exists

Source: Adapted from Blackie and Appleby *Community Health Care Nursing*, Churchill Livingstone (1998).

rightfully a part of the human condition, 'care' being defined as 'having concern for another/others, appropriate regard; a preparedness to act, and, sometimes properly, not to act' (p. 8). The implication here is that this is a planned response, not dependent completely on the emotional involvement, but demanding what they describe as 'serious mental attention'. Recognising stressors, which may lead to occasional vulnerability, and also the fact that some will be permanently vulnerable, should lead to the facilitation of appropriate protection for those concerned. The connection with altruism, and the recognition that the development of a capacity for concern, or care, needs to be fostered from infancy through a facilitating environment are issues which Hennessy and Swain (1997) see as having the potential to be positive contributors to health status generally. Because of the nature of activities which take place in the community, the term 'care' holds clear connotations, not only for the statutory and voluntary services on offer, but for the large army of informal carers who are responsible for 'care by the community'. The neglect of these long-suffering informal carers has been targeted by all the legislation as needing clear action to redress the lack of recognition of their invaluable contribution (DHSS, 1983; DoH, 1998).

Finally, the term 'health' is notoriously known to carry a range of varied meanings, many of which are familiar to most of us. Seedhouse (1986) argues that considering health as a foundation for human achievement provides the scope to ensure that, on a continuum, everyone has an opportunity to achieve, regardless of physical, mental, spiritual emotional or social state. This, of course, lacks the complete balance suggested by the original WHO (1946) definition, which talks about health as being a complete state of physical, mental and social well-being not necessarily always excluding disease. The influences on the capacity of an individual or community to achieve health must be understood and recognised within their context, along with their potential to contribute to unequal outcomes for health within communities. Blackie's (1998) list of factors, which identify groups (Table 1.1), similarly may also serve to identify those specific issues which could militate against individuals and communities and severely undermine their health status. At the very earliest, the Black Report (DHSS, 1980) and, more recently, the Acheson Report (1998) continue to identify health inequalities as a perpetual factor influencing health outcomes. Identifying and tackling inequality in health care must be a major remit for all primary care workers and has to be put in the context of true social justice, which together contribute to a clearer awareness of professional responsibilities (Hennessy and Swain, 1997).

A healthy community should have specific identifiable factors, which, to some extent should be measurable. Hunt and Zurek (1997) identify features of a healthy community, which will have direct impact on health outcomes for individuals and the community (Table 1.2).

Table 1.2 Features of a healthy community

Awareness that we are 'community'	Communication through open channels
Conservation of natural resources	Resources available to all
Recognition of, and respect for, the existence of subgroups	Settling disputes through legitimate mechanisms
Participation of subgroups in community affairs	Participation of citizens in decision making
Preparation to meet crises	A high degree of wellness among its members
Ability to problem solve	

Source: Adapted from Hunt and Zurek *Introduction to Community Based Nursing*, Lippincott-Raven (1997).

Student Activity 1.3

After reading the above points carefully:

◆ Identify those areas that may not be realistic in a community, and give reasons.

◆ Compare the factors identified with the community in which you live now, and have lived before, if they are different.

◆ To what extent are the points also applicable to your community placement?

◆ Discuss these points with a group of your peers, and with your assessor.

◆ Write down the outcomes of your discussion in your portfolio.

Understanding the historical context: 'nursing' versus 'care'

The development of care in the community and community nursing have separate histories, each contributing in different ways to the present state of affairs. It is, however, expedient to recognise that the origins of the community care debate started with the Mental Health Act 1959, which had its concerns not in the care of the physically sick, but for mentally ill and learning-disabled individuals who had long been kept away from the community in institutionalised care environments. We will come back to this later, but at this point, it is worth noting that, long before this development, the care of physically sick individuals had been pioneered from a number of sources. These were mainly informal (that is, provided by people without formal training, such as family members or members of religious bodies) beginning with the priest St Vincent DePaul (1580–1660). He not only undertook this task of caring for the poor, but encouraged his parishioners to do the same by organising them and defining their roles once they had visited a home (Allan and Jolley, 1982). This scheme was quickly extended to other parishes, and the scene for organised care was set.

In 1840, the Deaconesses' movement of Kaiserwerth pioneered the building of a hospital under the direction of Theodor and Frederick Fliedner. This had a cascading effect, which resulted in the setting up of numerous other hospitals and the extension of the service of caring for the sick in their own homes.

In 19th century England, Poor Law committees undertook the task of employing parish nurses to care for sick paupers in their own homes. This was seen as cheaper than transferring them, while they were sick, to the work-houses. Those who were not classed as paupers were cared for by visiting societies or charities and, in 1840, Elizabeth Fry set up an institution based on the concepts of the Deaconesses' movement of Kaiserwerth. The aim was to introduce women of the upper classes to training to care for their own sick. The success of this venture was limited, however, by poor structure and unclear goals (Fraser, 1980).

The present-day service of district nursing is considered by many to have, as its major early source, the work of William Rathbone. This Liverpool resident had been very pleased with the level of care provided by a St Thomas' nurse to his dying wife at home. After her death, he was happy to pay for the services of this nurse to care for poor sick people in his parish. Following consultations with Florence Nightingale, the Liverpool Infirmary was persuaded to train nurses to work in hospital and in the home, with the first batch starting work in Liverpool districts in 1863. Again, good practice was recognised, and many other schemes were set up across the country. In 1874 the Metropolitan Nursing Association was formed, and district nursing became a part of daily care in London. Training was for just over two years, and with strict rules of behaviour, especially regarding the acceptance of gifts, and a wide working remit. District nurses had to be prepared not just to 'nurse', but to cook, clean, wash, or undertake whatever other tasks might be needed within a home to promote recovery of the sick.

Notice here the early recognition of the link between health and social care and the lack of demarcation in the role of the nurse at that time. Note also that using these concepts showed recognition of the health-promoting role of the DN. In fact the role of the DN then was quite extensive, as they undertook work across the ages and in a range of activities relating to the care and health of families.

By 1887, the Queen's Jubilee Institute became the major provider and trainer of district nurses, with all other bodies being asked to amalgamate, but with strict criteria and inspection processes. Of course, this added to the prestige, as DNs became the 'Queen's nurses', if they joined up.

The late 19th and early 20th centuries saw major and rapid changes taking place in the developments within health and social care. Midwives were regulated in 1902, and the National Insurance Act was launched in 1911. Notification of births became compulsory, and by 1911, State Registration for nurses was introduced, becoming the accepted route for entry into district nursing. Note here that by the time the National Health Service (NHS) was introduced in 1948, the title 'home nurse' was also being used to refer to DNs, who were being trained by a number of routes, not necessarily just by the Queen's Institute. Alongside these developments was the recognition of the vast expanse of the DN's work, and the need to assess its feasibility.

By the time these discussions started, the introduction of health visitors in Manchester had already taken place, and school nurses had been introduced in some authorities. By 1968, when the Queen's Institute surrendered its responsibilities for training, the length of this training had been reduced from six months to four months. This drop from two years, to six, and then four months, did not help the professional status of district nurses. But, by 1979, the appointment of a panel of assessors eventually led to a new curriculum being established, with DN training becoming a one-year course, and moving from certificate to diploma level. The recent move of nursing education into the higher education (HE) sector now means that the DN is able to undertake graduate studies in community nursing, enabling the acquisition of skills and knowledge which contribute to the role of a specialist practitioner in community nursing. This should equate their role with those of the school nurse, health visitor and practice nurse, in terms of its importance. The Cumberlege Report (DHSS, 1986) on 'Neighbourhood Nursing' recommended far-reaching reforms of community nursing services, and health needs were considered to be inclusive of the following five key areas:

1. The elderly
2. The disabled
3. The chronically sick
4. The terminally ill
5. Preventive care.

This was a more inclusive approach to the needs of different groups in the community. Identifying them all as 'health needs' may have emphasised the 'nursing' perspectives and increasing focus on the vast numbers of people in the community needing health services. The management of illness has changed, with shorter stays in hospital and longer periods of recovery taking place at home. The implications for this in terms of the increasing demands on community health services are clear.

The purpose of this review was to help you to put within their appropriate context the developments which led to the establishment of the present DN role, and to be able to recognise the early lack of distinction of what is now seen as health versus social care. The concept of 'nursing' for the sick is certainly clearly identifiable from that of 'care', which we will now go on to explore.

Community care developments, as noted above, started with the Mental Health Act of 1959. This was concerned with the need to look at the institutionalised structure of care in which many mentally ill and learning disabled people were incarcerated. The need to identify ways of improving their care moved onto the government agenda, argued by some to have not just 'care' as its focus, but the appropriate use of resources. The use of the term then was meant to imply a plan of moving away from the emphasis on institutionalised care, and making efforts to move individuals closer to the community. By 1971, the DHSS Report on 'Better Services for the Mentally Handicapped' was meant to clarify the concepts, in order to reduce the level of mistrust as people saw a mass closing down of large mental health and learning disabled institutions. The occupants of these institutions had to return to their homes, or move into specially designed community homes alongside ordinary families. The resulting public outcry could have been due, in part, to a lack of proper consultations with communities, combined with a lack of understanding by the public about ways of dealing with the problems being presented by the newcomers into community life.

The Briggs Report (DHSS, 1974) attempted to clarify further the issues for formal providers by suggesting appropriate structures for financing and arranging the services. By 1982 however, the outcry of carers, those forced to look after family members when they had little understanding of their illnesses and little support, was taken up by the Equal Opportunities Commission. (The majority of these carers, of course, were women.) In 1983, the government was forced to restate the aims of the initiative, and explanatory notes on care in the community were published. It had become clear that much controversy existed between the perceptions of policy makers, carers, and the general public, regarding the practicalities of care in the community.

The perception that this was really 'care by the community' implied policy makers' willingness to use the informal goodwill of family and friends, mainly women, in caring for mentally ill and learning disabled people. During 1988 and 1989, two further reports were published, laying the way for major reforms of community care, but still in effect providing confusing perspectives which forced some to ask whether the term 'community care' had in fact become a meaningless slogan (Short, 1989).

The publication of the NHS and Community Care Act (NHS and CCA) in 1990, led the way for a much clearer understanding of how the then government wanted the services to be structured and delivered. This Act introduced a number of fundamental changes in the organisation and delivery of care, with the internal market and contract culture being key features. The NHS and CCA identified clear responsibilities for DNs, which made them accountable for delivering care that is inclusive of the wishes and the needs of patients and their carers. Care planning processes were specific, and the need to work in close partnership with other providers of care services, such as the private and voluntary sectors, along with closer collaboration of the members of the primary health care team, were clear statements of the Act. In effect, the NHS and CCA 1990 consolidated the historical developments of community (district) nursing, and community care, bringing them under the same umbrella. (See Chapter 4 for further discussion on the legislation.)

Student Activity 1.4

- Choose a patient from your assessor's caseload.

- Consider how he or she is being supported within the community, as identified by past and present policy initiatives. Use the aspects of a) independent living, b) patient participation and consultation, c) involvement of carers, d) partnership with other service providers.

- Identify, with reasons, whether the patient's care package represents an example of good practice.

- Discuss the case with your assessor.

- Make notes for your portfolio.

Early factors contributing to the changing focus of care

As discussed above, the process of shifting the emphasis of care from the acute sector (hospital and institutionalised settings) to the community has a long and sometimes controversial history. The setting up of the National Health Service in 1948 had specific aims: the promise to the nation was the provision of a comprehensive service, free at the point of delivery, to all. Over the years, however, major political issues have affected the service, with perhaps the main ones being a lack of resources, declining economy, and overuse, possibly abuse, of the service (Fraser, 1980). The unfortunate situation of demand increasing rather than decreasing, as had been envisaged by the planners, may have been as a result of more people actually being ill in post-war Britain than had been originally anticipated. Added to this was the emergence of new types of disease due, for example, to lifestyle factors, which became an added burden.

With a population that was living longer due to advances in medicine, and a resultant increase in older people in the society, recession and economic crisis had the inevitable result of forcing policy makers to look again at what the NHS was actually offering, and its capacity. The introduction of the internal market by the Conservative government was a major political turning point, emphasising individualism as a key feature of what became known as the 'Thatcherite era' (Blackie, 1998).

Student Activity 1.5

- ◆ Make a list of health services for which you have to pay as an NHS patient.

- ◆ Compare your list with the early NHS list of paying services.

- ◆ Has the number of services for which payment is needed gone up or down?

- ◆ Discuss this with your peers.

- ◆ Make notes in your portfolio.

The focus of the service in the early days on the acute sector meant that the major resources went into hospital services, with only a minimal focus on the community. The legislative frameworks which started the discussions, initially led to the perception that 'care in the community' really meant 'care by the community' as informal carers, mainly women, were seen to be available to undertake most of the caring tasks. It was not long before the issues were recognised for what they were, and eventually governments were forced to respond to the growing unrest with what was happening. The introduction of the health care 'market' was considered to be a key factor in moving away from the original traditional values of the NHS, and was not without its own brand of controversy, especially regarding standards of care and services. The introduction of The Patient's Charter (1992) and the emphasis on the central role of primary care in the NHS (DoH, 1990, 1997) began the redefinition, which was meant to be reflected in the way resources were allocated, and also ensure clearly defined quality of services for users.

More recently, the 1997 election of a New Labour government, and the publication of *The New NHS: Modern, Dependable* (DoH, 1997) have led to the introduction of a new Health Act (1999). The abolition of the internal market is a key feature of the new legislative framework (see Chapter 4), with the introduction of Primary Care Groups (PCGs) and Primary Care Trusts (PCTs) and a clearer focus on Health Action Zones. These developments are designed to ensure that formal nursing carers of adult patients are central contributors to the care policy and planning processes, and that the issues of equity and access are recognised as important areas of action for all concerned.

The organisation and delivery of health care in the community

Provision and providers of health care in the community are as variable as the adult clients themselves, the main focus of the DN's role. The needs for seamless provision and collaboration between providers have been identified as major aspects of the legislative frameworks, beginning with one of the earliest (NHS and CCA, 1990), through to one of the most recent (DoH, 2000). The provision can be categorised as in Table 1.3.

Seamless care delivery practices are a central feature, and this needs to be examined in terms of the benefits and possible problems of the approach. The legislation identifies as major benefits, the economical aspects of services not being duplicated but rather becoming more effective if all providers work together. However, where providers have always worked independently, with services being fragmented in the process, it is easy to understand the problems which are likely to occur as they try to combine their interests for the benefit of their patients. Wilson (2000) points out that there are profound differences in the way that different professionals view the same problem. Furthermore, the health/social care divide has always been disputed. The approach is by no means straightforward, neither is it standardised. It is therefore arguable whether real success has been achieved in the collaboration process between all the providers (see Chapters 4 and 13). Health and social care services, as statutory providers, still have a requirement to continue fostering good partnerships. Different professionals find this hard because of their varied cultural and professional perspectives. The situation is not helped by the diverse approaches to training and education. Interprofessional education still features insufficiently in the way members of the PHCT are prepared for their largely similar roles in meeting the needs of the community they all serve. This is further complicated by organisational and departmental differences which can effectively deter even those with the best will (Wilson, 2000).

The same is true of voluntary provision, the main source of services before the introduction of the welfare state. Because of gaps in welfare services, the need for the voluntary sector remained. Voluntary groups have again become major providers of services, mainly initiated by small pressure groups, which

Table 1.3 Health care provision in community settings

Health care provision	Examples of providers	Type of provision
Statutory provision	NHS and social services, via the PHCT	Formal care, required by legislation
Voluntary provision	Voluntary organisations	Formal care, not legislated
Private provision	Private entrepreneurs	Formal care, regulated
Carers	Family, friends, neighbours	Informal care

have gone on to become well organised voluntary groups. The back-up services provided are funded largely by individual contributions. The services have expanded to include, for example, the hospice movement as key providers of palliative and terminal care, and organisations (such as Age Concern) dealing with the welfare of older people. While the services on offer are well known, and can be accessed directly by patients, or on behalf of patients, by professionals, the extent to which there is real collaboration in terms of care planning and delivery, is not well researched.

Many local areas now have a co-ordinated approach to voluntary services, with representation across the health and social care divide. So it could be argued that structures are in place to encourage closer links, which work well in some settings. Funding from central government, encouraged by the Conservatives, was designed to encourage the voluntary sector in terms of enhancing and expanding their roles as key providers, an aspect of enabling the 'market concept'. Health authorities were made to consult with the sector through statutory requirement.

Private providers of health care have featured largely in residential care services, especially for older people. Again they were encouraged in their entrepreneurial activities, and became considered as mainstream providers of services in the community. Many issues have been raised, again regarding standards of care, which have featured regularly in the press. The resulting regulatory efforts by Social Services are meant to safeguard vulnerable patients and ensure minimum standards of care.

Student Activity 1.6

- ◆ Negotiate with your DN assessor to:
- ◆ Spend some time walking around in the locality of your placement.
- ◆ Identify all the voluntary and private facilities in the locality, which support positive health outcomes for people in that community. For example, who runs the fitness clubs? What voluntary services are there?
- ◆ Keep a record of your findings in your portfolio.

Perhaps the largest provider of care services in the community is the army of family, friends and neighbours who are reported to number over six million people (Twigg, 1994). The majority of these carers are women, and over the years they have been able to build and maintain a strong voice. This has resulted in greater legislative awareness of their needs, with the Carers (Recognition and Services) Act 1995 being the most recent. This puts a statutory duty on health and social care providers to ensure that carers' voices are heard, through independent assessments of their needs, alongside those of the person they are caring for. How this works in actual practice is not well researched.

You should not forget to be aware of your potential to contribute to increasing the literature base through small scale research. For example, case studies of individual patients and their carers may be done individually, in conjunction with your assessor and course tutors, once the procedures have been followed. Assumptions about the caring role of carers were made by the former Tory government regarding individual responsibilities (care by the community), but carers were not recognised in terms of the financial savings they were contributing to statutory spending.

Student Activity 1.7

♦ After reading the above section, consider the extent to which you think it is possible for collaboration to take place in the delivery of community health care.

♦ What examples of good practice have you seen in your placement?

♦ Were there examples where the process could have been improved?

♦ You may wish to comment on this in your portfolio.

Primary health care and the PHCT

In order better to understand the PHCT, it may be useful to talk a bit about the concept of primary health care. The move towards the present emphasis on primary health care has been influenced by a number of significant changes that have occurred over the years. Some of these have already been discussed. However, in the context of changing social, demographic, epidemiological and economic factors, primary health care began to gain momentum. As the population becomes older, the majority of people will have to be cared for in the community. Although many people may go into hospital for a short stay, it has now been recognised that 95 per cent of the population would be looked after within their community (Office for Central Statistics, 1991).

The increasing demand for a primary care led service has been heavily influenced by these changes. In particular, economic factors had a major role in focusing policy makers on the reality of a declining economy, coupled with ever increasing costs of funding services through the NHS. The use of high technology hospitals was absorbing major slices of the budget, and building new ones was getting more expensive. So, exploring new ways of becoming economically effective became a high priority. Emphasis on institutionalised care had started to decline, and certain types of care were seen as being unsuited to a hospital setting. Evidence was emerging of an increase in the numbers of infections and other complications, acquired as a result of admission to hospital and subjection to excessive bed rest and psychological stress. There was also more advanced knowledge of what was possible with early discharge and intensive therapy in the home. Home based technology and better standards of living were contributory factors here. It was also becoming important to ensure that consumer choices were possible and encouraged, especially given the emphasis on the rights of the individual through The Patient's Charter (Danning and Needham, 1994).

The Cumberlege Report (DHSS, 1986) identified a range of groups of individuals with health needs in the community. It specifically mentioned a 'hospital at home' scheme in Peterborough which was very successful. Other initiatives have developed across the country. The popularity of these schemes suggested that patients value the choice of place of care, and, where possible, will always opt to be cared for at home or as close to their community as possible. The implications for nursing are quite clear, the increasing demands on the role of, for example, the DN and other specialist nurses supporting patients at home, call for adaptability, flexibility and responsiveness to current changes. Continuous professional development (CPD) of both hospital and community nurses becomes imperative. Given the increasing workloads resulting from having to deal with more patients at home, primary care workers have to be proactive in ensuring that they are able to make time to keep ahead of rapid changes in care delivery practices. The recognition of the importance of ensuring that patient care meets the highest standards, and the legislative drive to foster greater nursing involvement across all aspects of patient care, are factors which should help to encourage greater interest in ensuring that all practice is driven by the evidence. This will only be possible through a regular programme of CPD.

Primary care, therefore, is about the provision of health services which are as close as possible to the patient's home and community, in order to respond to these changing factors. WHO (1978) identified primary care as:

essential care based on practical, scientifically and socially acceptable methods and technology, made universally accessible to individuals and families in the community throughout their full participation and at a cost that the community and country can afford to maintain at every stage of their development, in the spirit of self reliance and self determination. It forms an integral part both of the country's health system, of which it is the central function and main focus, and of the overall social and economic development of the community. It is the first level of contact for individuals, the family and community with the national health system, bringing health care as close as possible to where people live and work, and constitutes the first element of a continuing health care process. (Clause VII, Declaration of Alma Ata)

This all-inclusive definition provides the basis for a variety of approaches based on the individual country's system of care. It may now be better understood why general practice has been the key focus. In practice, and traditionally, this may be considered to be the first official point of call by most, if not all patients, although in principle this may not always need to be the case. Certainly, changes such as NHS Direct, walk-in centres, and Internet access, may mean that referral points will slowly change, so that the general practitioner (GP) will not necessarily be the very first point of contact with patients in the community.

There are specific factors, which underpin the concept of primary care. These are identified by the RCN (1992), as follows:

- Accessibility: health care being provided as close as possible to where people live and work.
- Acceptability: appropriate health care, provided in ways which people can find acceptable.
- Equity: the right of everyone in the community to health and health-care on an equal basis.
- Self determination: individual right and responsibility to make own health choices.
- Community involvement: individual and collective rights and responsibilities to participate in planning and implementing their health care.
- A focus on health: the promotion of health, as well as the care of those who are sick, frail or disabled.
- A multi-sectorial approach: the need to recognise the impact of housing, food policies and environmental policies, on outcomes for health and health care.

Within the community, primary health care services are provided by a number of professionals who offer a wide range of care, which is required by statute. The two key providers involved here are the NHS and Social Services. Services are organised through a system of referrals, which now tend to be reasonably flexible, the main aim being to foster easier access for patients and carers. Essentially then, the PHCT (Table 1.4) comprises a group of professionals from a variety of disciplines who work together to jointly deliver a service to patients in the community. This interprofessional partnership is supposed to ensure that care delivery is as seamless as possible, so that patients can benefit from, and have access to, the services when they are needed. Blackie (1998) argues that the need for the team to be seen as a daily resource for clinical practitioners should override any urges to move towards politically correct definitions. While the team has a core and an ancil-

Table 1.4 The primary health care team (PHCT)

Core team	Ancillary team
Nursing: District nursing team, including RGNs and health care assistants (HCAs)	Community medical specialists, for example, paediatricians and so on
Medical: General practitioner	Specialist nurses, for example Macmillan, continence, stoma, school, diabetic, asthma infection control, tissue viability, psychiatric nurse. Ability specialist/key workers (may become core members, depending on input)
Practice management: Managers, receptionists	Social worker, counsellor, dentist, pharmacist, optometrist
Practice nurse	Audiologist, speech therapist
Health visitors and their teams	Chiropodist, dietitian, physiotherapist
Midwives – where appropriate	

lary (extended) element, Blackie (1998) thinks that the inclusion of all and sundry is unrealistic, and could contribute to a team which is too large to be appropriately functional. However, it is imperative that the contribution of the ancillary team members is recognised, as patients sometimes have as much, or even possibly more, contact with these members. This, of course, depends on which service is being mostly accessed at any particular time.

Student Activity 1.8

◆ From your observations since starting your community place-ment, make a list of core members of the PHCT in your locality.

◆ Who are the ancillary members?

◆ Give reasons why you think this is the situation in your location.

◆ Discuss with your assessor.

The core team

The main skills of the core team are in the direct delivery of patient care, acting as autonomous clinical practitioners, and being prepared to work collaboratively to ensure the highest possible outcomes of care. Interprofes-sional collaboration is a key requirement of all the legislative frameworks, as discussed earlier. This would imply that this method of working was not always a strong feature of the services, and there are still some problems that need to be overcome. The need to ensure that fragmented services are a thing of the past is now considered as important as the actual provision of those services. Professionals who enter patients' homes should know which of their colleagues may also be visiting to provide help or care. Being able to co-ordinate dates and times of visits, for example, and sharing documentation relating to a patient (within the constraints of confidentiality) ensures a reduction in possible overlaps, or even unnecessary overloading of services to a particular patient.

The ancillary team

The ancillary team of the PHCT consists of those members who may be practitioners, but to whom the core team may have to refer patients. In many cases, their input to care may be limited. However some could have long-term contact, making them key participants in care planning and delivery processes. It is imperative that confidential aspects of collaboration, which could present as a problem, are explored, and agreed frameworks determined with patients' awareness. Blackie (1998), however, identifies primary health care as not being mainly about teamwork, as the majority of care is delivered by the core members of the team (general practitioners, practice nurses, district nurses and health visitors). Even so, the advantages must be explored – especially given the legislative emphasis on the need for a more effective process.

Multidisciplinary and interdisciplinary teamwork

Differing perspectives relating to 'multidisciplinary' as opposed to 'interdisciplinary' teamwork, have been discussed by Blackie (1998) (see Table 1.5). Multidisciplinary teamwork involves the application of individual professional skills by a particular practitioner. This is usually done without necessarily consulting with other team members, even though there may be an awareness of their input. The consequences could be that care being delivered to the client by these different professionals is not seamless, but could have varying perspectives in terms of, for example, symptom relief. An example is in the case of the GP who may use a particular approach to dealing with the patient's illness, while the DN or other specialist practitioner may have other perspectives. The widespread acceptability of this model may lie in the fact that it is seen as showing respect for professional boundaries. However, this may lead to actions not always being challenged or dealt with appropriately, so as to avoid crossing these boundaries. The approach is heavily medicalised, and will rarely, if ever, reflect the holistic approach needed if the patient is to be the main beneficiary of the process.

Table 1.5 Multidisciplinary and interdisciplinary teamworking

Multidisciplinary teamworking		Interdisciplinary teamworking	
Advantages	Disadvantages	Advantages	Disadvantages
Disease process measured reliably, hence simpler evaluation of outcomes	Medical model, with the disease process being used as the definitive factor	Hierarchy of professions absent	Role blurring may result in problems, or be uncomfortable for some
Respect for existing role boundaries, with clear expectations of each	Patients' problems limited in definition to particular professional input	Full holistic view taken to patient health outcomes	Requires highly developed teamworking skills
Easy to grasp, as learning new behaviours is not necessary	Some problems could be overlooked and slip through the net	Patient likely to have a clearer understanding of teamworking, hence be more involved and motivated	

Patients want more say in how they are treated and who manages their care (Wilson, 2000). Flexible interpretation of professional roles would indicate the centrality of the needs of the patient to the process, enabling professionals to apply complex interpretations to the problem, as opposed to a more restricted narrow, individualised view. Implicit within this concept is the need to respect individual professional values, and the contribution they bring to the ultimate goal of promoting the best health outcomes for the patient.

Student Activity 1.9

♦ Are you able to identify the referral routes between the core and ancillary teams? What are these?

♦ Identify the main roles of the core team, and confirm these with your assessor.

♦ What do you think should be the main features of team collaboration?

♦ What practical problems have you encountered with the way the PHCT works? And how do you think this will change with primary care groups (PCGs) and primary care trusts (PCTs)?

♦ Discuss these with your assessor, and keep notes in your portfolio.

The application of an interdisciplinary model to meeting patient needs implies a more sophisticated understanding of the process, and carries the potential of a much improved and better integrated professional delivery for the patient. This approach necessitates team contact on a regular basis for review and evaluation, and emphasises the need to value and respect the professional roles of all concerned, irrespective of the hierarchical position. The added dimension here is the involvement of the patient as a valued participant in his or her care, and the involvement of the patient's 'significant others', whoever they may be. The outcome, according to Blackie (1998), will be care which is co-ordinated, non-hierarchical and holistic. This is perhaps an idealistic model, but one which (while it may be difficult to achieve in practice) ought to be the one for which professionals strive.

Student Activity 1.10

♦ Reflect on the above models of teamworking and try to apply them to your placement setting.

♦ Which of these two models can you recognise in practice?

♦ What are the specific benefits or problems you have observed?

♦ Discuss these with your peers from another placement setting, and see if you can identify any similarities or differences.

♦ How do the models in practice, in your view, affect patients?

♦ Make notes on the above in your portfolio/notebook.

Primary care, as defined by WHO (1978), is seen to revolve around general practice. Perhaps this may have contributed to the perception of the role of GP as the most important in the equation. Although the agenda specifically stresses the centrality of the team approach and a move away from the old power bases, the evidence of problems in actual practice would indicate this to be easier said than done. Pearson and Spencer (1997) argue that, while the PHCT is a major strength of primary care, there are still many barriers to the positive outcomes that should be possible. The effect of primary care trusts (PCTs) and primary care groups (PCGs) in terms of raising the levels of positive outcomes is something you should try to observe while you are in the community.

The latest round of NHS reforms should make a visible contribution to the role of the PHCT, and a number of initiatives are aimed at strengthening the role of all nurses. These include clinical governance and the participation of nurses in the new PCGs and PCTs (see Chapter 15). It has been suggested that all these developments may have the potential to contribute to a shift in the power base, with hierarchical structures being replaced by more participative approaches. Nurses must now take responsibility for ensuring that they grasp the opportunities being presented to them for active contribution to policy development, based on their expert knowledge of the patient and the patient's community. After all, they make up the professional group with whom patients arguably have the most contact. They should therefore be able to help ensure that community health care reflects patients' individual and community circumstances.

The PHCT, therefore, represents the patient's first contact with statutory health care in the community setting. The role of the team is extensive, and usually dependent on the nature of the problem that led to the contact in the first place. The following is a summary of the major aspects of their role:

- To encourage contact as early as possible, where needed, for advice or help relating to health, or social aspects, preventive or curative.
- To ensure that the need is met either directly, or by referral to other team members.
- To foster, as far as possible, the well-being of the community, by recognising the family and carers as important contributors to care delivery processes.
- To maintain continuity of care and ensure that patients are educated on matters to do with their health.
- To gather data on the demographic and epidemiological aspects of disease transmission and the relationship to the population.
- To ensure that patient care in the home or other community setting is promoted.

Turton and Orr (1993) summarise the main advantages of teamwork in primary care, as follows:

- Care being provided by a group is greater than the sum of an individual delivering care.
- Skills which are not common can be used more appropriately.
- Informal learning and peer influence within the group help to raise the standard of care.
- Job satisfaction is increased among team members.
- Co-ordinated health education is encouraged.
- The prevalence of disease in the community is lowered.
- Individual patients become more efficient in their understanding of treatment during their illness.

In spite of the possible problems the team may encounter, it is generally agreed that this method of working has the best chances of providing the most positive outcomes – both for the health of the individual patient, and for the community as a whole.

The role of the nurse is a major one in the team, and this has been affected by many sociopolitical, professional and educational changes. For example, the development of Project 2000 which heralded the arrival of specific pathways in nursing (for adult nurses, children's nurses, mental health and learning disability nurses) meant that post-registration education and practice needed to be re-evaluated. Community nursing was discussed by the UKCC (1992a), and it was agreed that the work of community nurses was complex. Hence a range of nurses would have to continue to provide for the health care needs of individuals and communities. The effect on educational preparation was that a core programme would prepare all community practitioners, with add-on modules for a particular speciality. As a result of the UKCC report, Project 2000 nurses were also able to work as first level nurses under the direction of qualified community nurses. This allowed for a more varied skill mix and what Turton and Orr (1993) describe as 'a rational and cost effective framework' in order to ensure that resources are appropriately utilised. The new curriculum in nursing, with its one-year Common Foundation Programme (CFP) followed by two full years in the Branch Programme, was aimed at enhancing the experiences and clinical expertise of first level nurses. This should contribute eventually to a much more clinically confident practitioner who is fit for practice. *The Scope of Professional Practice* (UKCC, 1992b) introduced greater autonomy and made all nurses more directly accountable for their professional practice. The removal of restrictions on practice meant that qualified nurses became responsible for ensuring that their practice is evidence based. Being able to identify the limits to individual practice, and act on these accordingly, removed the ability to blame others for any deficits in practice, which had not been responsibly identified. For example, a qualified nurse who is asked to undertake a procedure for which there has been no preparation, must be responsible for declining to participate until appropriate preparation has been received. The introduction of nurse prescribing was as a result of the Cumberlege Report (DHSS, 1986), which recommended this extension of role for community nurses to be in the best interests of health outcomes for the patient. All community nurses are now able, following a period of training and preparation, to administer from a defined range of substances, based on the individual needs of patients in their care. The examples for DNs include dressings, stoma care and continence products, bandaging and other appliances. Where patients are terminally ill, or suffer from diabetes, DNs may be able to alter doses in consultation with the GP if the patient's condition demands this.

The increase in size and complexity of the community nurse's role has been heralded by many of the factors identified above. The demographic and

Student Activity 1.11

◆ Ask to see the nurse prescribing protocol, and consider how this compares with what you have seen in practice.

◆ While you are with your assessor, make a note of substances/appliances etc, which you see being prescribed.

◆ Ask your assessor to tell you the benefits of this to patient care.

◆ Discuss your findings with your peers from another practice placement, and check for similarities and comparisons.

◆ Keep a record of your views in your journal/portfolio.

epidemiological changes have been the main contributors, along with other factors such as the increasing demand for care to be given as close to home as possible. The community nurse will see and care for patients in a variety of settings; not just patients' homes, but residential accommodation, GP surgeries and health centres. The main focus of the work is with older people, the chronically sick and those who are terminally ill. You will see them involved in other ways too, however, as the type of population and the community being served will influence the caseload.

The nature of the care needed by patients of the DN could mean that those patients are usually on the caseload for a very long time. This care may sometimes appear repetitive and uninteresting to a new student who has not been in this setting before. Ask your DN assessor to help you identify patient improvement, as this may not always be obvious.

The role of the DN has been summarised as follows (adapted from Turton and Orr, 1993):

● To assess, plan and provide for the nursing needs of patients in the community, ensuring a holistic approach is being utilised.

● To recognise the continuity of role over time, even when being absent from the care setting.

● To lead the DN team, delegating, liaising and co-ordinating with other members of the PHCT to provide an effective interrelated service. To ensure appropriate communication, education and support of patients and their significant others, those people who care for them, whether family friends or neighbours.

DNs along with other community nurses are independent practitioners, with a high level of autonomy in practice. This makes for above average levels of responsibility, as their work is not directly observable by anyone other than patients and carers (unlike the acute hospital settings). This also makes them powerful practitioners (Miers, 1999) about whom patients may be loath to complain if there are any problems with care assessment or delivery. Is it possible that patients of negligent DNs may not feel able to complain because of the nature of the relationship? The level of skills required is wide ranging and, while you are visiting with your assessor, it would be useful to try and identify the kind of skills which are being used in various settings. Some may be simple, others complex. In particular, you may want to look for examples of multiprofessional skills, and how these are applied.

Conclusion

This chapter has explored the varied meanings which may be encountered in the literature, and the way they have influenced present concepts relating to the care of sick adults in the community. It has looked at the contribution of the historical events from 'care' and 'nursing' perspectives, and their influences on the organisation and delivery of health care in the community today. The issues which have been responsible for the shift from acute settings to the care of people as close to their homes as possible have been identified and discussed, and the roles of primary care and the PHCT have been examined. Throughout the chapter, you have been provided with the opportunity to reflect on some of the issues raised and to discuss these with your peers and/or your assessor. You should have been able to identify and clarify roles and responsibilities, and be able to compare the information provided with practice experiences in placement. On completion of this chapter, you should have a good overview of the development of health care for sick adults in the community, and on the way the PHCT strives to function for the benefit of the patient. This will provide you with a sound basis from which to build for your future learning.

Further reading

Hennessy, D. and Swain, G. (1997) Developing community healthcare. Chapter 1 in Hennessy, D. (ed.) *Community Health Care Development.* Basingstoke, Macmillan – now Palgrave.

Hunt, R. and Zurek, E.L. (1997) *Introduction to Community Based Nursing.* New York, J.B. Lippincott. Chapter 1.

Twinn, S., Roberts, B. and Andrews, A.S. (1996) *Community Health Care Nursing.* London, Butterworth Heinemann. Chapter 20.

References

Acheson, E.D. (1998) *Independent Inquiry into Inequalities in Health*. London, HMSO.

Allan, P. and Jolley, M. (1982) *Nursing, Midwifery and Health Visiting Since 1900*, 2nd edn. London, Faber & Faber.

Blackie, C. and Appleby, F. (eds) (1998) *Community Health Care Nursing*. London, Churchill Livingstone.

Danning, M. and Needham, G. (eds) (1994) *But Will it Work, Doctor?* London, King's Fund.

Department of Health (1990) *The NHS and Community Care Act*. London, HMSO.

Department of Health (1992) *The Patient's Charter*. London, DoH.

Department of Health (1997) *The New NHS: Modern, Dependable*. London, HMSO.

Department of Health (1998) *Our Healthier Nation*. London, DoH.

Department of Health (1999) *The Health Act*. London, HMSO.

Department of Health (2000) *The NHS Plan*. London, HMSO.

Department of Health and Social Security (1959) *The Mental Health Act*. London, HMSO.

Department of Health and Social Security (1971) *Better Services for the Mentally Handicapped*. London, HMSO.

Department of Health and Social Security (1974) *Report of the Committee on Nursing* (The Briggs Report). London, HMSO.

Department of Health and Social Security (1980) *Inequalities in Health* (The Black Report). London, HMSO.

Department of Health and Social Security (1983) *Explanatory Notes on Care in the Community*. London, HMSO.

Department of Health and Social Security (1986) *Neighbourhood Nursing* (The Cumberlege Report). London, HMSO.

English National Board (1992) *ENB News*. Issue 6, Autumn. London, ENB.

Equal Opportunities Commission (1982) *Who Cares for the Carers?* Manchester, EOC.

Fraser, D. (1980) *The Evolution of the British Welfare State*, 6th edn. Milton Keynes, Open University.

Gallen, D. and Buckle, G. (1997) *Top Tips in Primary Care Management*. Oxford, Blackwell Science.

Hennessy, D. and Swain, G. (1997) Developing community healthcare. Chapter 1 in Hennessy, D. (ed.) *Community Health Care Development*. Basingstoke, Macmillan – now Palgrave.

Hunt, R. and Zurek, E.L.(1997) *Introduction to Community Based Nursing*. New York and Philadelphia, J.B. Lippincott.

Miers, M. (1999) Health care teams in the community. In Wilkinson, G. and Miers, M. (eds) *Power and Nursing Practice*. London, Macmillan – now Palgrave.

Office for Central Statistics (1991) *Population Statistics and Surveys*. London, HMSO.

Pearson, P. and Spencer, J. (1997) *Promoting Teamwork in Primary Care*. London, Arnold.

Royal College of Nursing (1992) *Powerhouse for Change*. London, RCN.

Seedhouse, D. (1986) *Health: the Foundations for Achievement*. Chichester, John Wiley.

Short, R. (1989) Is community care a meaningless slogan? In *Nursing Management*, 1(13): 221–7.

Tadd, W. and Tadd, V. (1997) *The Ethics of Community Care*. London, Arnold.
Turton, P. and Orr, J. (1993) *Learning to Care in the Community*, 2nd edn. London,
    Arnold.
Twigs, T. (1994) *Carers Perceived*. Milton Keynes, Open University Press.
Twinn, S., Roberts, B. and Andrews, A.S. (1996) *Community Health Care Nursing*.
    London, Butterworth Heinemann.
UKCC (1992a) *Code of Professional Conduct for the Nurse, Midwife and Health
    Visitor*. London, UKCC.
UKCC (1992b) *The Scope of Professional Practice*. London, UKCC.
Wilson, T. (2000) Human information behaviour. In *Informing Science*, **3**(2): 49–56.
World Health Organization (WHO) (1946) *Alma Ata Declaration*. Geneva, WHO.
World Health Organization (WHO) (1978) *Alma Ata*. Geneva, WHO.

2

Preparing to nurse in the community

DONNA YOUNG, JENNY DOWLING
and PAULA HEIGHTON

Learning outcomes

By the end of this chapter you will be able to:

- Describe the role of a district nursing team, and its function within multi-disciplinary care provision.
- Discuss the services available to people being cared for in the community setting.
- Discuss the similarities and differences between a community placement and an acute hospital placement.
- Discuss the ethical and legal issues relating to the health care of adults in the community.
- Identify your own responsibilities when undertaking a placement in the community.

Introduction

Now that you are beginning your community placement, what thoughts are going through your mind? What does 'community' mean to you? What will be expected of you? How will you fit in? Are you looking forward to the experience or dreading it? All these emotions are quite normal. All you need to remember is that the care you are about to participate in is provided in the patient's own environment. You will be guided and supported by experienced staff in adapting to a variety of primary care situations, which differ considerably from the more formal hospital setting.

The purpose of this chapter is to help you, as a student, make the transition from classroom or hospital ward into the wider community setting. This will require a transferral of your current knowledge and clinical skills into a different working environment, and will provide you with the opportunity to widen and develop those skills as well as encounter new practices.

Throughout the chapter, use will be made of a variety of typical care issues relating to people in a community setting. Opportunity will be given for you the student to undertake some exercises to assist understanding of the principles and practice of nursing in the community and primary care setting.

The placement you are about to undertake may be described by a one of a variety of terms, for example:

- Community placement
- District placement
- Primary care placement.

Whatever the terminology the principle of the learning experience remains unchanged. While you will get the opportunity to work with a variety of care workers in this setting, the majority of your time will be spent with the district nurse (DN) who looks after the care of sick adults in the community.

For many years authors have tried to define the term 'community', describing its function as being either the location of activities, for example community nursing, or the placing of values or worth on feelings and sentiments as in 'community spirit' to describe the feelings shared by people in a particular area (Turton and Orr, 1993) (see Chapter 1 of this text for further discussion on meanings).

In the context of community nursing, the term 'District' relates to an original practice of community nurses working within a defined geographical area, hence the title 'district' nurse (Baly, 1980). 'Primary care' relates to general practitioners (GPs) and practice staff, who as part of the primary health care team (PHCT) provide the scope and basis of the placement caseload.

Within this chapter we will be referring to a defined geographical area and considering the need to study environmental aspects of that area. We will also be referring to social relationships and networks contributing to the lives of residents in that area. Therefore the terminology used will be 'community'. For the sake of simplicity 'community' refers to all health care provision outside the acute hospital setting. 'District nurse' is used in its generic form, covering district nursing sisters and district charge nurses.

Preparing for your first day: some helpful hints

Your community placement will be agreed between your educational establishment and the community or primary care trust in which you are placed. As a student registered with a university or higher education establishment, you will be made aware of guidance relating to your personal safety. This may be found in your student's handbook; if not please ask your tutor. The following are some simple, practical steps, which will contribute greatly to ensuring that your placement in the community is as smooth as possible. They should also help you to overcome some of the concerns you may have.

- Ensure you have the name, telephone number and working base address of your supervisor.
- It would be useful to contact your supervisor prior to your placement to confirm your starting and finishing time, ensuring that these are understood within the overall guidelines from course/module teachers.
- Bike riders should check security and parking arrangements.

- If you own a car, ask about availability of car parking, charges, and arrangements for use of your own car while you are on placement.
- Ensure that you have local bus and train timetables where appropriate, with added time as needed to travel between the bus stop, train station and your community base.
- Most district nursing services start at 8:30am, so give yourself plenty of time, and be sure to negotiate and discuss any actual or potential problems with your supervisor and the university.
- An A–Z street guide is an absolute must for finding your way around the locality.
- Plan your clothing. Summer uniform can be worn with a cardigan, but in winter and on wet days an outside coat will be required. Discuss this with your district nurse supervisor prior to placement. Remember that a professional appearance is essential, hence uniform codes should be followed at all times.
- Even though district nursing teams have transport, there may be times when you will be required to spend time walking to visits, and so on. So plan your footwear – it should be comfortable and sensible.
- Keep a list of phone numbers with you, together with change and/or a mobile phone, in case you need to ring your supervisor or tutors in an emergency.
- Lunch times on your community placement may vary. Make sure you either take lunch with you or are able to buy something nearby. Again your supervisor can advise you.
- Personal belongings, ideally, should remain with you. Where this is not possible, it is advisable to ensure they are stored securely at the base.

If you follow the above suggestions you should be able to relax and enjoy your placement.

What is a district nursing team?

A district nursing team will be led by a qualified nurse who has undertaken a district nursing course, leading to a degree in Community Health Studies, within an institute of higher education. Therefore, district nurses are recognised as specialist practitioners:

> This education, with integrated taught and supervised practice, enables the nurse to give skilled research based nursing care to the patient within a community setting (home or residential home), and to offer appropriate support to relatives and carers. (Skidmore, 1997)

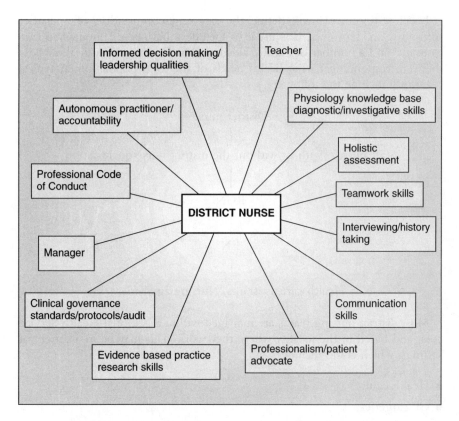

Figure 2.1 The core elements of the function of a district nurse

The district nurse is professionally accountable for assessing the needs of the patient and family, for initiating programmes of care, ensuring their implementation and for the continual evaluation and reassessment of such programmes (Skidmore, 1997). The varied nature of the district nursing teamwork requires district nurses to have all-round generalised skills, with a sound evidence base. The core elements of the district nurse's role are summarised in Figure 2.1.

Student Activity 2.1

◆ Make a list of the duties and responsibilities you associate with the district nurse's role. How does this role differ from other members of the primary health care team?

◆ Discuss these with your assessor/supervisor.

◆ Keep notes in your portfolio.

Local requirements will define the size and composition of a district nursing team. However, it is usual to include a balance of unqualified care assistants and a number of highly skilled qualified practitioners to allow flexibility in responding to the health needs of the local population. A typical team may include the following:

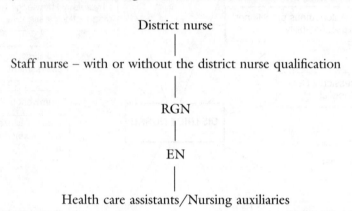

District nurse
|
Staff nurse – with or without the district nurse qualification
|
RGN
|
EN
|
Health care assistants/Nursing auxiliaries

Most district nursing teams are managed within a National Health Service trust and based in the locality where they work. This may be in a variety of settings, which could include:

- Health centres
- GP surgeries
- Community hospitals
- Community centres
- In some rural areas the district nurse's base may well be his or her own home.

The District Nursing Service is available 52 weeks of the year, seven days a week. The nature of the service varies according to the local policy and local health care needs. Therefore service provision may vary throughout the country, some providing a 24-hour nursing cover seven days a week while others provide nursing cover until 10 or 11pm. With the advent of more individual treatment regimes and better care packages (including symptom control), district nursing teams are not required to be available to provide four- or six-hourly visits as in the past. However, when more intensive care is required, it may be provided by specialist services, for example 'Hospital at Home'. Many areas now have an 'On Call' night service in place which responds to nursing requests from GPs, patients or concerned carers and relatives.

In some areas integrated nursing teams have been established to provide a seamless service to the patient. Ask your supervisor about integrated nursing teams, or integrated working.

Student Activity 2.2

♦ Negotiate some time with your assessor to visit the locality in which you are placed.

♦ Find out who are the other providers of statutory services in the area.

♦ Make notes on what they do.

Arrangements for providing health care over seven days can vary. Some trusts favour a rota system for staff to work five days out of seven, covering weekend work, while others employ dedicated staff to work weekends and bank holidays. In some areas an evening or twilight service is also provided. The arrangement for staffing this service varies from flexible working arrangements to employing staff specifically to work the necessary hours. During your placement you may have the opportunity to work with staff within one of these systems. Discuss with your supervisor the opportunities available, and what you would like to take advantage of to maximise your learning within the community.

Student Activity 2.3

♦ Find out what types of out-of-hours services are available in your placement area.

♦ Who provides these, and what do they do?

♦ If possible, find out if you will be able to spend some time with the out of hours team.

♦ Keep a record for your portfolio.

Referrals

Patients will normally be referred to the district nurses by the GP, or by the local hospitals. They may be referred directly from the hospital ward, or through a district nurse liaison system, requesting assessment or follow-up care. Referrals for assessment can also be accepted directly from patients themselves, carers or families and a variety of other agencies. Social workers frequently request a district nursing assessment when their own involvement has discovered actual, or potential, health care needs. This may result in a decision to undertake a joint assessment. In this situation a social worker and district nurse will visit a patient together so that a full assessment of health and social care needs can be made. It is then possible to design and agree a 'joint package' of care for a particular patient, taking into consideration the needs of carers and families. To assist in this process, many areas will have developed a 'Health and Social Care Protocol' document to guide staff from the various statutory agencies when negotiating responsibilities within such packages of care. The benefits of joint assessments have led to some areas progressing to joint funding of specific equipment for issue to patients being cared for in a community setting.

The criteria for referral to the district nursing service differs across the country, due to local agreements with other services and agencies. It would be useful to understand the referral criteria in your local area, and the means by which patients/carers are referred on to other agencies when appropriate.

Your supervisor can discuss with you the local policy for referral to the service, admission onto caseload, management of caseload and discharge from the service, for example: service eligibility criteria, setting out the patients who would be eligible for the district nursing service.

• The process by which district nurses prioritise care within their caseload.

• Identification of levels of response linked to caseload management.

• What criteria are used when discharging patients from the caseload.

Communication and interaction with all relevant people and agencies is important to achieve the best possible health care for patients in the community. This will enhance the process of assessment – planning – implementation – evaluation.

An example of a simple referral onto a district nurse caseload and the action taken is illustrated in Case Study 2.1.

Case Study 2.1

Mr and Mrs Harris were on holiday in Cornwall when Mr Harris had a cerebral vascular accident and he was admitted into the local hospital and then transferred to a hospital near his home.

His wife wants him to come home as soon as possible.

He weighs 19 stone and is six foot tall. He is unable to walk due to a left sided weakness that is not improving although he has started a regime of

Case Study 2.1 continued

physiotherapy. He is losing weight because he has difficulty in swallowing and his speech is very slurred.

What should be done to help with the discharge of Mr Harris? Consider which services might be needed.

Solution

In order to discharge Mr Harris from hospital, a case conference would be convened with all professionals involved in Mr Harris's care package, to empower communication and interaction and enable a smooth discharge.

Factors that should be taken into consideration include:

Environment
Assessment of his home environment to look at access, equipment and adaptations, to allow Mr Harris to be independent and safe from hazards.

Social care needs
If identified, this could involve personal hygiene needs, taking into account what Mr Harris could do independently.

The outcome of this should be negotiated as to whether it is 'health care' or 'social care' that is involved.

Physical needs
Mobility factors should be taken into consideration due to Mr Harris having a left sided weakness following his CVA. Advice from the physiotherapist would be taken into account regarding the risk assessment of moving and handling issues, and appropriate equipment provided.

The speech therapy involvement would include swallowing reflex and nutritional status.

Health needs
District nursing involvement may be indicated if there are identified problems in relation to elimination needs and skin integrity.

Psychological needs
Consideration to Mrs Harris is paramount, taking into account the carers' strategy which would enable the care team to assess her needs with regard to caring for her husband. However, Mr Harris has problems with his speech, but would still need to be involved with all of the assessments.

The planned case conference allows communication and decision making to be initiated prior to discharge. This prevents complications arising when Mr Harris returns home.

District nurses, as leaders of the district nursing teams, are professionally accountable for assessing and reassessing the nursing needs of the patient and family. The process used for assessment may vary. It may include the use of one of the established models of nursing care, such as, 'Orem', or 'Roper, Logan and Tierney'. The rationale for the application of a conceptual model of care to the assessment and care delivery process may vary across trusts. Be sure that you are aware of why and how these decisions are made, and are able to recognise their effectiveness or otherwise, in actual practice. Models applicable to community care delivery are well represented in the literature (Walsh, 1991; Fraser, 1996). They are also responsible for monitoring the quality of care provided by other members of the nursing team. An effective assessment will ensure that help, both financial and social, is made available as appropriate. In order to do this efficiently, liaison links with other agencies such as social services departments, welfare rights and voluntary agencies are essential. This is a theme which will be developed later in the chapter.

Student Activity 2.4

 ◆ Discuss the nursing documentation that is used in your locality.

 ◆ What conceptual frameworks are used to assess, plan and deliver care?

 ◆ Why are these used, and would you say they were effective?

 ◆ Discuss your views with your assessor.

Caseload

During your placement you will begin to recognise the various categories of care that make up a district nurse caseload. A major part of the caseload revolves around the care given to patients with complex needs, often with a multiplicity of health problems, who require nursing care. Modern medical technology and improved treatments lead to shorter hospital stays and, combined with continuing developments in day case surgery, increase the number and nature of the referrals. As a result, DNs routinely use a wide range of skills to provide the necessary high level of care. These skills are used to:

● Provide care to patients who are in the terminal stage of their illness, this could be cancer, or some of the chronic illnesses.

- Assist and support patients who require technical equipment to enable them to stay at home.

- Help people who have continuing care needs, and require intensive packages of care from the district nurse and other agencies involved in that care.

Every caseload will, at some time, include elements of caring for children, young adults, middle aged and elderly people in response to acute, shorter term care needs. However, the major part of most district nursing caseloads relates to long-term care of the elderly and other patients with chronic health care needs. A typical daily caseload for the district nurse and members of the team may include:

- Holistic assessment of patients newly referred.

- Reassessment of ongoing care needs.

- Visits to administer insulin to patients who, through disability or advancing age, are not able to administer their own.

- Nursing care to the acute and long-term sick, the terminally ill and the disabled, some of which may be shared with social service staff.

- Administration of a wide range of injections, for example antibiotics, controlled drugs and other prescribed drugs.

- A variety of wound dressings ranging from surgical dressings to four-layer bandaging for leg ulcers.

- Post-surgical administration of eye drops.

- Health education and health promotion activities.

- Health assessments for those aged over 75.

- Nurse-led clinics for, for example, leg ulcers, continence, minor treatments.

An underlying principle of district nursing is maximisation of independence and self-catering for patients in their own home. Caseload management therefore requires maintaining a balance between meeting the needs of individual patients and cost effective use of time.

Role development

It is recognised that throughout the centuries there have been a variety of people who have provided 'care', either in the home, institutions or poor houses. Examples of this care can be found in the literature of this time and portrayed in fictional characters like Dickens's Sarah Gamp.

This sort of 'care' provision was seen to be of a lowly status, many 'care givers' being dirty, unkempt and often inebriated. This stereotyping remained for many years, even after Florence Nightingale had successfully demonstrated that cleanliness was linked very closely to health and healing. It was William Rathbone in the 1800s, a Newcastle businessman, who recognised the benefit of employing a 'nurse' to care for his ailing wife at home. Following her death he continued to support the concept of caring for people in their own home. They became known as welfare workers and continued their work until the Queen's Nursing Institute recognised the need for a formal training (see Chapter 1).

From that time district nurses have been portrayed in a number of guises by the TV producers. The popular media image of district nurses is that they are 'round', white, female, middle aged, used to riding a bicycle, and that they attempt to care for everything and everybody. The reality is that in the 21st century the role has developed to provide high quality care for people at home. The future of care is focused within the community in which people live. The community services, and district nurses in particular, are trained to a high level of expertise to enable them to meet that challenge.

The district nursing role has needed to respond to developments in various aspects of health care provision, which were dictated by:

- Early discharge
- Technical developments, such as blood transfusions
- Day case surgery
- Primary care provision of minor surgery
- Nurse-led clinics
- Demands for evidence-based practice
- Enteral feeding
- Intravenous therapy.

Part of the continuing development of the district nurse's role has involved prescribing. Community nurses with either health visitor or district nursing qualifications are now able to undertake a course enabling them to prescribe from a limited formulary of drugs, dressings and appliances (DoH, 1999). It was envisaged that this initiative would improve patient care, save nurses' time and strengthen professional relationships with the primary health care team (DHSS, 1986; DoH, 1989b). The effectiveness of nurses as prescribers has led to extending the groups of nurses eligible to prescribe, and increasing the items identified within the formulary of drugs, dressings and appliances (UKCC, 1992; DoH, 1999; 2000).

Although the district nurse is seen as a specialist practitioner this title relates to the generic role undertaken in providing evidence-based and high quality care in the community. District nurses are not, however, able to be expert in all areas of specialised care. Within your community placement you may well meet or become aware of input from specialist nurses, who provide advice and care in a very specific area. Specialist nurses in palliative care, for example, include Macmillan nurses, and Marie Curie nurses.

There are a number of other specialists that you will need to become familiar with:

- Tissue viability nurses
- Infection control nurses
- Continence specialists
- HIV/AIDS specialists
- TB specialists
- Nurses specialising in the haemoglobinophathies
- Asthma and respiratory nurses.

In many areas of the community you will also become familiar with the nurse consultants who work in a variety of specialities, for example rehabilitation, primary care, intermediary care. Should the opportunity arise it would be beneficial to request some time with one or more of these specialists.

To support these developments, clinical supervision has played a major part with audit frames to identify areas of good practice (see Chapter 3). District nurses are encouraged to continue to research projects, thereby establishing a sound basis for future clinical practice.

Working relationships

The district nursing team is part of a larger team providing holistic care to people in the community. Their closest working relationship is with the various members of the primary health care team (PHCT), as discussed in Chapter 1. They will link closely with social services, learning disability and mental health services and with school nursing.

The majority of people spend most of their lives within their own communities, where their health needs are met by the PHCT. This care may need to be supplemented by services provided within the acute hospital service, for example x-ray or pathology, without actual admission to a hospital ward. The philosophy of this team is to enable people to remain within their 'homes' by provision of care and support as required. The term 'homes' is used to describe a variety of settings which includes:

- The patient's own home
- Sheltered accommodation
- Residential care homes

- Nursing homes
- Day care facilities, including community hospitals.

Such broad based provision enables management of chronic illness, rehabilitation and terminal care to be provided in that home setting. Those people who do require care within an acute hospital setting, will normally be discharged back into their home, for their ongoing care to be provided by the PHCT.

Working environment

One of the strengths of the effective district nurse is an ability to adapt to ever changing environments. This could mean working within a densely populated area of an inner city or in a rural setting consisting of scattered villages and isolated farms. Although vastly different, each of these settings requires the ability of the nurses to work on their own initiative without the close proximity of other medical or nursing colleagues.

The situations district nurses find themselves in could be very different from their own living environments, in so much as they are required to work within a wide range of social bands, from the very deprived to the more affluent households.

The types of living conditions can also vary from the more formal home or flat, to caravans, huts, and hostels for the homeless.

Wherever their work takes them, and in whatever condition they provide care, district nurses are required to maintain a non-judgemental approach, respecting the individual and their circumstances regardless of their personal views about particular situations (see Chapter 11).

As a student nurse on a community placement you will be expected to respect the rights of the individual and the circumstances in which they live. Many of these circumstances are not by choice, although a small number of people will make their own choices which influence their living conditions. However, district nurses will endeavour to provide help and guidance to those patients whose health and social welfare suffers due to those living conditions. Chapter 5 should help you to identify some of the reasons, which may be influencing the way some people live in the community. Poverty is an enduring problem, which you will need to be aware of (Acheson, 1999).

Figure 2.2 illustrates the variety of settings in which a community nurse may be required to undertake various duties. However, superimposed upon this are a variety of factors, which influence the means by which the patient/users can access the service (Figure 2.3) and conversely, by which nurses can effectively deliver the care required.

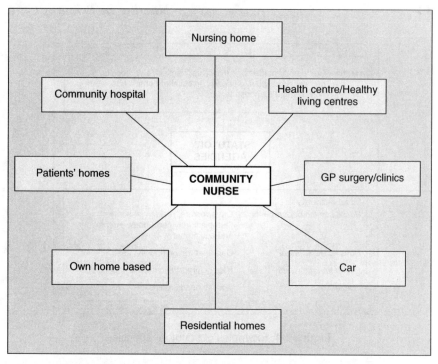

Figure 2.2 The working environment of the community nurse

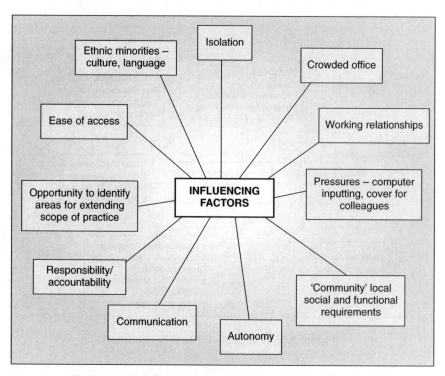

Figure 2.3 Factors influencing the delivery of nursing care

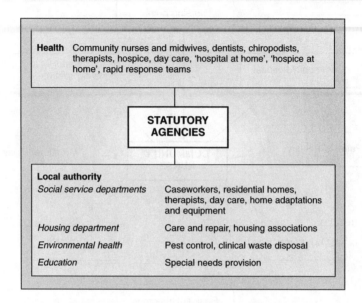

Figure 2.4 Examples of statutory agencies

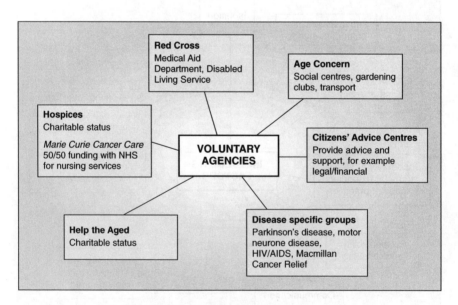

Figure 2.5 Examples of voluntary agencies

Services available for people being cared for in the community setting

Within each geographical community setting there may be different social and functional requirements. One of the district nursing skills when assessing patient and family needs is to have a local knowledge of other sources of support. This could be achieved by knowledge of local 'informal' support or the recognised statutory and voluntary agencies.

Within each area there may also be a variety of local support groups and facilities established in response to local cultural, social or religious needs. These facilities can range from sitting services, interpreters and befrienders to practical provision such as luncheon clubs, day care and respite care.

Statutory agencies are established through government legislation created by an Act of Parliament. Such agencies are, therefore, required to act in response to current government policies and objectives. Examples of such agencies can be seen in Figure 2.4.

Because government policies are subject to constant review and change, the focus of health care will change in response to new legislation. Government-led initiatives on reducing waiting lists in acute hospitals affected the financial allocation for community care, restricting developments of new services.

Voluntary agencies are independent of the State and are supported by voluntary contributions, but may be registered as charities for taxation purposes (Figure 2.5).

Challenges of working in a community setting

The majority of people, as seen above, are cared for within the community setting where their health care needs are met by the members of the PHCT. This approach is in contrast to the acute hospital setting (secondary care) which is accessed at times of acute episodes of health need, planned admission following diagnostic tests or treatment pathways which could include more complex procedures.

The community role has evolved in response to:

- Earlier hospital discharge.
- Advancing surgical and medical techniques.
- Research evidence.
- Government-led initiatives – *Care in the Community* (DoH, 1989a); *Making a Difference* (DoH, 1998).
- Levels of education and training.

District nurses are autonomous practitioners, making decisions regarding patients' care on the evidence available, and in the light of professional experience. You will become aware that all members of the district nursing team work largely unsupervised. An underlying principle of community nursing is maximisation of independence and self-caring for patients in their own home. Caseload management therefore requires maintaining a balance between meeting the needs of individual patients and cost effective use of time.

Some of the major challenges faced by district nurses relate to their ability to respond to the continuing care of patients discharged from hospital and requiring increasingly high-tech treatment regimes.

There is also the consideration of caring for the long-term sick and disabled whose needs are ongoing. The challenge in caring for this group of patients is to ensure continuity of that care in a dynamic way, taking advantage of any appropriate new developments in the care techniques and equipment required. Relationships with the patients/carers are crucial to the process of agreeing individual care programmes, which may include a number of agencies. In many instances the nursing auxiliary/health care assistant will be the most frequent giver of care, and will be relied upon to observe and report any changes of condition to the district nurse for the appropriate action to be taken.

Student Activity 2.5

♦ Find out what discharge planning arrangements exist between the community services and the acute sector.

♦ Ask your assessor for help with this activity.

♦ Keep notes in your portfolio.

In Britain we have an increasing elderly population which has an effect on the health care needs of the general community (Donnellan, 1995). Older people are often discharged from hospital more speedily and in poorer health than formerly. This consequently places extra pressure on community services, including district nursing. Effective communication between acute and community health settings is essential to ensure discharge planning facilitates the provision of appropriate ongoing care.

To meet these increasing challenges, district nurses have a personal responsibility for their own professional development and that of their team. You may find it interesting to discuss with members of the nursing team their personal profiles compiled as evidence of achievement.

Legal and ethical issues relating to nursing adults in the community setting

Patients being cared for in the acute hospitals are usually required to comply with the rules of that particular establishment. In contrast to this, patients being cared for within a community setting are in a position to choose their degree of compliance with proposed care provision.

Many of these patients will be cared for within their own home, and supported by partner or family, therefore any community services involvement in that home will need to be negotiated and agreed by the individuals concerned.

Within this framework the particular issues to be considered include:

- Documentation
- Provision of drugs and dressings
- Health and safety and risk assessment.

Documentation

There is a legal responsibility to ensure that all care providers document their involvement with individual parties. Within the community the nursing responsibility to provide that record of care lies with the district nurse. This record is kept by the patient and informs other members of the nursing team of the care to be provided. It also acts as a communication link between other members of the primary health care team, and may be used as evidence in an investigation into care provision. While the records remain legally the property of the health care trust, they are available to the patient and carers for information and reference throughout the period of treatment. It is important to explain the purpose of these records and who is entitled to read and write within them to ensure confidentiality is maintained. An example of a misunderstanding is shown below.

> A district nurse, after explaining to an elderly lady that the nursing notes would be left in the home and signed by everyone coming to the house, returned two days later to find that the notes contained signatures of the postman, the milkman, and the window cleaner!

Record keeping is an integral part of good nursing practice. There are a number of factors which contribute to effective record keeping. The following have been taken from the UKCC's *Guidelines for Records and Record Keeping* (1998). According to this document, a nursing record must:

- Be factual, consistent and accurate.

- Be written as soon as possible after an event has occurred, providing current information on the care and condition of the patient.
- Be written clearly and in such a manner that the text cannot be erased.
- Be written in such a manner that any alterations or additions are dated, timed and signed in such a way that the original can still be read clearly.

Good record keeping is a mark of a skilled and safe practitioner and helps to protect the welfare of the patient.

Student Activity 2.6

◆ There are twelve factors identified in the UKCC's (1998) *Guidelines for Records and Record Keeping*. Identify the other eight.

◆ Can you think of some examples from practice, which illustrate the importance of good record keeping?

◆ Keep notes in your portfolio.

Provision of drugs*

Within the community settings drugs are legally the property, and remain the responsibility, of the patient named on the dispensing label. Prescriptions are usually written by the GP and dispensed by a community-based pharmacist. (An exception to this would be a person attending a hospital outpatient appointment when the hospital may provide both the prescription and the necessary drugs.)

Recognising that some patients may have difficulty collecting prescriptions and drugs, many pharmacists provide a collection and delivery service. In selected rural areas GPs may still prescribe and dispense drugs to their patients.

Administration of drugs by the district nursing team

Most patients taking drugs at home are able to self-administer, though some may require a prompt from a carer or friend.

Procedures for administration of drugs may vary between different institutions and organisations. Within the community setting, qualified nurses from

---

* For the sake of simplicity the word 'drug' is used throughout this chapter to cover all types of medication.

the district nursing team will work unaccompanied to administer all categories of drugs, as prescribed, including controlled drugs.

District nursing documentation is designed to demonstrate compliance with the legal requirements surrounding the administration of drugs, particularly scheduled and controlled drugs.

As opposed to hospital practice where all drugs are a ward resource, drugs no longer required by patients in the community setting should be disposed of by the patient or a relative. In the case of controlled drugs, the District Nurse has a responsibility to ensure they are destroyed, having gained consent from the patient or a responsible relative.

All qualified nurses are expected to abide by the UKCC's current Standards for the Administration of Medicines.

Provision of dressings

The majority of dressings required by patients in the community are available on prescription. However, non-prescribable items for specific conditions will be obtained to ensure the necessary care is given.

Health, safety and risk assessment

Employers are required to have a written Health and Safety policy which must be readily available to all employees (Health and Safety at Work Act 1974). This document also states the responsibilities of employees to comply with regulations relating to their place of work.

Areas of particular concern for community include:

- Fire regulations
- COSHH (control of substances hazardous to health)
- Moving and handling
- Needlestick injuries
- Infection control
- Risk assessment.

You will be expected to familiarise yourself with the policy surrounding fire, health and safety and the procedure for reporting accidents within the locality which will be your base. This information should be made available to you as part of the introduction to your placement base. If it is not please ask.

Personal responsibility of students undertaking a community placement

The beginning of this chapter highlighted some responsibilities for preparing to undertake a community placement. Some thoughts should now be given to the responsibility within the placement itself.

The district nurse has a responsibility to ensure that, where care is provided, the environment for patients, carers and members of staff alike is safe. However, you will need to be aware of possible security risks for personal items such as bags, purses, and so on. Ask your district nurse about a safe and secure place to keep personal belongings. It will also be important to arrange for car parking if that is appropriate as not all health centres or GP surgeries have that facility.

The district nurse, or named nurse assessor, has the overall responsibility for you during your placement, but there are some areas where you must be totally responsible. These relate to the following.

- *Punctuality* The community teams work under certain pressures, one being to deliver care at appropriate times. For example, to diabetic patients requiring insulin injections, to terminally ill patients for pain-relieving drug administration, or to patients waiting for the dressing of a wound. All these care packages have been agreed with individual patients, and include an expected time band for the visit. Therefore you will need to confirm the time you need to be starting duty. If at any time you are unable to attend your placement, the district nurse will need to be informed at the beginning of the working day.

- *Appearance/attitude* As district nursing is a uniformed service you will probably be required to wear a uniform while visiting patients. An outdoor coat would also be advisable – it may be appropriate to discuss this with your district nurse. The wearing of jewellery is limited to a wedding ring or signet ring and watch, though in some areas earring studs are acceptable. As you will be visiting a wide range of patients, you will need to be mindful of cultural and social expectations regarding the attitude and appearance of health service staff. Your attitude to learning needs to be positive, regardless of your views about the placement. Not everyone will like the community setting. Some find it interesting, even exciting. Others find it slow and tedious. As a student, however, you have to be mindful of the need to meet expected learning outcomes, as well as of the present emphasis on primary care in the policy agenda. You should be prepared to put into your placement as much as you wish to get out of it. If you choose to practise in the acute sector when you qualify, you will find that your experience in the primary care setting will have contributed to a better understanding of where your patients in the acute sector are being admitted from, and being discharged to.

- *Confidentiality* While visiting patients and being involved in their care, you will be party to information that could be of a sensitive nature. It may be helpful to discuss any matters of concern or interest within the nursing team, but you should remain within the bounds of confidentiality. Such discussions should not take place outside the immediate professional team.

During your placement there should be the opportunity to develop new skills, and build on previous experience. However, this development will need to be supervised by the district nurse who retains overall responsibility for the patient's care.

Whatever your skills or experience in a previous position, it should not be assumed that those skills can be used without first agreeing with the district nurse, who may wish to assess your competence. Your nurse assessor will be aware of your expected learning outcomes, and should be supportive in helping you meet those outcomes. However, you will have a personal responsibility to take up opportunities, actively, as they arise. This could involve negotiating with your supervisor to visit a location outside your original placement, so that you can observe new or innovative practice.

Student Activity 2.7

Reflect on the following questions and write notes in your portfolio. You may also find it helpful to discuss these issues with your peers or tutor/supervisor.

◆ What are your potential fears and how would you overcome them?

◆ What issues are particularly relevant to your personal situation?

◆ Can you think of other issues that may be important that you would wish to discuss with your supervisor prior to your placement?

As an ongoing part of your community placement, you will be expected to review and evaluate your own learning progress, in the form of reflective practice.

Conclusion

Your community placement can be anything you wish it to be; it can fulfil your learning outcomes, provide you with the opportunity to investigate different organisational cultures and structures, and provide you with an understanding for a potential career pathway.

The roles of the various district nursing team members are challenging and far reaching. The need to identify and work within the local cultural and social environment adds an exciting edge to the requirement for a high level of professional skill and expertise.

However, a career working in the community will not be right for every nurse. Some students will respond enthusiastically to the challenges offered, while others may feel they prefer the different structure and relationships within the accute sector. This is a very normal response when deciding on your future career, and provides the health service with staff who are enthused and motivated about their own particular area of work.

Regardless of your feelings about a future career in the community, from a potential patient's point of view one of the most successful outcomes from your placement will be the knowledge you take back into the acute setting. A closer understanding and appreciation of the different nursing roles will help to ensure a smoother transition between the various elements of health care services.

The intention of this chapter was to provide you with a practical insight into community nursing and its relationship to the academic framework and the wider scenario of health care. This should help you deal with the everyday issues as they crop up on your placement, so that you will be able to get the maximum benefit from your experience.

As you begin your community placement, take this opportunity to further enhance your learning experience and appreciation of the wider aspects of care. You will find that district nurses are very enthusiastic about their unique role, and this is likely to contribute to your enjoyment of your placement.

Further reading

Skidmore D. (1997) *Community Care: Initial Training and Beyond.* London, Arnold. Chapter 2.

USEFUL WEB SITE

Journal of Community Nursing www.jcn.co.uk

References

Acheson, E.D. (1999) *Inequalities in Health: The Evidence Presented to the Independent Inquiry.* Bristol, Studies in Poverty and Social Exclusion.
Baly, M. (1980) *Nursing and Social Change*, 2nd edn. London, Heinemann.

Cain, P. and Hyde, V. (1995) *Community Nursing – Dimensions and Dilemmas.* London, Arnold.

Department of Health (1989a) *Caring for People: Community Care in the Next Decade and Beyond.* London, DoH.

Department of Health (1989b) *Working for Patients.* London, DoH.

Department of Health (1998) *Our Healthier Nation.* London, DoH.

Department of Health (1999) *Review of Prescribing, Supply and Administration of Medicines, Final Report.* London, HMSO.

Department of Health (2000) London Standing Conference for Nurses, Midwives and Health Visitors: Response to Consultation on Proposals to Extend Nurse Prescribing. London, DoH.

Department of Health and Social Security (1986) *Neighbourhood Nursing* (The Cumberlege Report). London, HMSO.

Domant, M. (1990) *The Challenges of Primary Health Care in the 1990s: A Review of Education and Training for Practice Nursing, the Substantive Report.* London, English National Board for Nursing, Midwifery and Health Visiting (ENB).

Donnellan, C. (1995) *Our Ageing Generation.* Cambridge, Independence Educational Publishers.

Fraser, M. (1996) *Conceptual Nursing in Practice: A Research-based Approach*, 2nd edn. London, Chapman & Hall.

Groves, E. (1997) *Community Care: Initial Training and Beyond.* London, Arnold.

Hunt, G. and Wainwright, P. (1994) *Expanding the Role of the Nurse. The Scope of Professional Practice.* Oxford, Blackwell Science.

Johnson, S. (1997) *Pathways of Care.* Oxford, Blackwell Science.

Ross, F. and Mackenzie, A. (1996) *Nursing in Primary Health Care: Policy into Practice.* London, Routledge.

Skidmore, D. (1997) *Community Care: Initial Training and Beyond.* London, Arnold.

Smith, M. and Maurer, F. (2000) *Community Health Nursing. Theory and Practice.* London, W.B. Saunders.

Turton, P. and Orr, J. (1993) *Learning to Care in the Community*, 2nd edn. London, Arnold.

Twinn, S., Roberts, B. and Andrews, S. (1996) *Community Health Care Nursing Principles into Practice.* Oxford, Butterworth Heinemann.

United Kingdom Central Council for Nursing, Midwifery and Health Visiting (1992) *Code of Professional Conduct.* London, UKCC.

United Kingdom Central Council for Nursing, Midwifery and Health Visiting (1998) *Guidelines for Records and Record Keeping.* London, UKCC.

Walsh, M. (1991) *Models in Clinical Nursing. The Way Forward.* London, Baillière Tindall.

3

Student supervision in community nursing practice

DANNY PERTAB

Learning outcomes

By the end of this chapter you will be able to:

- Describe the historical development of supervision in nursing education.
- Define 'supervision' as a formal, structured and purposeful activity in relation to your own learning as a student.
- Identify the purpose and benefits of student supervision in community nursing practice.
- Describe various methods of supervision.
- Delineate the roles, responsibilities and necessary attributes of the supervisor and the supervisee.

Introduction

With constant change in the health service, nurses face an increasing challenge to respond rapidly and work flexibly. They must provide high quality nursing care, often with limited resources. They encounter complex problems, requiring imaginative measures to maintain standards, alleviate stress and raise morale in the profession. Irrespective of their position in the hierarchy, all nurses need a degree of support to function effectively. Support provision is patchy. Investing in staff welfare is rarely popular and has little hope of immediate 'returns'. There are no 'quick fixes' to current difficulties and strategies for lasting success rest on a clear vision, long-term planning, not on short-term expediency measures. Assisting nurses to develop, both personally and professionally, is a necessary prerequisite to stability and happiness in the nursing workforce and the delivery of optimum care. Supervision is recognised as supporting practice, enabling nurses to maintain and promote standards of care (UKCC, 1996). Nursing, however, requires a radical change in culture matched with the necessary resources to embed the practice of supervision in a meaningful way. This chapter is a small step towards this ambition. It is designed to help you, as a student nurse in the community, to understand the meaning, rationales, principles, practice and limits of supervision in community nursing. This input on the topic will equip you to work in partnership with your named supervisor and fulfil your needs for learning, development and support.

Popularisation of supervision in nursing

The concept of supervision for qualified nurses is currently very popular. With a few exceptions, current nursing publications on the subject appear to concentrate mainly on the needs of these nurses. The bulk of the material comes from eminent sources, strongly weighted towards psychiatric nursing and intangible psychological constructs, rather unfamiliar to novices and adult branch nurses educated in the pre-Project 2000 era. Clinical supervision, as a topic for discussion and academic interest, has made a major impact. Regrettably, however, the practice of supervision for qualified nurses in the workplace is lagging behind (Bishop, 1998). While being recognised as essential, supervision for student nurses also has its problems. This may be symptomatic of a combination of factors, linked to unclear understanding of the phenomenon, the complexity of nursing in a modern context, nurses as diverse occupational groups with differing needs, the lack of genuine commitment and suitable role models, and shortage of essential resources. However, nurses at all levels must contribute to the development of the practice of supervision. The current opportunities must be seized with all vigour, to serve nurses and ultimately to benefit patient care. As a student, you should recognise and be aware of your own responsibilities to the process. This will help you to get the most out of the experience.

Student Activity 3.1

◆ What do you think your responsibilities are as a student to your supervision in the community?

◆ Make a list of these.

◆ Discuss these with your peers.

◆ Make notes in your portfolio.

Precursors to supervision in nursing

There are a number of factors, which have provided the basis for a clearer concept of supervision, relating to qualified nurses in particular, but also forcing a closer look at student supervision, albeit at a slower pace.

These factors, most significantly the publication of *Vision for the Future* (NHSME, 1993), have contributed to the rapid development of clinical supervision in nursing. Fowler (1996) notes that the 'vision' was founded on four major initiatives launched in the health service – *Caring for People* (DoH, 1989), *The Health of the Nation* (1992), The Children Act 1989 and The Patient's Charter (DoH, 1993) – all concerned with safety and standards of care in the health service. It also acknowledges the Project 2000 initiatives (UKCC, 1986) for basic nurse education. The tenth target of *Vision for the Future* sets the impetus to further develop clinical supervision. Other momentous events supporting the case of supervision for nurses are the Allitt Inquiry (House of Commons, 1994) and the Health Ombudsman's successive reports on the standards of nursing. Supervision is considered to be a necessary safeguard against malpractice and to guarantee high quality care. It is also timely to underpin the UKCC's *Code of Professional Conduct* (1992a) and *Scope of Professional Practice* (1992b). More recently the Department of Health (1999) in its publication *Making a Difference* and the UKCC (1999) report *Fitness for Practice* have both endorsed supervision and mentorship.

Student Activity 3.2

◆ Can you think of some reasons why safety and high standards are such key considerations affecting the debate on clinical supervision?

◆ Discuss and compare these with some of your peers.

◆ Make notes in your portfolio.

Supervision in clinical nursing education

The supervision of nursing students in clinical practice goes back to the Nightingale system of nurse training. Students worked as apprentices to qualified nurses and this approach had stood the test of time until the advent of Project 2000 courses. Supervision was informal and students learnt by 'sitting next to Nellie' although Nellie was often juggling with the competing tasks of patient care and student teaching. In practice, the pressures of work meant there was shortage of quality time to look after and teach learners properly. Students could hardly reap the full benefit of the apprenticeship system. They were counted as part of the nursing workforce, recruited primarily to deliver routine but essential patient care. In the order of priority, student learning came second to patient care and a significant part of students' work was unsupervised and stressful. This state of affairs took its toll and student support became a running theme of debate in the late 1970s and early 1980s. Such concern contributed to the most radical review of nurse education in Great Britain. The Diploma in Higher Education in Nursing Course is a result of this review. However, the debate still continues, and questions are still raised about the effectiveness of student supervision under the present system (Watson, 1999).

Student Activity 3.3

- ◆ Describe your early experience of clinical supervision in the community.

- ◆ Ask one or two of your peers to do the same.

- ◆ Compare and discuss the reasons for similarities and/or differences in your experiences.

- ◆ Make notes in your portfolio.

Supervision: a problem of definition

'Supervision' is a complex phenomenon open to wide interpretations. The term was imported in nursing from other caring disciplines such as social work, psychotherapy and counselling. 'Supervision' in the context of clinical practice is a confusing concept (Goorapah, 1997), a confusion perpetuated by nurses in their indiscriminate use of other equally vague schemes of support: mentoring and preceptoring. A lack of consensus on meaning makes supervision difficult to translate in practice (Watson, 1999). However, this quagmire also presents an opportunity for nurses themselves to critically examine the phenomenon and reach a composite view to suit their particular work settings. A consensus is paramount to make progress in the practice of supervision.

Definitions of supervision

There are several definitions of (clinical) supervision in the available literature. A selected number of examples are presented here for the purpose of study. Activity 3.4 is designed to help you search for meaning and formulate your own view of supervision as applied to student learning in community nursing.

Student Activity 3.4

The search for meaning

Step 1:
You have already written down and discussed with your peers, your own experiences of supervision in your placement.

Student Activity 3.4 *continued*

◆ Now, using those statements, see if you can formulate your own meaning of supervision.

◆ Ask one or two of your peers to do the same, and write down your conclusions in your portfolio.

Step 2:

Below is a sample of definitions on clinical supervision from various perspectives.

◆ Study them carefully and identify the main points.

◆ Identify their similarities and differences.

Step 3:

◆ Compare the above definitions with your own.

◆ Identify areas of similarities and differences.

◆ Which of these definitions most closely matches your view of supervision?

Step 4:

◆ Having studied the various definitions, are you now inclined to change or adapt your views in any ways? Give rationales for your particular stance.

Step 5:

◆ In the light of your newly acquired knowledge revise your definition as appropriate, and make notes in your portfolio.

Clinical supervision, in the context of student learning, is a planned activity to enable the student to learn and practise safe, evidenced-based (where appropriate) and quality nursing care with a level of support, commensurate with caring abilities and experience. It also provides planned moments to reflect on nursing situations and uncover or tap potentials for learning:

> Clinical supervision is an exchange between practising professionals to enable development of professional skills. (Butterworth et al., 1998)

> An intensive, interpersonally focused, one to one relationship in which one person is designated to facilitate the development of therapeutic competence in the other person. (Loganbill et al., 1992)

Clinical supervision is a formal arrangement that enables nurses, midwives and health visitors to discuss their work regularly with another experienced professional. Clinical supervision involves reflecting on practice in order to learn from experience and improve competence. An important part of the supervisor's role is to facilitate reflection and the learning process. (Kohner, 1994)

Clinical supervision is a formal process of professional support and learning which enables individual practitioners to develop knowledge and competence, assume responsibility for their own practice and enhance consumer protection and the safety of care in complex clinical situations. It is central to the process of learning and to the expansion of the scope for practice and should be seen as a means of encouraging self-assessment and analytical and reflective skills. (NHS Management Executive, 1993)

The above definitions suggest that supervision embodies:

- Certain values and assumptions
- A formal, deliberate and purposive activity
- A methodology of practice
- A process of learning, development and support
- An interpersonal relationship
- A sharing of responsibilities
- A context and boundary of practice
- A set of desirable outcomes.

The emerging view of supervision

The meaning of supervision is changing. Supervision, by tradition, involves inspecting the work of junior staff by managerial staff usually in higher positions of the organisational hierarchy. However, the current view of supervision departs from this narrow managerial perspective. Unlike its policing or punitive focus, supervision is an enabling activity. Its main purpose is to assist a person to realise his or her full potential as a fully functioning individual and professional. In the context of nurse education, supervision is designed to enable students achieve their optimum performances as learners and developing professional carers. It is potentially a 'shock absorber' against stress. The supervisor–student relationship is based on mutual respect and reciprocity and both individuals are beneficiaries. Students receive support, and are able to acquire practice and refine their knowledge base and caring skills. Supervisors become more accomplished helpers in the process.

Embracing values and assumptions

Introduction to supervision should begin in professional training and education, and continue thereafter as an integral part of professional development. (Butterworth, 1998; Cutliffe and Proctor, 1998).The practice of supervision in the context of pre-registration nurse education implies that the nursing profession holds a particular set of values about its new recruits. These assume that students are:

- An important asset and resource to nursing
- Valued and respected as adult learners
- Individuals with developmental and support needs
- Individuals with rights to high quality service
- To be nurtured into the profession
- Entitled to learn from competent role models
- Allowed to work at their appropriate levels of competence.

Models of supervision

Models of supervision fall into three main categories (Ayer et al., 1997; Butterworth et al., 1998). These are:

1. Those which describe supervision in relation to the supervisory relationship and its main constituents.

2. Those which describe the elements of the main function or role of supervision.

3. Developmental models that emphasise the process of the supervisory relationship.

Functions of supervision: a theoretical perspective

Supervision serves various functions including educational, management, supportive and the development of self and self-awareness (Bodley, 1992). Proctor (1986) contends that supervision serves three main functions: formative, restorative and normative. In nurse education, this can be interpreted as follows:

● *Formative:* the educative process that enables students develop the requisite knowledge, skills and attitudes for their professional caring role.

● *Restorative:* the supportive function that equips students to effectively manage the stresses associated with learning and nursing.

● *Normative:* the managerial function that provides the critical quality control element and helps students to practise safe, ethical and high standard nursing care, deal with human failings and prejudices, and achieve appropriate educational and developmental outcomes.

The goals of supervision, therefore, are to:

1. Expand your knowledge base as a student

2. Assist in developing your clinical proficiency

3. Help autonomy and self-esteem (Platt-Koch, 1986)

4. Deal effectively with stress

5. Develop self-awareness through reflection and self-evaluation (Johns, 1993)

6. Receive support, ultimately leading to improved standards of care (Westheimer, 1977).

Student Activity 3.5

◆ Using point number three, above, identify ways that you feel you have become more self-aware while undertaking your community experience.

◆ You can refer to examples relating to one or more specific events from your experience, for example dealing with a difficult situation, and so on.

◆ Discuss with one or more of your peers, and your assessor.

◆ Make notes in your portfolio.

The need for student supervision in community nursing practice

Irrespective of contexts, learning and nursing are stressful and demanding. All nurses need a level of support to function optimally and students are no exception. In practice professions including nursing, the importance of learning in the practical setting is well established (CCETSW, 1987; Thompson et al., 1999). Students learn their nursing from practice models, rather than educational input, both in the institutional setting (Fretwell, 1982) and community setting (Baillie, 1993; White et al., 1994). Clinical nursing is paramount for students to gain exposure to 'real' nursing, acquire professional role and identity, apply theoretical knowledge actively into practice settings for effective learning and to become confident.

Merely placing students in practice settings does not guarantee skills acquisition and effective learning however (UKCC, 1999). There are various difficulties in providing a conducive learning environment. Stress, student status, support systems, clinical staff and their ability to identify learning opportunities all affect learning (Powell, 1989; UKCC, 1999). The lack of supervision in itself is linked with student dissatisfaction with nursing and the inability to maximise clinical learning. Students can be expected to be worried for a number of reasons (McAllister et al., 1997) These include:

- Students' own expectations

- The expectations that others have of them

- The learning and working environment

- Patients' problems, such as illness, pain, accidents, poverty or neglect

- Their relationship with the supervisor and others

- The level of confidence they have in their abilities

- Worries concerning their own reactions, such as a fear of panicking if anything goes wrong

- Support provision.

Yet in spite of these difficulties, community nurses still provide educational experience that is highly valued by students (Jowett et al., 1992; Hallett, 1997). Clinical supervision is increasingly seen to provide some possible answers to problems associated with student learning in community nursing. Thompson and colleagues (1999) state that student satisfaction appears to be related to supervision, particularly to the length of time students spend on one-to-one contact with their practice supervisors and to the supervisors' breadth of experience. Thus student supervision appears to pay dividends when it is given over consistent periods of time, and particularly by supervisors who are experienced community nurses. This has clear implications for training and preparation, both for supervisors themselves and for their employers.

Good clinical supervision in your community placement may enable you to:

- Fit in smoothly in your designated community placements

- Develop professional caring skills

- Learn and practise nursing skills safely
- Develop self-confidence
- Bridge theory to practice, expectations to realisation and past to present experience (Holloway, 1994)
- Develop reflective skills (Severinsson, 1998)
- Be taught effectively by competent supervisor-carers
- Receive ongoing feedback on progress
- Identify and address areas of deficit
- Develop an enquiry based approach to nursing
- Identify and emulate suitable role models
- Define your own high standards of care
- Achieve personal and course objectives
- Manage stress effectively
- Enjoy learning and working in the community
- Experience caring supervision
- Learn the knowledge and skills of supervision.

Ogier and Cameron Buchierri (1990) hold that:

> Supportive, competent supervision is essential if nurses are to give their best care to the ill, frail and vulnerable.

Student Activity 3.6

- ◆ Use one or two examples to identify how you have been able to develop an enquiry based approach to your learning and to nursing from your community experience.
- ◆ How did your assessor/supervisor contribute to this?
- ◆ Discuss with your assessor/supervisor.
- ◆ Make notes in your portfolio.

The ultimate goal for your supervision in practice is to enable safe and high quality client care. Students nurtured under caring supervision may be more likely to develop as good supervisors, and thus be able to provide support for prospective learners. Student supervision bodes well for student learning in the future, as caring supervision becomes, from the very outset, integral to one's nursing career.

Supervision: a methodology of practice

Supervision follows a deliberate, goal-orientated and systematic approach. Nicklin (1997) conceptualised a six-stage cyclical model of supervision (Figure 3.1). The cycle consists of the following stages: practice analysis, problem identification, objective setting, planning, implementation and evaluation. Experienced learners should identify with these stages, as these are akin to the problem-solving steps of the nursing process. This cycle is equally applicable to student supervision, with perhaps one minor modification, that is the use of the term 'needs assessment' instead of 'practice analysis'.

Supervision in clinical nurse education

Supervision is an integral part of your whole educational package. It requires time and energy and is not an incidental event (Butterworth, 1998). Careful planning and co-ordination of activities between educational and practice providers are paramount, so that you can get the maximum benefit from your experience (Coates and Wright, 1991). Preparation of students for placements begins in the educational setting, before you embark on your designated locality. Several factors must be considered at this stage, including:

• The allocated placement
• The orientation programme
• Learning in clinical practice.

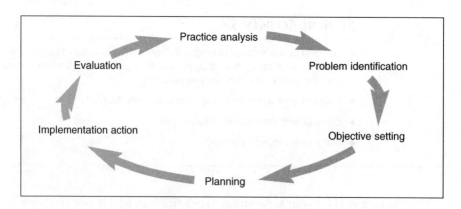

Figure 3.1 Supervisory cycle
Source: Adapted from Nicklin 'A practice centred model of clinical supervision'. In *Nursing Times,* **93**: 52–4, 12–18 November 1997.

Case Study 3.1

Jane is about to commence her first community nursing experience. She is rather apprehensive but looking forward to learning and caring for patients in the community setting. Jane lives 20 miles from her designated health centre (placement), which is situated outside the normal bus route. She has therefore some concerns about travelling to and from her placement.

What are the various needs that Jane may have in terms of learning, support and delivery of patient care:

(a) in her first week of allocation?

(b) by her second week of allocation?

(c) by mid-allocation?

(d) by the end of her allocation?

Identify ways in which the designated supervisor, and the district nursing team, may help Jane to fulfil these needs.

Give rationales for your answers based on reasoned judgement.

Discuss your answers with one or more of your peers.

Make notes in your portfolio.

Allocated placement

Details such as location of placement, ease of access, transport facilities, travelling expenses, basic amenities, contact person/named supervisor should be provided. The placement co-ordinator (allocation officer) will usually consider the circumstances of each student prior to allocation. Students' place of residence, travelling facilities, family commitments and other limiting factors should be carefully assessed. Flexible rostering may be necessary to ensure individual ability to attend placements without undue hardship. Placing a large number of students in a limited number of placements is understandably a major logistical 'nightmare' for placement co-ordinators. However, failure to consider students' individual circumstances may present severe difficulties later. Your own role and responsibility in this process includes appropriate forward planning by ensuring that you make the allocations officer aware, in advance, of personal factors which could impact negatively on your learning and where you are placed. Experience suggests that students who do not drive, cannot secure 'lifts' from peers to attend placements and have no alternative modes of travelling other than public transport

services have added stress when expected to travel 20–50 miles return
journey from base, in certain areas. Single parents, those with young children
or with sick family members and international students are particularly
vulnerable. During winter months you can be allowed to work shifts, which
are convenient to ensure that you return home in the safety of daylight
without being stranded in darkness at bus stops or railway stations. Sensitivity
and a caring approach is possible. As a learner, you must remember that you
have a role in helping practitioners understand your particular circumstances,
and negotiating placements and shifts that will help to optimise your learning
capacity in practice.

Learning in clinical practice

Information will usually be provided on:

- Organisations providing placements
- Uniforms and dress code
- Orientation to clinical placements
- Meeting with supervisor or mentor
- The purpose of your allocation
- Learning objectives and their relation to the course curriculum
- Availability of appropriate resources
- Clinical supervision and mentorship
- Teaching and learning opportunities
- Placement visits from designated module teacher
- Assessment scheme
- Planned reflection on learning and feedback: techniques and frequency
- Dealing with any difficulties.

If you are to get the most out of a supervised community placement you
should, if at all possible, sit down together with your supervisor, at appropriate intervals, in order to:

- Negotiate the content, method and process of supervised practice
- Accommodate your past learning and caring experience
- Focus on relevant areas of practice
- Identify learning objectives in tune with perceived areas of needs
- Identify areas of perceived weakness

- Match theory with relevant practical skills
- Negotiate choice, participation and autonomy in learning
- Make learning efficient in terms of limited resources.

Methods of supervision

Houston (1990) proposed five main methods of supervision:

1. One-to-one sessions between two individuals of the same discipline

2. One-to-one sessions between two individuals of different disciplines

3. One-to-one peer sessions

4. Group supervision

5. Network supervision.

One-to-one sessions

There are two different types of one-to-one method. In the first instance, the learner and the supervisor come from the same discipline. This approach is common in pre-registration nurse education, where you will be supervised by registered nurses, who meet the necessary requirements. The second approach also involves two individuals; but in this instance, the student and the supervisor come from two different disciplines. One example is where a professional carer allied to nursing supervises a student nurse. This is common practice in aspects of shared care. For example, when a physiotherapist teaches a student nurse skills of physiotherapy or a medico-social worker assists the learner on conducting a home assessment.

One-to-one peer supervision

In this approach, supervision takes place between people of similar grades and expertise. It is more in tune with learning and working between equals. This usually occurs by default in pre-registration nursing where a student turns to his or her peer for help, particularly during periods of intense activity or when the named supervisor is unavailable or perceived to be unhelpful. Learning from your peers can, however, be a positive experience if it is approached appropriately. Notice that in some of the activities, in this chapter and others, you have been asked, at different points, to discuss issues with your peers. This can help you to gain comparative and contrasting perspectives on clinical situations. In most instances, you will be in a different team from your peers, which could indicate differences in caseload. The potential for learning should not be undermined. You may even wish, at an appropriate time, to negotiate an exchange of placement with one of your peers from a different placement or in a different team, to help give you another view. This may be for a day or a week, depending on the overall length of your placement. Certainly if you have a twelve-week placement, which is usual in some areas, a week in an alternative placement is a good way of enhancing your learning.

Group supervision with a supervisor

Here, a group of students come together to learn and seek help from a designated supervisor. In education, lecturers commonly use this approach in guiding small groups of students in essay planning, seminar preparation and other small group activities. Such a forum enables you to seek clarification on title, presentation style, use of learning resources and other skills. It is also useful in allaying anxiety at individual or group levels. This method can be, and is, used effectively by supervisors in practice settings to demonstrate specific skills to a small group of students. It can be very efficient in the use of limited time and resources. It also helps to ensure that where large numbers of students are placed within some areas, the use of clinical workshops ensures that everyone benefits from the skills of all the specialist practitioners, whom they may not have been able to access individually. The role of the supervisor here includes group facilitation, helping students to clarify and share ideas and allaying anxieties.

Network supervision

In network supervision a group of people with similar expertise and interests who do not necessarily work together on a daily basis, meet for supervision. Network supervision has the advantage of linking professionals, community wide, to explore issues of common interest. These may include any aspects of community nursing such as policies on tissue viability, clinical supervision, development of clinical governance and primary care trusts (PCTs), on which different professional groups share joint responsibilities. Such forums may help to find answers to problems from differing perspectives. In areas where shared learning between medical and nursing students is beginning to happen, network supervision may enrich learning for both groups, in addressing overarching issues from their differing worldviews.

Deciding on an appropriate method of supervision depends on many factors. The 'perfect model' is still in the making. For the vast majority of nurses, models used stem from working with, adapting and refining existing ones. However, a 'good' model must be simple, user-friendly, compatible with prevailing values, context relevant, yet flexible and fit for purpose.

Community nursing may provide the flexibility to practise wide-ranging methods of supervision to suit the differing learning and working conditions. These methods may be used either singly or in an eclectic manner for maximum gain provided each approach is carefully considered and organised with due care.

In the community district nurses generally work independently caring for their specific caseloads. They work with clients on a one-to-one basis, mainly in the patients' own homes, although they also provide care from other settings such as the health centre, the GP surgery and nursing homes. You are assigned to individual community nurses for community experience. Such condition makes the one-to-one approach between student and the community nurse rather attractive. Students find this close one-to-one working relationship in the community is highly conducive to learning (Hallett, 1997). This dyadic relationship brings three advantages: every student knows who his or her designated supervisor is; there is continuity in learning; and the length of time student and supervisor spend together helps to develop close interpersonal relationship, which Hallett (1997) claims is one of the most important characteristics of the community placement. The supervisor may also organise the student to work with other professionals, and other members of the district nursing team in order to learn related caring skills.

The attributes of student supervision

Supervision as an activity takes place in relational terms. It involves two or more persons coming together to serve their mutual interests. There are three basic requirements for effectiveness in this kind of relationship: attraction, action and affect (Darling, 1984). For this relationship to thrive, good communication is paramount. It is the vehicle by which all supervisory activities take effect. An enduring, close but non-toxic relationship is important for a successful outcome.

As with any other forms of human relations, student supervision calls for certain attributes if it is to be positively meaningful. Faugier (1998) identifies these supervisory qualities as:

- Generosity
- Reward
- Openness
- Willingness to learn
- Thoughtful and thought-provoking
- Humanitarian
- Sensitive
- Uncompromising
- Personal

- Practical
- Orientated
- Relationship-centred
- Trust.

Supervisors who respect and value students and put themselves out to help learners are perceived as good supervisors. Credible supervisors are able to communicate freely, make students feel comfortable, build trust, inspire confidence, put commitment into concrete actions, engage students in decision making, respond appropriately to students' concerns, and are themselves competent nurses (Fowler, 1996; Sloan, 1998). These qualities are equally important to nursing and teaching. Nurses who openly express these qualities in their daily work with students are appreciated and perceived as good supervisor–practitioner–teachers. Enabling students to learn and function at their very best, and with the right support, is an essential component of supervision. The partnership necessary for this to work rests with your understanding of the processes and your contribution to ensuring positive outcomes (Twinn and Davies, 1996; Durrari and Kendrick, 1999).

Contractual dimensions

Student supervision in nursing is a formal process based on ground rules between supervisor and student. The contractual framework embraces the educational institution (university), practice providers (community health trusts) and the profession's code of conduct (Nicklin, 1997). A contract helps to set the supervisor–supervisee relationship on a professional footing. It serves to negotiate the agenda, scope, levels and boundaries of supervisory practice and where appropriate frequency, dates, locations and duration are set. The contract should cover such issues as:

- Privacy, confidentiality, trust and veracity (Nicklin, 1997)
- Support, teaching and learning plan
- Learning and practice environments
- Frequency of access and interaction
- Opportunities for reflection
- Provision of feedback
- Assessment procedure and charting a profile of progress
- Documentation procedure and completion of reflective diary
- Contingency plan for mitigating circumstances

● Integrity: honouring contract and appropriate recourse of actions for breach of contract.

Supervision is no panacea to all ills in nurse education and must be placed in context. There are several problems that may determine outcomes. Nurses must pitch their expectations of supervision on a realistic basis to avoid disillusionment with its practice.

Conclusion

This chapter has explored the concept of supervision and its various dimensions, with particular reference to your learning during your community placement. For your supervision to work successfully, it must be clearly defined to fit the contextual reality and provide a measurable yardstick for practice. The benefits of supervision must be pitched at a realistic level. It will not compensate for poor commitment, inadequate resources, and the lack of managerial support for practising supervisors, who may be juggling with the competing needs of learners and patients in a demanding work environment. Supervision of learners grounded on a sound foundation and actively supported by community nurse managers holds great promise for community nurse education in the future. The supervisor–student relationship in practice is special and must be actively encouraged to flourish. It may prove to be the single most important factor determining success in student learning and development. It is a major protection against stress, and potentially may make student learning experience worthwhile against all the possible odds. To this end, your supervisor and you must work actively and in the spirit of true partnership to achieve your mutual goals. Hopefully, your own positive experience of supervision, along with the knowledge and skills learned during your community experience, will help you to contribute positively to the process when this becomes appropriate, following your completion of your programme.

Further reading

Butterworth, T., Faugier, J. and Burnard, P. (1998) *Clinical Supervision and Mentoring in Nursing*, 2nd edn. Cheltenham, Stanley Thornes.
Fowler, J. (1996) How to use models of clinical supervision in practice. Professional development. *Nursing Standard*, **10**(29): 42–7.
Hawkins, P. and Shohet, R. (1992) *Supervision in the Helping Professions*. Milton Keynes, Open University Press.
Kohner, N. (1994) *Clinical Supervision in Practice*. London, King's Fund.
Morton Cooper, A. and Palmer, A. (1993) *Mentoring and Preceptoring, A Guide to Support Roles in Clinical Practice*. London, Blackwell Science.

References

Ayer, S., Knight, S., Joyce, L. and Nightingale, V. (1997) Practice-led education and development project: developing styles in clinical supervision. *Nurse Education Today*, 17: 347–58.

Baillie, L. (1993) Factors affecting student nurses learning in community nursing placements: a phenomenological study. *Journal of Advanced Nursing*, 18: 1043–53.

Bishop, V. (1994) Clinical supervision for an accountable profession. *Nursing Times*, 90(39): 35–7.

Bishop, V. (1998) *Clinical Supervision in Practice*. Basingstoke, Macmillan – now Palgrave, Chapter 1.

Bodley, D.E. (1992) Clinical supervision in psychiatric nursing: using the process record. *Nurse Education Today*, 12(2): 148–55.

Butterworth, T. (1998) Clinical supervision as an emerging idea in nursing. In Butterworth, T., Faugier, J. and Burnard, P. (1998) (eds) *Clinical Supervision and Mentorship in Nursing*, 2nd edn. Cheltenham, Stanley Thornes.

Butterworth, T., Faugier, J. and Burnard, P. (1998) *Clinical Supervision and Mentorship in Nursing*, 2nd edn. Cheltenham, Stanley Thornes.

Central Council for Education and Training in Social Work (1987) National Nursing Conference, Ulster. *Care for tomorrow: the case for reform of education and training for social workers and other care staff.* CCETSW, London.

Coates, H. and Wright, J. (1991) *The Integration of Work-based Learning with Academic Assessment, Guidelines for Good Practice. A User's Guide.* Coventry Polytechnic.

Cutcliffe, J.R. and Proctor, B. (1998) An alternative training approach to clinical supervision: 1. *British Journal of Nursing*, 7(5): 280–5.

Darling, L. (1984) What do nurses want in a mentor? *Journal of Nursing Administration*, 14(10): 42–4.

Department of Health (1989) *Caring for People – Community Care in the Next Decade and Beyond*. London, HMSO.

Department of Health (1989) *The Children Act*. London, HMSO.

Department of Health (1992) *Health of the Nation: A Strategy for Health in England*. London, HMSO.

Department of Health (1992) *The Patient's Charter*. London, Department of Health.

Department of Health (1999) *Making a Difference: Strengthening the Nursing, Midwifery and Health Visiting Contribution to Health and Health Care*. London, HMSO.

Durrari, W. and Kendrick, K. (1999) Update: Implementing clinical supervision. *Professional Nurse*, 14(12): 849–52.

Faugier, J. (1998) The supervisory relationship. In Butterworth, T., Faugier, J. and Burnard, P. (eds) *Clinical Supervision and Mentorship in Nursing*, 2nd edn. Cheltenham, Stanley Thornes.

Fowler, J. (1996) The organisation of clinical supervision within the nursing profession: a review of the literature. *Journal of Advanced Nursing*, 23: 471–8.

Fretwell, J.E. (1982) *Ward Teaching and Learning: Sister and the Learning Environment*. London, Royal College of Nursing.

Goorapah, D. (1997) Clinical supervision. *Journal of Clinical Nursing*, 6: 173–8.

Hallett, C. (1997) Managing change in nurse education: the introduction of Project 2000 in the community. *Journal of Advanced Nursing*, 25: 836–43.

Holloway, E.L. (1994) A bridge of knowing: the scholar–practitioner of supervision. *Counselling Psychology Quarterly*, 7(1): 3–15.

House of Commons (1994) *Independent Inquiry Relating to Deaths and Injuries on the Children's Ward at Grantham and Kesteven General Hospital During the Period of February to April 1991* (The Allitt Inquiry). London, HMSO.

Houston, G. (1990) *Supervision and Counselling*. London, The Rochester Foundation.

Jardine, J. and Asherton, J. (1992) Development of community practice teaching in Swindon. *Health Visitor*, 65: 88–9.

Johns, C. (1993) Professional supervision. *Journal of Nursing Management*, 1: 9–13.

Jowett, S., Walton, I. and Payne, S. (1992) *Project 2000 Research: Interim Papers 4 and 5*. Slough, National Foundation for Educational Research.

Kohner, N. (1994) *Clinical Supervision in Practice*. London, King's Fund.

Loganbill, C., Hardy, E. and Delworth, U. (1992) Major contribution, supervision: a conceptual model. *The Counselling Psychologist*, 10:1.

McAllister, L., Lincoln, M., McLeod, S. and Maloney, D. (1997) *Facilitating Learning in Clinical Settings*. Cheltenham, Stanley Thornes.

NHS Management Executive (1993) *A Vision for the Future: The Nursing, Midwifery and Health Visiting Contribution to Health and Health Care*. London, Department of Health.

Nicklin, P. (1997) A practice-centred model of clinical supervision. *Nursing Times*, 12(46): 52–4.

Ogier, M. and Cameron Buchierri, R. (1990) Supervision: a cross-cultural approach. *Nursing Standard*, 4(31): 24–6.

Platt-Koch, L. (1986) Clinical supervision for psychiatric nurses. *Journal of Psychosocial Nursing*, 26(1): 7–15.

Powell, J. (1989) The reflective practitioner in nursing. *Journal of Advanced Nursing*, 14: 824–32.

Procter, B. (1986) Supervision: a co-operative exercise in accountability. In Marken, M. and Payne, M. (eds) *Enabling and Ensuring*. Leicester, Leicester Youth Bureau and Council for Education and Training in Youth and Community Work.

Severinsson, E. (1998) Bridging the gap between theory and practice: a supervision programme for nursing students. *Journal of Advanced Nursing*, 27: 1269–77.

Sloan, G. (1998) Clinical supervision: characteristics of a good supervisor. *Nursing Standard*, 12(40): 42–6.

Sloan, G. (1999) Understanding clinical supervision from a nursing perspective. *British Journal of Nursing*, 8(8): 524–9.

Thompson, A., Davies, S., Shepherd, S. and Whittaker, K. (1999) Continuing education needs of community nurses, midwives and health visitors for supervising and assessing students. *Nurse Education Today*, 19: 93–106.

Twinn, S. and Davies, S. (1996) The supervision of Project 2000 students in clinical setting: issues and implications for practitioners. *Journal of Clinical Nursing*, 5(3): 177–83.

United Kingdom Central Council for Nursing, Midwifery and Health Visiting (1986) *Project 2000: A New Preparation for Practice*. London, UKCC.

United Kingdom Central Council for Nursing, Midwifery and Health Visiting (1992a) *Code of Professional Conduct for the Nurse, Midwife and Health Visitor*. London, UKCC.

United Kingdom Central Council for Nursing, Midwifery and Health Visiting (1992b) *The Scope of Professional Practice*. London, UKCC.

United Kingdom Central Council for Nursing, Midwifery and Health Visiting (1996) *Position Statement on Clinical Supervision for Nursing and Health Visiting*. London, UKCC.

United Kingdom Central Council for Nursing, Midwifery and Health Visiting (1999) *Fitness for Practice*. London, UKCC.

Watson, N. (1999) Mentoring today – the students' views. An investigative case study of pre-registration nursing students' experiences and perceptions of mentoring in one theory/practice module of the Common Foundation Programme on a Project 2000 course. *Journal of Advanced Nursing*, 29(1): 254–62.

Westheimer, I. (1977) *The Practice of Supervision Within Social Work, A Guide for Supervisors*. London, Ward Lock Educational.

White, E., Riley, E., Davies, S. and Twinn, S. (1994) *A Detailed Study of the Relationships Between Teaching, Support, Supervision and Role Modelling in Clinical Areas within the Context of Project 2000 Courses*. Report from the English National Board for Nursing, Midwifery and Health Visiting, London.

4 The legislative basis of community nursing

CAROL WILKINSON

Learning outcomes

By the end of this chapter you will be able to:

- Recognise the historical and contemporary legislation affecting community nursing.
- Discuss the impact of the NHS and Community Care Act 1990 on health care provision.
- Briefly examine the most recent health reforms.
- Analyse the impact of legislation on patient care.

Introduction

This chapter is intended to provide a brief overview of some of the issues that you may encounter as a student during your placement in the community. Some will have a bearing on your rights and obligations as a nurse in terms of professional accountability and confidentiality. This is coupled with late 20th-century political reforms in health and health care in Britain.

History and background

Policies during the 1980s largely reflected an inability of central government to provide leadership in developing community care (see Chapter 1 for background information on the pre-1980s history and development). The 1985 House of Commons Select Committee Report criticised the slow movement of people being discharged into the community, stressing that community-based services cannot be established on a cost neutral basis. At the same time it inherently confirmed the status quo underlining the salience of the family as prime carer. In addition, these policies rarely included carers and merely referred to supporting families, interweaving statutory formal with informal care, working in partnership or complementing the role of the family. Family care was taken for granted. The Audit Commission's *Making a Reality of Community Care* (1986), while admitting that policies placed an additional burden on relatives at a time when the whole concept of a supporting community is breaking down, still took the view that support from relatives and even neighbours remained at high levels in the form of dispersed extended families, and by implication that this was not necessarily a source of concern. Assuming a high level of support from carers represented a highly cost effective strategy. Social care agencies only needed to contribute minimal amounts of formal resources to ensure extensive inputs from the informal sector (Twigg and Atkin, 1994).

Increased reliance upon the family to provide care (through reducing the proportion of public expenditure going to personal social services) was set (Qureshi and Walker, 1989). At the same time, however, a range of the government's own economic and social policies were undermining the ability of families to shoulder such responsibilities. It was not until the publication of *Community Care: An Agenda for Action*, better known as the Griffiths Report (1988), that recognition of the role of unpaid carers and the broader notion of community care began to emerge.

Griffiths considered that the modernising of management of community care was more important than altering its organisation. The report empha-sised a mixed economy of care. The emphasis rested with social services acting as the designers, organisers and purchasers of non-health care services and not primarily as direct service providers. Emphasis was placed on making the maximum possible use of voluntary and private sector bodies to widen consumer choice, stimulate innovation and encourage efficiency.

It was argued that the role of social services would become one of case management, assessing the gap between resources and individual needs, targeting funds to devise cost effective care packages and regularly reviewing priorities. Radical change in the workforce was needed, involving significant changes in role for a number of professional and occupational groups. There was a further argument taken up from the earlier Audit Commission Report (1986), namely the creation of a new occupation of community carer to undertake the front line personal and social support of dependent people (Griffiths, 1988). This provided a case for developing new skills among existing staff to enable them to tackle the new tasks proposed, developing completely new roles and replacing those that no longer appeared to be necessary.

The report sought to eliminate the perverse incentive towards residential care, which the system had created by making both local authorities and social security responsible for funding residential and domiciliary care in an ad-hoc manner. It was argued that a unified community care budget be allo-cated to local social services authorities in the form of a specific grant, prin-

Student Activity 4.1

◆ Discuss with a group of your peers whether the burden of responsibility for the care of sick relatives should be the responsibility of the state or the individual.

◆ Provide reasons for and against.

◆ Keep notes in your portfolio.

cipally composed of resources transferred from the social security system. This principle was adopted by the government and formed the basis for the financial arrangements ultimately introduced in 1993.

Residential and nursing home residents in the public, private and voluntary sectors received public funding support only after separate assessments of the financial means of the applicant and of the need for care made known.

The process was inclined to begin with an assessment of whether residential care was an appropriate way to meet the need of people. The social security system should then contribute a financial assessment but the resultant benefit, the residential allowance, would be set in the light of the average total of income support and housing benefit to which someone living other than in residential care would be entitled. This would leave social services authorities in the position of making up the balance of the contribution.

The Griffiths Report – recommendations

The main recommendations of the Griffiths Report on Community Care were:

- The appointment of a Minister for community care.
- Social services should act as lead agents of community care.
- There should be continuing collaboration of agencies involved in care and the development of case management.
- New financing methods should be made available for community care, including grants to local authorities.
- There should be a single path towards publicly financed residential care.
- Joint and shared training between different professional groups should be encouraged.
- More consumer choice should be encouraged.
- The responsibilities and role boundaries of health and social care agencies should be encouraged.
- Availability of resources should be balanced against political aspirations.
- Independence for the consumer should be encouraged, with an emphasis on home-based care, personal development and a greater consumer voice.

The 1989 White Paper *Caring for People* became the government's response to Griffiths. Not all of Griffiths' recommendations were adopted, and so a shortfall was left in aspiration of community care in years to come. The paper underlined the issues of promoting choice and was immediately followed with *Working for Patients* published in the same year. Both papers formed the basis of the NHS and Community Care Act 1990.

Caring for People

The main objectives of the paper were to:

- Promote domiciliary, day and respite services to enable people to live in their own homes wherever feasible and sensible.
- Make practical support for carers a high priority by service providers.
- Encourage needs assessment and a case management approach to enable the process of high quality care.
- Ensure that the independent sector was developing alongside quality public services.
- Clarify the responsibilities of agencies and to enable performance accountability.
- Introduce a new funding structure for social care.

NHS and Community Care Act 1990

Prior to 1989, health ministers were afforded full responsibility for health policy formulation but had very limited control over activities within the NHS. Power and service developments at local level lay in the hands of doctors, who were not accountable to ministers for their actions or for the resources they used. There was increasing pressure from Parliament to improve central monitoring of the NHS. Indeed, this is highlighted in the works of Culyer (1988), and Klein and Day (1988). The arguments were initially put forward by Enthoven (1985) who observed that:

(a) There was poor matching of funding to workload. The 'Resource allocation working party' (RAWP) system of allocating funds was inadequate, for example day and outpatients were not included in the calculation although this may be the most cost effective form of treatment.

(b) There were inappropriate incentives for managers and clinicians. Reputations for shorter waiting times or clinical excellence attracted more referrals but no extra money. Cost effective behaviour such as prevention work and carrying out more minor surgery was not rewarded.

(c) A lack of responsiveness to consumers was evident. Curative hospital-based medicine dominated at the expense of prevention, health promotion and community services and high priority was given to the treatment of short-term episodes of acute illness to the detriment of care and rehabilitation of the chronically ill.

(d) Continued and persistent inequalities were still apparent between classes in health status despite the availability of a free health service.

(e) Cost data services were largely unavailable.

(f) Outcome measurements of services and treatment were largely absent.

(g) Decision-making was fragmented rather than based on evidence about the cost effectiveness of treating full patient episodes of care.

(h) The medical profession has remained dominant. Service quality and efficiency measurement are inadequate and carried out strictly by the medical profession.

(i) There were few incentives to innovate.

Enthoven (1985) concluded that health planning in the NHS required some attention.

So what is health planning?

Planning per se is required to prevent waste, make full use of scarce resources, contain costs to what is affordable and see that they are distributed geographically on an equitable basis. This is in effect a rationing process.

Health planning aims to ensure the necessary services, of the right quality, are provided at the right place, at the right time; that the health services have a balanced relationship with other social services and that this is achieved at the lowest possible cost in real resources and is affordable. Thus health planning relies on the availability of information about the service, treatment and cost, guaranteed efficiency and equity. In order to ensure quality within a given service, there needs to be:

- *Specification of objectives:* what type of service is needed? What evidence is available to support demand? How is the service to be delivered?

- *Evaluation of outcomes:* have objectives been achieved? Is any modification required?

- *Measurement of present and future cost:* cost of labour per hour/day, equipment, hidden costs accounted for, possible expansion, charges of competitor taken into consideration?

- *Evaluation of alternative courses of action:* is there another method of treatment as beneficial in terms of financial and human cost?

Enthoven saw the need for such a rationing process to occur in the NHS and offered a solution; the separation of the purchasing of health care from its provision and management and subjecting providers to an element of competition for contracts. This would mean that providers would have a financial incentive to cut costs, improve quality and be more responsive to what consumers wanted. Purchasers in turn, as they would be cash limited, would have an incentive to bargain for improved value for money.

Support for Enthoven's views of the internal market came from the British political right and was introduced in *Working for Patients* (DoH, 1989b).

Student Activity 4.2

♦ £3 million has been allocated to your primary care trust for two consecutive years to set up services to improve ethnic health within your area. Within this time, the Trust will be expected to demonstrate the effectiveness of the service, and establish the means to secure additional income to pursue and continue the projects started.

♦ Using the notion of health planning as discussed above, iden-tify the best ways of utilising funds for this community project.

♦ Discuss this activity with a group of your peers.

♦ Make notes in your portfolio.

Other developments in health planning were also taking root in the NHS:

● The Welsh Health Planning Forum produced a consultative document, *Strategic Intent and Direction for the NHS in Wales* (WHPF, 1989), the central theme of which was the notion of health gain.

● *Promoting Better Health* (DoH, 1990b): in this document, the govern-ment gave an undertaking of its commitment to health promotion and improvement of primary health care services; followed later by the publi-cation of the *Health of the Nation* (DoH, 1992) which set out specific targets in health promotion to achieve health gain with the undertaking of achieving health for all.

The relevance of these documents directed intentions for investment, disin-vestment, and concentration of specific service delivery in health. Community health promotion was one of the first areas to experience the difficulties emerging between free market intentions and central planning. Decisions had to be made in the continuation as service provider or contractor of services. It was assumed that community nurses continued to be providers of care under the new regime.

The purchasor/providor split

The contracting process (Figure 4.1) required publicly funded purchasers to contract with providers. These could be private or public firms. The purchaser was required to assess the needs of the local population, and to purchase those services which met these needs cost effectively. If related to the notion of planning, in order to operate efficiently, the purchaser required information about the cost effectiveness of competing procedures. Information facilitated prioritisation, which reflected both efficiency and social values. The primary purchaser was the District Health Authority. However, general practice fundholders (GPFH) also purchased services. The aim was to enhance primary and secondary care in terms of service provision. Like the notion of planning, the contractual process aims to make the best use of scarce resources through deciding priorities for their allocation.

Resources are allocated in such a way as to maximise health gains in society. This was in an attempt to achieve efficiency. Efficiency is about comparing costs or resources spent and benefits to well-being produced by competing

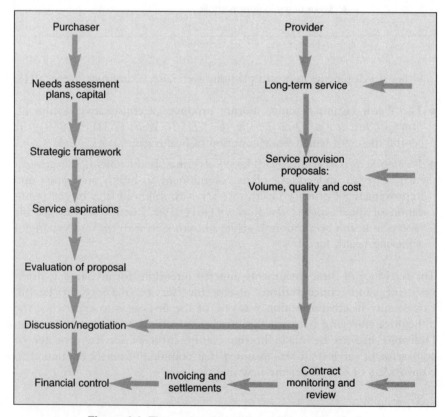

Figure 4.1 The contracting process (internal market)

health care interventions. Operative and allocative efficiency is based on the assumption that the care considered is effective, that is, actually produces health gain.

Health gain

There are two components to the notion of health gain:

- Adding years to life, and
- Adding life to years.

Whether or not the former part is necessarily desirable, it is at least generally measurable. Adding years to life is seeking to improve the quality of a person's life by improving his or her health status. Adding life to years is measured in QALYs, that is Quality Adjusted Life Years. The QALY developed by Professor Alan Maynard, is a method of assessing the health benefits of a given procedure against the resources used to achieve it. For example, the cost of achieving one QALY for renal dialysis might be equal to 190 preventive advice sessions on smoking by GPs. Benefits are defined as improvements in life expectancy adjusted for changes in four key indicators of quality of life: physical mobility, capacity for self-care, freedom from pain or distress and social adjustment. The value of extra years of life diminishes if one or more of these quality factors declines or cannot be assumed. Hence the need for quality adjusted life years.

The health reforms of the 1990s were designed primarily to improve efficiency and effectiveness in health care, alongside improved service provision for the consumer. Aspects of the NHS and Community Care Act 1990 affecting nurses in the community came into force from 1 April 1993. This response was the culmination of earlier reforms under the Griffiths Report (1988) and *Caring for People* (DoH, 1989a).

The Act specified the following:

1. Provision of community care plans

Section 46 of the Act stipulates that the local authorities in conjunction with health authorities and the voluntary and private sector must prepare plans for the provision of services in the community and revise them annually. This intended to make clear specific intentions of the services to encourage greater coherence.

2. Assessment of need

Section 47 requires local authorities to carry out an assessment of needs for community services on any individual in its catchment area who would appear to be in need of any services that it provides or for which it arranges the provision. Where appropriate, the health authority and/or the housing authority may be required to be involved in the assessment (the concept of joint assessments). In urgent situations community care services can be provided temporarily and an assessment should take place as soon as possible thereafter.

3. Finances: nursing and residential accommodation

Responsibility for purchasing accommodation for clients became the domain of the local authority in April 1993. Those residents moving into local authority accommodation after 1st April 1993, may purchase a place at a nursing or residential home and recover the fees from residents, who can claim means-tested Income Support from the Department of Social Security but only at the ordinary level.

4. Powers of the State

Persons can be authorised by the Secretary of State under Section 48 to inspect premises used for the provision of community care services. Local authorities have inspection units. The Secretary of State can issue directions as to the exercise of social services functions (Section 50) and has required all local authorities to establish a procedure for considering any representations, including complaints about a failure to discharge local social services functions.

5. The Act also makes provision for the transfer of health service staff to local authorities (Section 49)

The legislation enabled the progression towards greater development of care in the community.

Rights and charters

The reforms in the NHS in the early part of the 1990s brought with it a series of concerns about the issue of quality. The purchaser–provider split was a result of introducing market economics and ideologies into a service that was unaccustomed to competition among the professions, let alone among individual hospitals within the same community.

The patient factor was one area of health care that gained increasing prominence as there became greater choice in terms of selecting where to place their custom, starting with the choice of GP, then to the hospital for the routine test or major surgery. This was also the case in dental services. Indeed, researchers in the field saw the patient factor being linked to the giant issue of quality for fear that custom might be taken elsewhere, be it to another NHS Trust or the private health sector. There were wide variations under the early contractual arrangements relating to quality standards, including issues around patient requirements and satisfaction. It transpired that there was little data to make adequate comparisons across the range of services.

Student Activity 4.3

◆ Find out if there is an annual community care charter produced for the community in which you are placed.

◆ Is this a health and social care plan?

◆ Discuss it with one or two of your peers.

◆ Ask your assessor the extent to which the plan reflects what happens in the community.

◆ Make notes for your portfolio.

The Patient's Charter, introduced in October 1991, became a part of the process in accumulating information about the consumer and also in instituting quality standards in care provision.

The Patient's Charter initially introduced ten rights, nine national standards and four local standards. Seven of the rights were enshrined within the various NHS Acts and three new rights were subsequently introduced in The Patient's Charter of 1993 (Tschudin, 1995; Ryland, 1996).

Student Activity 4.4

◆ Discuss with a group of your peers your rights as a citizen, and ways in which you exercise them.

◆ What are your rights as an employee? Locate the sources of law, which give you these rights.

◆ Make notes on the above in your portfolio.

What is a right?

A right is any claim or title that is morally just or legally granted as allowable or due to a person. A standard is an accepted or approved example of something against which others are judged or measured. Rights should be inalienable and enforceable by law, standards are aspirations which will not always be reached (Plant, 1989).

The Department of Health defines a right as *a level of service to which the patient is entitled and which must be delivered.* The official definition of a right is that patients will receive 100 per cent compliance. It is in effect an absolute guarantee. The guarantee of admission for treatment within two years in The Patient's Charter is called a right, waiting times in outpatient clinics or for an ambulance are standards. Both depend on resources and other health service priorities. The issue of rationing and responsibility comes under the notion of The Patient's Charter. It is against common sense and morality to treat someone for a minor problem simply because they waited two years and fail to treat someone with a serious problem, in order to comply with this right (Hogg, 1994).

There are few rights in health care enforceable in law. However, an individual does have the right to health care. While the Secretary of State has a duty to provide a comprehensive health service, this right is not enforceable in law. For example, if a relative attends court to argue for life saving treatment for a spouse where the health authority lacked the funds, the court would decide that funding was a matter of politics rather than law (Hughes, 1992).

Other rights have restrictions on them, often because of a lack of commitment to them. The restrictions are justified on the grounds that the professional is in a better position to judge the best interests of patients than patients themselves (see chapter on needs assessment). Examples include the issue of access to health records, informed consent and the right to refuse treatment as well as confidentiality. Some rights are hard to define. The right to give consent based on information has been established in court, but there are still problems of defining informed consent in practice. The right to privacy and to be treated with dignity is hard to define and definitions will depend on the quality of existing services. The expectations of what is considered acceptable standards as services improve, are variable (Hogg, 1994).

Implications of The Patient's Charter for nursing

The document itself was seen as politically motivated, it aims to move the NHS towards a market economy in line with the rest of the public sector and, as such, must be viewed in conjunction with the other government initiatives such as *Caring for People* (DoH, 1989a) and *Working for Patients* (DoH, 1989b).

The Charter was an opportunity for nurses to strengthen their position and for them to actively participate in the development of service delivery for their patients. The Charter provides health care workers and users of health care services with a formal quality monitoring tool. Despite the fact that nurses and health workers as well as patients were crucial in the operation of The Patient's Charter, they were not consulted prior to its introduction. It is also acknowledged that the managerial sector of the NHS received little opportunity to assimilate the implications before the Charter was introduced.

Under The Patient's Charter, the issue of quality within the NHS became a live one. Wilson-Barnett (1981) states that quality concerns itself with the value of benefit that can be derived from care. Quality is the degree of success which is achieved in reaching goals; it assumes evaluation of care. The definition focuses on the outcome or product of care. The definition can therefore be seen as acceptable when looking specifically at tasks, knowledge base, efficiency and the results or products of care. All these things can be measured, and as such, can satisfy the nurses' role within The Patient's Charter. Statistics can be produced in relation to the Charter's rights and standards.

The issue of quality is broadened by Ellis (1988) who suggests that quality is the totality of features or characteristics of a product or service that bear on its ability to satisfy a given need, suggesting that quality is that which gives complete customer satisfaction. Such a definition considers both the process of the service and its outcome. However, confusion arises when attempts are made explicitly to identify the customer. Patients receive direct care. That is, the services provided by nurses, and could, therefore, be considered, as the recipients of a service, as customers. However, the purchaser provides the finance necessary to offer the services and could, therefore, also be reasonably considered as the customer, as the services nurses provide are identified in contractual agreements.

Nursing is perhaps the most developed health care profession in considering process standards (Ellis and Whittington, 1993). This is essential in order to ensure that patients have a better understanding of the process of health care, and are able to relate this information to their own individual experiences. For the benefit of both nursing and the patient, it is essential that standards continue to develop. It is not the purpose of The Patient's Charter to direct nursing care delivery, as this is inclined to constrain the role of the nurse and reduce creativity in developing new models of care.

Student Activity 4.5

◆ Read Chapter 7 of Brigit Dimond's (1999) *Patients' Rights, Responsibilities and the Nurse*, 2nd edn, Quay Books.

◆ Discuss with one or more of your peers.

◆ Make notes in your portfolio.

The notion of the named nurse was to provide a focal point for nursing care provision, for working in partnership with patients, their relatives and friends and in resolving problems. This was a crucial aspect of the standard, enabling the patient and significant others to identify a single nurse who could provide specific care and information about that care (Ellis and Whittington, 1993). The named nurse enabled the continuity of care and acted as an anchor point when the patient met with a series of busy health care professionals. In this sense, the named nurse could be seen as the nursing team's representative to the patient or rather an advocate (Tschudin, 1995).

The nurse's role is to care (Tschudin, 1992). The Patient's Charter, by its implication, stipulated that nurses must become involved with the patients they are responsible for in responding to their needs while in their care. This is not new and has been inherent in the role of the nurse for decades; therefore The Patient's Charter simply underlined this factor. Peplau (1952) suggested that nurses could only work with the information that patients gave them. Information gathering and exchange through the process of observation and communication is necessary in meeting the needs of patients in an effective and beneficial way (see Chapter 8).

For nurses, the inextricable link between responsibility and accountability is also identified by Manley (1991) who believes that accountability is characteristic of a profession. Leddy and Pepper (1989) take the notion one step further and state that the concept of the professional includes both legal and moral accountability as a characteristic of a profession. Burnard and Chapman (1988) suggest that being accountable is not only answering for one's practice but also understanding its origins and powers of carrying it out. Alternatively, Marks-Maran (1993) believes accountability to be justifying actions by understanding the rationale behind them and the possible consequences of such actions.

Is The Patient's Charter enforceable and effective in law?

Currently, it appears that it does not provide any enforceable rights in health care although there is provision in other service industries such as the railways for financial compensation (under the Citizen's Charter). There are issues around waiting times for treatment, which have become established in acute care settings. The only grounds upon which the patient can establish medical negligence would be in the civil courts. This may also include the application of the Bolam Test.

Patients have no legally enforceable right to seek alternative treatment in the private sector and then to invoice their local health authority for that care. They do, however, have a right to be registered with a GP and to have access to information regarding local services and treatment (Dimond, 1999).

The Patient's Charter

The Charter entitles individuals to:

• Receive health care on the basis of clinical need, regardless of ability to pay.

Bolam Test

This involved a case in 1957, Bolam vs. Friern Barnet HMC 1957 2 A11 ER 118:

If a situation involves the use of some special skill or competence, the test as to whether there has been negligence or not is ... the standard of the ordinary skilled person exercising and professing to have that special skill. If a surgeon failed to measure up to that in any respect, clinical judgment or otherwise, negligence is deemed to have occurred, and the situation should be so judged. (Dimond, 1995, p. 30)

- Be registered with a GP.
- Receive emergency medical care at any time through a GP or through emergency ambulance services and hospital accident and emergency departments.
- Be referred to a consultant acceptable to the patient, when a GP thinks this is necessary, and to be referred for a second opinion if the patient and GP agree this is desirable.
- Be given clear explanation of any treatment proposed, including risks and alternatives.
- Have access to health care records and to know that those working in the NHS are under a legal duty to keep their contents confidential.
- Choose whether or not to take part in medical research or medical student training.
- Be given detailed information on local health services, including quality standards and maximum waiting times.
- Be guaranteed admission for treatment by a specific date no later than two years from the date when a patient is placed on the waiting list. To have any complaint about NHS services investigated and to receive a full and prompt written reply from the Chief Executive or General Manager.

The New NHS

The White Paper *The New NHS: Modern, Dependable* was published in 1997, and was consolidated in the Health Act (1999). There were a number of issues and principles identified, which built on, and expanded the aims of the NHS and Community Care Act 1990, as follows:

1. Fair access to high quality, prompt and accessible services across the country.

2. Delivery of health care set against national standards with local responsibility. Doctors and nurses to be involved shaping services.

3. The NHS to operate in partnership. The needs of the patient to be at the centre of the care process.

4. Reduction of bureaucracy and monitoring of performance.

5. Quality to be central to decision making at every level of the service.

6. The patient as consumer. Ensuring their voices are heard and that the service is accountable to the consumer.

The principles defined under *The New NHS* have a series of implications concerning the way in which the professions are likely to work in future. This is still currently under debate and will continue as the professions change, adjust, extend and develop in their roles.

The New NHS: Modern, Dependable (DoH, 1997)

The commitments under this paper are:

- To provide integrated care based on partnership and driven by performance

- To encourage more investment and better technology

- Access to health care to be based on need as opposed to ability to pay, or location

- NHS Direct, a new 24-hour telephone helpline, to be staffed by nurses

- Each GP surgery and hospital to be connected to the NHS information superhighway

- Access to specialist services to diagnose and treat cancer within two weeks

---

Implications of joint working

Working together means acknowledging that all participants bring equally valid knowledge and expertise from their professional and personal experience (Davies, 2000). Nurses and doctors attempt to do this on a regular basis although their roles are markedly different. Their aim is to achieve the best possible outcome for their patients. Sometimes this causes tensions; joint working is not easy (see Chapters 1, 7 and 11).

To enable this process there needs to be support for joint working by all parties concerned. First, there needs to be an element of trust in working together. This means communication, understanding each other's individual expertise and encouraging openness where possible. Second, there must be ground rules. Somebody will need to act as facilitator to ensure that the focus is maintained and that powerful members do not dominate at the cost of quality service delivery. This may be difficult to achieve in light of the history of working together in the NHS.

In recent years community nursing as a specialism has emerged from community based nursing specialisms such as district nursing, health visiting and community psychiatric nursing and is gaining in importance in relation to the rest of the profession, although according to Twinn et al. (1996) community nursing has not yet established a clear and cohesive identity. The history of nursing has been characterised for decades by a struggle to mark out a role which does not consist of being a doctor's assistant or an attendant (Dingwall et al., 1988). At different times nurses have sought to develop their role by enhancing the technical and technological demands of their work on the one hand, and the interactional and person centred nature of their work on the other (Smith, 1993). The history of thirty years of nursing has been a move away from relatively hierarchical groups with formalised procedures and relationships towards a profession consisting of autonomous and self-responsible practitioners. The process has been particularly identifiable in community nursing where the autonomy of practitioners is less likely to be compromised than in the hospital setting (Nettleton, 1995). However, the enhanced role of GPs during this period means that medical power remains a major factor. Whether or not the emergence of primary care groups (PCGs) and primary care trusts (PCTs) will bring any significant shifts, remains to be seen.

The arrival of the community care reforms alongside the NHS internal market served to make the community nurse's position in the care system

---

Student Activity 4.6

◆ Get together with a group of your peers, and discuss the following statement:

Doctors and nurses have different systems of power, bureaucratic structures and ideologies regarding joint working, therefore joint working will always be problematic in the NHS.

◆ Make sure your debate contains constructive arguments for and against.

somewhat less secure than it had been beforehand (Owens and Petch, 1995). Nurses have experienced in a particularly acute way the ambiguity of the health and social care boundary, as they have had to negotiate a demarcation of tasks with social services employees, whose role is in some cases not professionalised to anything like the same degree (Higgins et al., 1994). This situation is likely to change under the most recent reforms where community nurses are likely to be empowered with the formation of primary care trusts (see Chapter 15).

The new National Institute for Clinical Excellence refers to health professionals rather than singling out any one group. It acknowledges that no one who works alone can stay at the forefront of knowledge, given the speed of organisational and clinical change (Davies, 2000). Considerable effort will need to be put into team building, communications and joint learning between the professions in order to achieve success (Doyal and Cameron, 2000).

Conclusion

NHS reforms have contributed to major changes to the delivery of health care in the community.

District nurses have a major role to play in ensuring that these reforms are reflected in the way needs are assessed and care is planned and delivered. As a student, you should look for opportunities to identify where the requirements of the legislation are a part of what actually happens. This is particularly important with regard to such issues as the support of people in their own homes, the need to consult with them and the need to ensure that their carers are integral to the process. Your contribution to the process will include talking to your assessor about these issues, and incorporating the evidence from practice and the literature, as part of your own future practice as a qualified nurse.

Further reading

Baggott, R. (1999) *Health and Health Care in Britain*, 2nd edn. Basingstoke, Macmillan – now Palgrave.

Davies, C. (2000) Getting health professionals to work together. *British Medical Journal*, **320** (15 April): 1021–2.

References

Audit Commission (1986) *Making a Reality of Community Care*. London, HMSO.

Burnard, P. and Chapman, C. (1988) *Professional and Ethical Issues in Nursing, The Code of Professional Conduct*. Chichester, John Wiley.

Culyer, A. (1988) *The Radical Reforms the NHS Needs – and Doesn't*. York, Centre for Health Economics, University of York.

Davies, C. (2000) Getting health professionals to work together. *British Medical Journal*, **320** (15 April): 1021–2.

Department of Health (1989a) *Caring for People: Community Care in the Next Decade and Beyond*. London, HMSO.

Department of Health (1989b) *Working for Patients*. London, HMSO.

Department of Health (1990a) *The NHS and Community Care Act*. London, DoH.

Department of Health (1990b) *Promoting Better Health*. London, DoH.

Department of Health (1992) *Health of the Nation*. London, DoH.

Department of Health (1992) *The Patient's Charter*. London, DoH.

Department of Health (1997) *The New NHS: Modern, Dependable*. London, HMSO.

Department of Health (1999) *The Health Act*. London, HMSO.

Dimond, B. (1995) *Legal Aspects of Nursing*, 2nd edn. London, Prentice Hall.

Dimond, B. (1999) *Patients' Rights, Responsibilities and the Nurse*, 2nd edn. Wiltshire, Quay Books.

Dingwall, R., Rafferty, A., and Webster, C. (1988) *An Introduction to the Social History of Nursing*. London, Routledge.

Doyal, L. and Cameron, A. (2000) Reshaping the NHS workforce (Editorial). *British Medical Journal*, **320** (15th April): 1023–4.

Ellis, R. (1988) *Professional Competence and Quality Assurance in the Caring Professions*. London, Croom Helm.

Ellis, R. and Whittington, D. (1993) *Quality Assurance in Health Care: A Handbook*. London, Edward Arnold.

Enthoven, A. (1985) *Reflections on the Management of the National Health Service*. London, Nuffield Provincial Hospital Trust.

Griffiths, R. (1988) *Community Care: An Agenda for Action*. London, HMSO.

Higgins, R., Oldman, C. and Hunter, D. (1994) Working together: lessons for collaboration between Health and Social Services. *Health and Social Care in the Community*. **2**: 269–77.

Hogg, C. (1994) *Beyond The Patient's Charter: Working With Users*. London, Health Rights Publication.

Hughes, D. (1992) A Question of Judgement. *Health Services Journal*, (102) 5 November: 11.

Klein, R. and Day, P. (1988) Future Options for Health Care in Social Services Committee Session 1987–1988. Resourcing the National Committee, *HC Papers* 284 – iv, pp. 48–51, London, HMSO.

Leddy, S. and Pepper, J.M. (1989) *Conceptual Bases of Professional Nursing*. Philadelphia, J. B. Lippincott.

Manley, K. (1991) Knowledge for Nursing Practice. In Perry, A. and Jolley, M. (eds) *Nursing: A Knowledge Base for Practice*. London, Edward Arnold, pp. 1–27.

Marks-Maran, D. (1993) Advocacy. In Tschudin V. (ed.) *Ethics: Nurses and Patients*. London, Scutari Press, pp. 65–83.

Nettleton, S. (1995) *The Sociology of Health and Illness*. Cambridge, Polity Press.

Owens, P. and Petch, H. (1995) Professionals and Management. In Owens, P., Carrier, J. and Horder, J. (eds) *Interprofessional Issues in Community and Primary Health Care.* London, Macmillan – now Palgrave.

Peplau, H. (1952) *Interpersonal Relations in Nursing.* New York, Putnam.

Plant, R. (1989) *Can There Be A Right To Health Care?* Occasional Paper, February 1989, Institute of Health Policy Studies, Faculty of Social Science, University of Southampton.

Qureshi, H. and Walker, A. (1989) *The Caring Relationship: Elderly People and Their Families.* London, Macmillan – now Palgrave.

Ryland, R.K. (1996) Guest Editorial. *Journal of Advanced Nursing,* **23**: 1059–60.

Smith, P. (1993) Nursing as an occupation. In Taylor, S. and Field, D. (eds) *Sociology of Health and Health Care.* Oxford, Blackwell.

Tschudin, V. (1992) *Ethics in Nursing, The Caring Relationship,* 2nd edn. Oxford, Heinemann.

Tschudin, V. (1995) *The Patient's Charter.* London, Scutari Press.

Twigg, J. (1994) *Carers Perceived: Policy and Practice in Informal Care.* Buckingham, Open University Press.

Twinn, S., Roberts, B. and Andrews, S. (1996) *Community Health Care Nursing.* Oxford, Butterworth Heinemann.

Welsh Health Planning Forum (1989) *Strategic Intent and Direction for the NHS in Wales.* Cardiff, Welsh Office.

Wilson-Barnett J. (1981) Janforum. *Journal of Advanced Nursing,* **6**(6): 503–14.

5

The impact of poverty in the community

CAROL WILKINSON

Learning outcomes

By the end of this chapter you will be able to:

■ Outline the concept of poverty and make clear its distinctions between absolute and relative poverty.

■ Assess the impact of poverty on specific groups of people within the community.

■ Discuss poverty in relation to health inequalities.

■ Examine the issue of poverty in light of historical and more recent government proposals.

Introduction

This chapter intends to make an assessment of some of the key issues relating to poverty within British society and its implications for nursing in the community.

The concept of poverty is defined within its historical context and draws on the notion of persistent inequalities. Indeed, inequalities within society as a result of economic factors and their impact on specific groups of people will be assessed. Key reports such as the *Independent Inquiry Into Inequalities in Health* (Acheson, 1998) will be brought under scrutiny alongside the Labour government's tax and benefits policies. The implications for children, lone parents, ethnic groups and the elderly will be highlighted. This will help you, as a student, to understand the relationship between health outcomes of individuals and groups and the poverty debate, which remains a persistent part of the equation.

The government of the late 1990s pledged to be a reforming government providing leadership on poverty not just nationally, but also on a global scale. Indeed, their 1997 Election Manifesto stated:

> The government will also attach much higher priority to combating global poverty and underdevelopment ... we will strengthen and restructure the British aid programme and bring development issues back into the mainstream of government decision-making. (The Labour Party, 1997: 39)

By the year 2000 policies and structures had been put in place to tackle this persistent problem. The approaches to tackling poverty operate at different levels as some of the problems are structural, others geographical or practical.

● *Structural:* If a person is born into poverty then their life chances are likely to place them at a disadvantage to those who are not. The means of escaping poverty for many is through the education system. However, poverty can also mean far less access to good education, and health care, as well as to resources such as libraries, water or food. Frequently there is also heavy reliance of parents on their children to leave school early, get a job and contribute to the household finances to maintain a standard of living where they just get by. Unskilled and low status occupations usually yield the lowest incomes for families, perpetuating subsistence standards of living.

- *Geographical:* The North/South divide in Britain is today regarded as a misnomer. Deprivation tends to exist in Britain alongside more affluent areas. There are various studies to indicate that deprivation exists in clusters across the country (Carstairs 1981; Mack and Lansley, 1985; Thurnhurst, 1985). Deprivation usually accounts for areas of high unemployment where industry and manufacturing has declined in the region. The consequence is that lack of investment means many people move out of the area to seek employment, homes, schools and amenities for their families. Those left behind see the general decline of their area. This is sometimes marked out by the rise in vandalism, theft and other crimes. The area may eventually be saved by short-term global investment or by newly arrived immigrant communities who bring business and their families to the community. This is by no means a certainty. Rural and urban communities alike experience poverty (Fox et al., 1984; Townsend et al., 1985, 1986). Indeed, the farming industry, with its problems of the late 1990s, and more recently with the foot and mouth crisis across the UK, has seen an increasing decline in food and livestock productivity, with the mass slaughtering of thousands of animals. This has had a major impact on the farming community specifically, and on British families generally. The rising costs of food, including meat and dairy products, will affect all families – especially those on low incomes. This crisis in the farming industry looks set to continue for some time, and the repercussions on the health of the nation may be long lasting. The repercussions for farming communities involve a consolidation of assets for some, and the loss of livelihood for others.

- *Practical:* The increase in separation and divorce have practical implications for families. Many people, especially women, find their standard of living greatly reduced when a partner leaves the household. The effects of their changed circumstances can be far reaching. It means going without and constantly attempting to make ends meet. It can lead to humiliation, and feelings of powerlessness. This in turn can contribute to strain manifested in physical and psychological problems in circumstances where there are limited social networks. This can include resorting to violence within families and the increasing reliance on alcohol or other addictive substances.

The cycle of deprivation

Lewis' (1965) study which continues to be quoted today was first published to outline the problems of deprivation in communities. It was immediately seized upon by politicians to blame individuals for their own circumstances. The cycle of deprivation began with the assumption of poverty arising from poor budgeting and socialisation. The ideological position states that this was passed on within families yielding poor social skills and education. There were low levels of attainment and achievement within the education system, hence poor employment prospects. These issues would in turn be transferred to the new generation of adults repeating the culture, thus creating a cycle of deprivation.

Poverty in Britain

Poverty in Britain has been cumulative over the last 20 years. The gap between rich and poor has increased considerably. For example, the share of income taken by the top fifth of earners before taxes and benefits rose from 43 to 50 per cent between 1977 and 1996; after taxes and benefits they rose from 36 to 40 per cent of all income. Conversely, the share of income distributed to the bottom fifth of the population has declined. Disposable incomes for those at the top of the hierarchy are on average five times greater than those of the bottom fifth (Office of National Statistics, 1998). In terms of average income per household, by the mid-1990s 14 million people were earning less than half the average income compared to less than 5 million people in 1979 (*The Economist*, 1997). This accounts for a quarter of the population of Britain.

Britain is now considered to be one of the countries in Europe with the greatest numbers of the population in poverty. Indeed it ranks eleventh out of 15 member states. During 1992, for example, 24 per cent were in poverty, children making up a large proportion of that number. In 1993, one in three children were living in poverty compared to one in ten during 1980 (Craven, 1998).

Currently, almost a quarter of all households include at least one person living on benefit or income support. Taken over a period of two years, this figure rises to more than a third. The number of people recorded as being on income support has increased more than twofold, from 4 million in 1979 to 9.6 million in 1996 (Acheson, 1998). This does not account for those who may actually be entitled to income support and for whatever reason do not claim.

Another factor relating to living standards of the poor is homelessness. During 1992 alone, although an estimated 400,000 people were registered as homeless, the actual figure was nearer to two million (Commission on

Social Justice, 1994). In 1995, a Joseph Rowntree Foundation report found that low income families often go without heat in cold weather, and shop daily so that family members do not eat the week's food too quickly (Joseph Rowntree Foundation, 1995; *The Economist*, 1997).

In addition to the points outlined above, we see an interesting picture emerging for specific groups of people in society. Although some 40 per cent of pensioners (mainly women) are a significant category of the poor, lone parents, ethnic groups, the unemployed and homeless have contributed to the feminisation and racialisation of poverty (Commission for Social Justice, 1994; Hutton, 1995). Findings from the Bristol Poverty Line suggest that more than a third of lone parent families, 28 per cent of single people, a quarter of pensioner households and more than one million couples with children are living in absolute poverty (Townsend et al., 1997). Pakistani and Bangladeshi communities, particularly, are over represented in the poorest fifth of the population when related to income distribution (Acheson, 1998).

Student Activity 5.1

◆ Discuss, with your assessor, the DN caseload to which you are attached.

◆ Find out whether there are any patients on the caseload who could be affected by poverty.

◆ Check with your DN assessor to see how this contrasts with other caseloads and other communities near your locality.

◆ Are there any measures used to assess deprivation individually or within the community?

◆ Make notes in your portfolio.

Clearly then inequality within British communities exists and has persisted and been sustained under many governments with detrimental consequences for some. Allied to these factors, the long Conservative government (1979–97) saw the results of a boom and bust economy with rising house prices, increase in interest rates, the highest rates of re-possession of mort-gaged property in history, the sale of council properties thus removing the safety net for those less well off. The rules for application for means tested benefits were tightened, and benefits cut for youths who refused to stay on in the education system or make themselves available for pre-employment training, steering them towards the poverty trap within a society that had become much more materialistic and self-interested. This subsequently made work and savings uneconomic, encouraging an increase in crime (*The Economist*, 1997).

Student Activity 5.2

Locate the most recent copy of *Social Trends* in a library, and find out:

♦ How many households are below average income in Britain.

♦ What reasons are given for this?

♦ Can you think of other reasons, other than the ones listed in *Social Trends*, that affect individuals and groups?

♦ Contact the local benefits office and find out what level of benefit is available for a lone parent with children under ten years. Are there any special clauses attached to what can be claimed? For example, what is the ceiling limit of income and savings?

♦ Add the information to your portfolio.

These effects were coupled with a world recession, reduction in the manufacturing base in Britain, and the reduced powers of the trades unions. This enabled employers to maximise their powers, instituting short-term contracts, longer working hours for fewer employees, and downsizing in the face of fierce competition in the pursuit of profit which generally contributed to the threat to the very fabric of society.

What is poverty? How is it measured?

The issue of poverty is not clearly defined although many have attempted to explain and analyse this phenomenon within particular frameworks.

From a historical viewpoint, early measurements undertaken by Charles Booth in the late 19th century demonstrated rather inadequate results for those living in poverty in London. Poverty was measured on the basis of weekly income of less than 21 shillings (approx. £1.05). This was followed up by Joseph Rowntree of York who was spurred on by his scepticism of Booth's findings. In *Poverty: A Study of Town Life* published in 1901, he found similar results concerning the level of *absolute poverty* (Blakemore, 1998).

Rowntree's investigation provided a rich source of evidence about the relationship between wages and patterns of expenditure. The evidence disputes claims that poverty was the result of individuals' own fecklessness and poor management of money. Instead, the primary indicator of widespread poverty in Victorian Britain was caused by low wages (52 per cent), family size (22 per cent), old age, sickness or disability (12 per cent).

Absolute poverty

Measures of absolute poverty are usually based upon the idea of subsistence. People are in poverty if they do not have the resources to physically maintain human life. The majority of measures of absolute poverty are concerned with establishing the quality and amount of food, clothing and shelter deemed necessary for a healthy life. This is also called *subsistence poverty* since it is based on assessments of minimum subsistence requirements. This means that those who use absolute measurements, are deemed to limit poverty to *material deprivation*. Absolute poverty is measured through pricing the basic necessities of life, drawing a poverty line in terms of price and defining as poor those whose income falls below that figure. People are considered to be multiply deprived if they experience inadequate educational opportunities, unpleasant working conditions or are powerless to improve their situation.

The notion of absolute poverty has been widely criticised, as the needs of people vary within and between different sectors of society. Work, cultural and leisure situations need to be taken into consideration. The context changes so frequently that having a fixed standard of subsistence is difficult to maintain or defend as a means of measuring poverty.

Relative poverty

Relative poverty is based on the living standards of the society at that particular stage in time. According to this view, the point at which the dividing line, which separates the poor from the other members of society, is drawn will vary according to how affluent the society is. Abel-Smith and Townsend (1965) looked at graduations of poverty in their influential study of 'The Poor and the Poorest'. As well as being involved in the preparation of the Black Report (DHSS, 1980), Townsend went on to contribute extensively to the literature on inequalities, including a major study of poverty in 1970s Britain (Townsend, 1979). His findings underlined the extent to which

Student Activity 5.3

♦ Find out the current state of pensions for a single elderly person. Using that figure, work out (in accordance with today's standard of living) the typical expenditure required for food, household and personal items.

♦ Discuss this with a group of your peers, taking into consideration how an individual would manage on a daily basis, and what would take priority.

♦ Keep notes in your portfolio.

society influences needs and expectations. This may include the ability or lack of it to participate in approved social activities, such as visiting friends or relatives, having birthday parties for children and going on holiday. He concluded that those most likely to be poor were elderly people who had been unskilled manual workers (especially those with substantial experience of unemployment, sickness or disablement) or those in one parent families.

The work of Townsend has been criticised on the grounds that the index on which he based his statistics was flawed. Piachaud (1981) argued that it was unclear what the items commented upon in the index (such as fresh fruit and vegetables or a Sunday joint) had to do with poverty. He argued that for other reasons, including culture, people may choose to be short of money or use it in ways that lead them into poverty. Piachaud has a point of view; whether it is agreeable will depend on your own perspective. As a student preparing for a career in nursing, you will find understanding the needs of people to be part of the role of community nurses, health visitors and social workers. But this understanding could be affected by your own, and your assessor's values as an individual. Understanding this is vital (see Chapter 8). The way people manage on a daily basis is something that can be observed by you. It may also be an issue for you to discuss and reflect upon with your assessor.

Student Activity 5.4

The film *Angela's Ashes* is based on a true story by the novelist Frank McCourt. It depicts a poignant portrayal of poverty and the consequences for families in Ireland during the last century.

◆ Obtain a copy from your video library and watch it with your peers.

◆ Afterwards, reflect upon it and consider how it might compare to the reality for some communities today.

Other measures of poverty

● The *European Union Measure* counts the proportion of households with income below half the average in each member state. The UK saw the largest increase between 1980 and 1985.

● *Income support:* The number of children in families on income support is currently in the region of 2,950,000. This accounts for nearly a quarter of all children. This figure represents a threefold increase to those children (923,000) on supplementary benefit, the precursor to income support in 1979.

Beveridge's principles

In legislative terms, developments before Beveridge were designed to contain rather than eradicate poverty. The emphasis was on national efficiency. The 1908 Old Age Pension Act, for example, was for the over 70s and supplementary rather than a subsistence benefit. In the drive towards efficiency, there was concern for war and peace, hence a necessity for a fit and healthy nation. This was channelled through the availability of maternity grants, subsidised school meals and free school medical inspections. The 1911 National Insurance Act also compelled workers, employers and the State to make contributions and entitled the sick or unemployed worker to draw benefit for a limited period of time. The measures did not drive poverty away, as the workhouse and debtors prison still beckoned for some well into the 1920s. This state of affairs continued up to and during the Second World War.

In 1944, Beveridge argued that a postwar objective should be to free Britain of 'Want' (a euphemism for poverty) alongside its other four evils: idleness, disease, ignorance and squalor. It is with this aim that a safety net provided by the new welfare state to eradicate these problems from society began to emerge. The 1944 Education Act and the National Health Service Act 1946 were introduced. Ridding society of squalor did not quite follow until the 1957 Housing Act, which defined minimum standards for the home. But nonetheless a reduction in want was expected as living standards rose and education became the norm within society.

Poverty was dealt with through the establishment of a compulsory social insurance scheme. This provided flat rate benefits for flat rate insurance contributions, so ensuring that no household fell below a minimum standard of living. The National Insurance Act passed in 1946 covered all full-time workers and any general risk that was involuntary, such as sickness, disability, maternity, old age, widowhood and unemployment. Child benefit (the family allowance) was paid to all families with dependent children to ensure that child poverty – which Beveridge (1944) called the worst feature of want in Britain before the war – would be ended. This legislation was underpinned by full employment, which drove the campaign against idleness.

Student Activity 5.5

- ◆ Discuss, with a group of your peers, what you think is meant by 'standard of living'.

- ◆ Compare and contrast your individual views on this topic.

- ◆ What would you consider to be a satisfactory standard of living?

- ◆ Compare today's standards of living with Britain in the 1970s.

- ◆ Keep notes for your portfolio.

Why does poverty persist at the beginning of the 21st century?

Beveridge achieved some qualified success in the provision of education for all sectors of society and a Health Service available to all at the point of delivery regardless of ability to pay. Over 50 years later, however, poverty remains an issue – especially among children. Indeed, at the end of the last millennium, the Social Security Minister, Alistair Darling, made the following point:

> Today as every other day, 2000 children will be born in Britain. And to this, the last six months of the twentieth century, a third of these children will be born into poverty. If we do nothing many of these children will not only be born poor but will live poor and die poor. (*Observer* 22 August 1999:20)

The issue is as relevant today as then. So what has happened to children since Beveridge's day and why does child poverty persist?

Child poverty

Between 1945 and 1979 successive governments provided greater universal access to education and health care by increasing contributions in public expenditure and nationalising services. This had the effect of availability of goods and public services for all the population regardless of ability to pay.

Changing family structures

Since 1971, there has been a marked decrease in families with dependent children who were married or cohabiting couple families, that is from 92 per cent in 1971 to 78 per cent in 1993. Over the same period, there was an increase in lone parent families from 8 per cent in 1971 to 22 per cent in 1993. Since 1993 there has been little change. In 1996, families headed by a lone parent formed 21 per cent of all families with dependent children, the majority of lone parents being lone mothers.

The proportion of all families with dependent children headed by:

- A *single lone mother* increased from 1 per cent in 1971 to 7% in 1996.

- A *divorced lone mother* increased from 2 per cent in 1971 to 6% in 1996.

- A *separated lone mother* increased from 2 per cent in 1971 to 5% in 1996.

The situation for lone fathers has remained unchanged since 1971 being 1–2 per cent (Office of National Statistics, 1998).

During the mid-1990s, a quarter of the total population were living in poverty (defined as 50 per cent of average income after housing costs). Among children, the proportion was one in three. By 1996, 2.2 million children were in a family receiving income support. Meeting the basic needs of children, according to recent studies, has revealed that the money provided by income support is insufficient, personal allowances for younger children in the family being less than that for the first child. Both expert and independent assessments of basic needs also indicate that the personal allowances paid to one- and two-parent families underestimate the relative costs of providing a basic standard of living for one-parent families.

It is estimated that a lone parent with two children would need 93 per cent of the amount required by a couple with two children to achieve the same moderate standard of living. The 1998 Budget with above inflation increases in the benefit rates for younger children, childcare tax credit for working parents and the working families tax credit should have contributed to the narrowing of these discrepancies (Acheson, 1998).

Student Activity 5.6

◆ Look at the book *The Five Giants: A Biography of the Welfare State*, by Nicholas Timmins (1996), Fontana Press. As it is a large book, you and a group of fellow students might like to take a chapter each to read and report back on.

◆ Discuss what you have read within the group.

Impact on health

Poverty is predominantly associated with those groups in the social context of either unskilled work or the unemployed. Standard of living is generally less than satisfactory. The impact on the health of children born into such circumstances can yield some of the following health problems. These often persist into adulthood:

● Babies born to fathers in social classes IV and V have a birth weight which is on average 130 grams lower than that of babies with fathers in social classes I and II. Babies whose mothers were born in the Indian sub-continent are on average 200 grams lighter than those born to mothers in the UK.

- Reduced growth in fetal life is associated with increased mortality and morbidity in the first year of life, and throughout childhood.

- People who had low birth weight, or who are thin or stunted at birth, are at increased risk of cardiovascular disease and disorders related to it in later life. Such associations are not explicable by confounding variables in adult life.

- Birth weight is determined by the weight and height of the mother, which in turn reflects her own growth in childhood. Children of women who are thin, that is with a low body mass index, run the additional risk of developing non-insulin dependent diabetes and hypertension in adulthood.

- Obese mothers are prone to the same health risks as the underweight which subsequently impacts on any offspring.

- Those children who have been or are in care are more likely to experience abuse, have high rates of alcohol, smoking and substance misuse, as well as mental health problems. They present with these difficulties in adult life (Buchanan and Brinke, 1997; Health Advisory Service, 1996).

Children in care

During 1997, 89,000 children were in the care of social services departments (SSDs) in England, and an estimated 30 per cent of youth who have been in care are homeless. An estimated one in seven young women who have been in care are either pregnant or are mothers. Over 75 per cent of those children leave care without any educational qualifications, and between 50 per cent and 80 per cent of those who leave care are unemployed (Office of National Statistics, 1998).

Examples of action by community nurses and health visitors

Community nurses are very much the eyes and ears of the health service in their local community. They are continually involved in raising standards of care and treatment as well as being advocates of health within the micro society. Through contact with families, they are able to detect whether a child is receiving adequate care and attention, whether a mother is getting enough rest or if there is tension within relationships. It is through observation and developing a rapport and trust with patients that the nurse will be able to provide that additional support or advice that families need. As you work with your assessor, look for examples of good rapport with families, and make sure you can identify how this contributes to improving health outcomes for all members of the family.

A group of health visitors has developed the Family Wise programme, a series of picture books designed to get the health messages across to mothers and their families. It was adopted by health visitors to supplement discussions with the families they visited on a range of subjects including positive parenting, budgeting, potty training, smoking cessation, healthy teeth and safety. An evaluation undertaken in Huddersfield (one of the original pilot sites) was very positive, for 97 per cent of mothers surveyed (HEA, 1999).

Children have also been heavily involved in health matters. The Landsdowne Infant School in Burton-on-Trent is one of eight pilot sites selected to develop and evaluate ways of improving health in schools, in an initiative to develop a National Healthy Schools Scheme. Its aim is to make every school a healthy school where health promotion is integrated into school life as a part of a drive to promote health and improve educational standards. Health is embedded in the curriculum, as well as other activities such as teaching healthy eating, importance of keeping fit and first aid training (HEA, 1999).

Women in poverty

Poverty is likely to affect women more than men, especially if they have been abandoned with children. Despite legislation, it is still the case that women who work generally receive lower rates of pay than their male counterparts. Employment is likely to be part time and, in some cases, during unsocial hours in order to fit in with raising a family (Land, 1987). Assumed dependence on men has been used historically to justify the family wage being higher for men, and was thus reflected in legislation. But family structures are changing, and more women are having to fend for themselves.

The disadvantages that women experience in the labour market are compounded by their lone parent status. Despite the capacities of women to cope in the face of adversity, to work and bring up children, some women may feel there is little economic advantage in doing so. The type of low paid work a woman may find, coupled with expenses of work and child-minding fees, mean that most lone mothers will not be better off than when drawing benefit. Previous governmental policies have limited the opportunities of women in terms of employment. Those dependent on benefit found it a disincentive to work part time as it reduced their benefit entitlements. The subsequent juggling brings with it stress, lack of fulfilment, and feelings of insecurity (Abbott and Wallace, 1997).

Women also are expected to be primary carers of children, but care of the elderly and other dependants is also within their domain. Women's poverty is underlined within the context of gender inequalities, which persist throughout life.

Impact on health

In 1996, the usual gross weekly household income was considerably lower among lone parent families than among either married or cohabiting couples. For example 33 per cent of families with a lone mother and 27 per cent with a lone father had a gross weekly income of £100 or less compared with 3 per cent of married and 6 per cent of cohabiting couples. The proportion of people living alone increased from 9 per cent in 1973 to 14 per cent in 1991, since then there has been little change. The group most likely to be living alone (58 per cent) were elderly women, particularly those over the age of 75 (Office of National Statistics, 1998).

Women in poverty shop frequently to prevent food being available at home and therefore at risk of being consumed before it is essential. Spending is reduced substantially during the second week of the benefit cycle. This is the same for the working mother on limited income. A mother often goes without in order to provide for her family, which subsequently leads to additional strain. Women are over represented in statistics for diagnoses of anxiety and depression. They experience greater psychiatric morbidity than men because of their role as wives, mothers, carers, lone parents (Gove, 1984). They are also more likely to find solace in the use of alcohol, tobacco or benzodiazepines as a 'prop' in the absence of emotional or financial support (Gabe and Thorogood, 1986). These substances predispose women to malnutrition, cirrhosis of the liver, and cancers.

Student Activity 5.7

♦ Get together with a group of your peers and discuss ways in which women can reduce social isolation in communities.

♦ Find out the leisure activities in your placement area, and identify those which are 'woman-centred', are available on concessionary rates, or free.

♦ Using computer technology, make a pamphlet to demonstrate the availability of these services.

♦ Discuss it with your assessor.

♦ Introduce it to women in your placement area, and find out whether it made a difference.

'Race', ethnicity and poverty

'Race' is a socially constructed phenomenon, which has been used historically to place groups at a disadvantage on the basis of specific features
including skin colour, language and communication skills. Those from
specific minority ethnic groups are more likely to be unemployed or on low
rates of pay in poor working conditions in Britain. Their treatment by the
welfare state institutions is significantly worse. These factors contribute to
poverty and reflect direct and indirect discrimination in society (Craig and
Rai, 1996). Much of the literature relates to the social security system and
structures within the employment system that reduce them to redundancy,
and the effects of being regarded as scroungers of the state, particularly if
they were employees in the low-skilled manufacturing sector (Gordon and
Newnham, 1985; Craig, 1992; Sly, 1994).

Socioeconomic status differs between ethnic groups. Labour Force Survey
estimates that in Britain rates of male unemployment are considerably higher
in African Caribbean (20.5 per cent) and Pakistani and Bangladeshi groups
(15.9 per cent). This compares to Indians of 7.45 per cent and the white
majority population which is 6.5 per cent (Sly, 1994). Surveys of minority
ethnic groups have higher absolute percentages of people out of work, but
the same pattern of differences between groups. Part of these differences are
due to the relative young average age of these minority ethnic groups and
associated high rates of unemployment in young age groups in general.

Social class distribution reveals similar patterns, with Pakistani and
Bangladeshi groups showing a more disadvantaged profile. Perhaps most
striking is the number of people from all minority ethnic groups who are
living in poverty, as defined by less than half the average income. Just under
a third of white households have incomes below this level, compared to a
third of Chinese, two-fifths of African Caribbean and Indian households and
four-fifths of Pakistani and Bangladeshi households. Minority ethnic groups
are also much more likely to be reliant on income support (DSS, 1995).

The population that arrived in Britain in the late 1950s and early 1960s
is now at retirement age. This has important implications for health care
and access to essential services, which they are likely to need as they advance
in age.

The age and gender distribution of minority ethnic groups is different
from that found in indigenous, white families. There is a higher proportion
of women and the mean age is relatively low. African Caribbean and South
Asian communities have a higher proportion of households with children
than the white population. Around three in ten households with a white head
of household contain children under the age of 16 years. Comparable figures
for minority ethnic groups are over four in ten for African Caribbean households, five in ten for Indian households and eight in ten for Bangladeshi
families. Bangladeshi families also have more children than families in the

Student Activity 5.8

In the ethnic community in Britain, there is a dearth of research documenting the experiences of older ethnic minority groups, their access to services within their communities, and how they cope on a limited pension, considering that many have spent half their working lives in another country, being unable to achieve their full potential here. If your placement has an elderly ethnic minority community (which could include refugee communities, or older people from other parts of Europe) try to find out the following:

◆ Do they manage on the pensions they receive, and are they supported by family members?

◆ To what extent do those living alone participate in the activities of their local communities? For example luncheon clubs, church outings and so on.

◆ What health and social and leisure provision is available to maintain their identity, culture and connection with other older people of similar backgrounds, if they so wish, and who are the services funded by?

◆ Do they experience isolation and alienation, and how can these be minimised? Are experiences similar among men and women?

◆ Once you have explored these questions, discuss them with your assessor, and find out whether they have a role in positively contributing to the needs of diverse groups.

majority white population while African Caribbean, Indian and Chinese families have similar numbers of children. It is recognised that African Caribbean households are more likely to be headed by a lone parent (Office of National Statistics, 1998).

Impact on health

Overall, people from minority ethnic groups are more likely than the ethnic majority to suffer from poverty or ill health. This difference comes from the poorer self-reported health of Pakistani and Bangladeshi people, and to a lesser extent African people. Chinese people consult their GP less often than whites, while African Asians are as likely to have consulted with their GPs as whites. All other groups consult their GP more (Acheson, 1998).

Peoples of South Asia have a tendency to central obesity and insulin resistance, which may pre-dispose them to conditions including diabetes and coronary heart disease. On the other hand, African Caribbean people have low death rates from coronary heart disease, despite the high prevalence of hypertension and diabetes. Depression appears to be more common in African Caribbeans than in whites. Tuberculosis is more common among Black Africans, Pakistanis, and Bangladeshis than whites, and the incidence of tuberculosis in all these groups is rising (Acheson, 1998).

The elderly

Since 1980, there has been a change in the profile of the elderly population living in private households in Britain. At the time of writing, the latest figures (Office of National Statistics, 1998) suggest the following:

- 21 per cent of people aged 65 years and over were in the 80 and over age category. This represents one in five of the population compared to 16 per cent in 1980 (see Chapter 13).

- 39 per cent of people lived alone in 1996. This is an increase of 5 per cent since 1980. There was also a decrease in the proportion living with others, including siblings or offspring, from 21 per cent in 1980 to 13 per cent in 1996.

- Elderly women were more likely than elderly men to live alone, now 49 per cent compared with 26 per cent in 1996.

Many of the poorest elderly are on benefit, and experience a reduction in their incomes and circumstances following retirement. Their changed circumstances can lead them to loneliness and isolation as they may feel unable to take advantage of leisure services and amenities in their localities. Their pensions compared to their counterparts in Europe are lower (Eardley, 1996) and fewer take full advantage of their entitlements. In fact, around one in four of the elderly population do not claim their state pension. Some factors for such reluctance include the perceived stigma that accompanies receipt of benefit from the state and wanting to maintain their dignity and independence. There may also be lack of knowledge of their entitlement, inability to collect their benefit because of poor access to transport or for physical reasons. Indeed, 14 per cent of elderly people living alone were unable to go out for a walk on their own and 12 per cent could not manage steps or stairs. Only 1 per cent or less of those living alone were unable to get about the house, get to the toilet or get in and out of bed (Office of National Statistics, 1998).

Student Activity 5.9

The 'pensioners' one stop shop': Acheson (1998) recommends the setting up of a pensioners' agency as a way of achieving 'one stop' provision of welfare or a welfare counsellor located in primary care centres in areas of disadvantage.

Supposing you were given the resources to develop and launch such an agency, how would you:

♦ Decide the underlying principles and aims of the agency?

♦ Form the structure of the agency?

♦ Plan and operationalise activities?

♦ Involve pensioners?

♦ Monitor and evaluate the service?

Impact on health

Apart from the prevalence of the usual physical problems of hypertension, mobility, heart disease and stroke among the aged in lower socioeconomic groups, factors such as poor diet, fuel poverty and limited access to services are also seen as real issues. The government intends to increase benefits and provide assistance for the poorest pensioners, as well as to contribute to the fuel bill. The impact on health as a result of these changes has yet to be assessed.

Some reflections on new issues related to poverty

The recommendations made in *Independent Inquiry Into Inequalities in Health* (Acheson, 1998) are wide ranging and ambitious. Closer attention to resources for specific groups within society to combat the problems of poverty is necessary to raise their health profile. Notwithstanding this:

1. More research into ethnic groups is required, especially the impact of poverty on health of pensioners who choose to live out their retirement in their host country, compared to those who return to their homeland. Close attention to be given to those women who arrived post war, and are still living in Britain. It must be emphasised that many, particularly from the Caribbean, India and Pakistan, will have spent half their working lives

in Britain in low status occupations with poor pay. Their benefit entitlement may be substantially limited (pre-1976) as a result of pension
contributions where married men and their partners' superannuation
contributions were joint.

2. Men have also shared a fluctuating relationship with the job market within
this time period. Their circumstances need to be investigated in comparison to indigenous Caucasian population of similar age and status and
recommendations made for improvement.

3. A greater understanding of the impact of poverty on women, not merely
through the ideologies of care and joint home and work domains. The
impact of divorce, multiple families (that is, women with children by more
than one partner) and whether the Child Support Agency has improved
their circumstances, or whether they continue in the cycle of poverty.

4. The government has pledged to assist 1.4 million families through the
working families tax credit scheme for those earning below £235 per
week. Encouraging lone parents to go out to work will need to be closely
observed in terms of impact on the family living situation and on the
children, and whether or not the fund is adequate to maintain a reasonable level of subsistence in comparison to their present situation.

There are many groups in society in need. New schemes to improve health
through, for example, healthy living centres must be monitored in terms of
the overall benefit to the community, to see whether they assist in creating a
better way of life for the poor.

Conclusion

Many groups in society experience poverty at some point during their lives.
Some are born into poverty, others encounter it for reasons relating to family
breakdown and changes in employment circumstances. The role of government is to find ways of tackling poverty, either through tax and benefits or
changes to the structure of welfare and work, to provide incentives which will
alleviate poverty in families and communities.

The contribution of community nurses to this process includes careful
observation of those factors, which affect individuals, families or communities, provision of care, which is sensitive to the findings from observations
made, and mobilising action for families and communities, using a sound
knowledge base from research in practice. As a student, you should have
participated in a range of observation techniques which will have helped you
to recognise good practice in action in the community. This involvement in
the decision-making processes should contribute to your development as you
move towards becoming a qualified nurse.

Remember to ensure that you use the available evidence to inform your practice, and look for new ways to contribute towards generating more of that evidence. This will have a crucial part to play in helping you identify new ways of tackling an enduring problem.

Further reading

Acheson, E.D. (1998) *Independent Inquiry into Inequalities in Health*. London, HMSO.
Donnellan, C. (1995) *The Poverty Trap: Issues for the Nineties*, Volume 9. Cambridge, Independence Educational Publishers.
Townsend, P., Gordon, D., Bradshaw, J. and Gosschalk, B. (1997) *Absolute and Overall Poverty in Britain 1997: What the Population Themselves Say*. Bristol, Bristol Poverty Line Survey, Bristol Statistical Monitoring Unit.

USEFUL WEB SITES

European Anti Poverty Network www.eapn.org

Comparative Research Programme on Poverty (CROP) www.svf.uib.no/helsos/crop/txtfile/crop.htm

Scottish Poverty Information Unit spiu.gcal.ac.uk/home.html

Child Poverty Action Group www.namss.org.uk/cpag.htm

Harvard University and NISSI Smart Library on Urban Poverty www.societyonline.org/partners/harvard/

1998 Index of Local Deprivation www.regeneration.detr.gov.uk/98ild/index.htm

Democratic Left www.democratic-left.org.uk/

References

Abbott, P.A. and Wallace, C. (1997) *An Introduction to Sociology: Feminist Perspectives*, 2nd edn. London, Routledge.
Abel-Smith, B. and Townsend, P. (1965) *The Poor and the Poorest*. Occasional Paper on Social Administration No 17. London, Bell.
Acheson, E.D. (1998) *Independent Inquiry into Inequalities in Health*. London, HMSO.
Beveridge, W. (1944) *Full Employment in a Free Society*. London, George Allen and Unwin.
Blakemore, K. (1998) *Social Policy: An Introduction*. Buckingham, Open University Press.
Buchanan, A. and Brinke, J. (1997) *Outcomes for Parenting Experiences*. York, Joseph Rowntree Foundation.
Carstairs, V. (1981) Multiple deprivation and health state. *Community Medicine*, 3: 4–13.

Commission on Social Justice (1994) *Social Justice: Strategies for National Renewal*. London, Vintage.

Craig, G. (1992) Managing the poorest. In Jeffs, T., Carter, P. and Smith, M. (eds) *Changing Social work and Welfare*. Buckingham, Open University Press.

Craig, G. and Rai, D.K. (1996) Social security, community care – and 'race': the marginal dimension. In Ahmad, W. and Atkin, K. (eds) *Race and Community Care*. Buckingham, Open University Press.

Craven, M. (1998) Poverty Undermines Rights in the UK. www.blink.org.uk/hrights/poverty.pdf.

Department of Health and Social Security (1980) *Inequalities in Health* (The Black Report). London, HMSO.

Department of Social Security (1995) *Family Resources Survey. Great Britain, 1993/94*. London, HMSO.

Eardley, T. (1996) *Social Assistance in OECD Countries: A Study Carried Out on Behalf of the Social Policy Research Unit*. London, HMSO.

Fox, A.J., Jones, D.R. and Goldblatt, P.O. (1984) Approaches to studying the effect of socioeconomic circumstances on geographic differences in mortality in England and Wales. *British Medical Bulletin*, **40**(4): 309–14.

Gabe, J. and Thorogood, N. (1986) Prescribed drug use and the management of everyday life: the experiences of black and white working-class women. *Sociological Review*, **34**: 737–72.

Gordon, P. and Newnham, N. (1985) *Passports to Benefits? Racism and Social Security*. London, Child Poverty Action Group and Runnymede Trust.

Gove, W. (1984) Gender difference in mental and physical illness: the effects of fixed roles and nurturant roles. *Social Science and Medicine*, **19**(2): 77–91.

Health Advisory Service Report (1996) *Children and Young People: Substance Misuse Services*. London, The Stationery Office.

Health Education Authority (1999) *Healthline 1998/99*. London, HEA.

Hutton, W. (1995) *The State We're In*. London, Jonathan Cape.

Jones, L. (1994) *The Social Context of Health and Health Work*. Basingstoke, Macmillan – now Palgrave.

Joseph Rowntree Foundation (1995) *Report of an Inquiry into Income and Wealth*. York, JRF.

Labour Party (1997) *Labour Party Manifesto*. London, Labour Party Central Office.

Land, H. (1987) Social policies and women in the labour market. In Ashton, F. and Whitting, G. (eds) *Feminist Theory and Practical Policies*. Bristol, School of Advanced Urban Studies.

Lewis, O. (1965) *La Vida: A Puerto Rican Family in a Culture of Poverty*. London, Panther.

Mack, J. and Lansley, S. (1985) *Poor Britain*. London, Allen & Unwin.

Office of National Statistics (1998) *Living in Britain: Results From the 1996 General Household Survey*. London, Stationery Office.

Piachaud, D. (1981) Peter Townsend and the holy grail. *New Society*, **51**, 10 September: 419–21.

Sly, F. (1994) Ethnic groups and the labour market, *Employment Gazette*. May.

The Economist 19 April 1997. Poverty: worse off but richer. Election briefing.

Thurnhurst, C. (1985) *Poverty and Health in the City of Sheffield*. Sheffield, Environmental Health Department, Sheffield City Council.

Timmins, N. (1996) *The Five Giants: A Biography of the Welfare State*. London, Fontana.

Townsend, P. (1979) *Poverty in the United Kingdom*. London, Penguin Books.

Townsend, P., Simpson, D. and Tibbs, N. (1985) Inequalities in health in the city of Bristol: a preliminary review of statistical evidence. *International Journal of Health Services*, **15**(4): 637–63.

Townsend, P., Phillmore, P. and Beattie, A. (1986) *Inequalities in Health in the Northern Region: An Interim Report*. Bristol, Northern Regional Health Authority/Bristol University.

Townsend, P., Gordon, D., Bradshaw, J. and Gosschalk, B. (1997) *Absolute and Overall Poverty in Britain 1997: What The Population Themselves Say*. Bristol Poverty Line Survey, Bristol, Bristol Statistical Monitoring Unit.

6

Equal value equal care: differences and diversity, primary care perspectives

NAOMI A. WATSON

Learning outcomes

By the end of this chapter you should be able to:

■ Define the terminology in use, and recognise the background and rationale for this.

■ Discuss the legislative historical and political basis of the equality debate.

■ Illustrate anti-discriminatory health care access and delivery as good
  practice.

■ Explore ways of delivering appropriate care to marginalised groups in the
  community.

■ Discuss those factors that contribute to inequality, which eventually has
  an impact on access to service delivery, and on health care practices of
  community nurses.

■ Recognise the role and responsibilities of the community nurse in
  contributing to, and promoting equality of access to, and delivery of,
  services.

■ Discuss the implications within the theoretical frameworks and apply
  these to examples from clinical practice.

Introduction

There is now a general agreement that British society currently consists of a
wide variety of divergent groups, with culturally contrasting perspectives.
While the use of the term 'multicultural' has been generally used to identify
the range of differences, it could be argued that its use has tended to restrict
its application to visible minorities in the society. Diversity, however, presents
itself in a variety of ways, many of which are not immediately recognisable.
The response to differences is usually similar once recognition has occurred.
Because discrimination is endemic in society, the subtle impact may not
always be acknowledged. This makes it the more necessary to ensure there is
clear understanding of the historical nature of the problem, the politico-social
responses, and the nursing requirements in terms of understanding and application to practice.

Delivering nursing care in the community exposes community nurses to
diversity. Inevitably, this has an impact on care delivery practices, with ethical
and other implications. In order to understand these implications, the theoretical, historical and legislative background must be explored, and the arguments considered. This will help to ensure that there is a sound knowledge
base from which appropriate care can be planned and delivered. The ultimate
goal is to ensure that services are not only sensitive, but responsive to differ-

ences, so that individual needs are recognised and addressed. A sound theoretical background should help to ensure that the positive nature of diversity is appreciated. In this context, community nurses have an active contribution to make to changing commonly held negative perceptions and assumptions which do not necessarily provide an accurate reflection either of a community or the lives of individuals within a community.

The use of conceptual frameworks within which the planning and delivery of care are now structured, can provide a good basis for the recognition of individual differences. Nursing models are meant to remind nursing caregivers of the need to use an individualised, systematic approach when assessing, planning and delivering care. While their use has been widely adopted, it is arguable whether or not they have contributed to equitable practices (Gerrish, 1999). Historically, the evidence has suggested that, while health inequalities are largely perpetuated by political and social factors, the nursing perspective has also made a contribution. The Black Report (DHSS, 1980) identified issues of access and actual treatment of patients. But even before the publication of this report, it had already been established that nursing care is delivered differentially, based on a variety of factors which served to make some patients more popular than others (Stockwell, 1972). The requirement within the UKCC's *Code of Professional Conduct* (1992), that nurses recognise and respect the uniqueness and dignity of each patient and client and respond to their need for care irrespective of ethnic origin or religious beliefs, is considered by some to be translated in actual practice only rarely (George, 1994). In this context, the challenge for community nurses is clear. Reading this chapter and working through the activities will give you the opportunities to explore the practice implications of differences in the community. This should help you to understand the importance of diversity, and your role in promoting positive understanding making a difference to negative perceptions.

It is worthwhile taking some time to explore our responses to those differences which are easily recognisable, as well as to those which we may not

Student Activity 6.1

◆ Jot down, in a notepad, those factors which make you different from other people.

◆ Are these differences visible or invisible? Would you say that they are generally considered negatively or positively?

◆ Share those differences which you are happy to disclose with a group of your peers.

◆ How did they respond to invisible differences which you disclosed? How did you respond to theirs?

have been aware of if we had not been told by someone else, or by the individual concerned. The responses to these disclosed differences could depend on a variety of factors, which will include your initial feelings about the individual or group, and the information which you may have acquired about them before their disclosure. You may have been shocked, surprised or indifferent – again, depending on your understanding of the issue disclosed and whether it is considered as negative or positive. Visible differences which are considered negatively may initiate responses within the subconscious, and these may affect our ability to interact appropriately, or to deliver care effectively. Rogers (1969) argues that our inner feelings are reflected in our behaviour, even subconsciously, and that recognising this fact helps to ensure a person-centred approach when delivering care. There is sometimes a tendency to deny this, especially where it may not be politically correct to be seen or known to think negatively or disapprove of certain differences, visible or invisible.

Rogers also states that showing unconditional positive regard for individuals does not necessarily imply approval of any behaviour, especially if it is destructive or hurtful.

Could there be a possibility that there is an overemphasis on understanding certain differences, or even approving them rather than unconditionally respecting them, regardless of our own views? Certainly, it is imperative that we take time to consider the implications for nurses and other health care workers, who must be seen not only to deliver care in a sensitive manner, but also to ensure that they have an understanding of the problems of inequality and access to care and services. These issues continue to be highlighted. The Black Report (DHSS, 1980) was followed by *The Health Divide* (Whitehead, 1987) and more recently, the Acheson Report (1998). Central to the evidence is a variety of new and continuing initiatives within the legislative framework (NHS and Community Care Act 1992) and *The New NHS: Modern, Dependable* (DoH, 1997a) which puts the onus on all nurses involved in direct patient care to demonstrate that they are responding to the government's wishes. As you reflect on these issues, use the next activity to explore your experiences of direct patient care so far.

Student Activity 6.2

◆ Make a list of other *visible* and *invisible* differences that you have encountered among the clients you have met in the community.

◆ What are the common perceptions that are held about them?

◆ Did they fit the common stereotype?

◆ If not, how did they differ from the common stereotype?

Issues of relevance in community care practices

When considering the relevance of these arguments in care delivery practices, there are three main issues that should be considered. These are:

- Access to care and services
- Inclusion in care planning processes
- Delivery of care and services.

Access

The debate about appropriate access to services is a long-standing one and, as mentioned earlier, dates back to the publication of the Black Report in 1980. It could be argued, however, that Stockwell's (1972) work, which identified nurses as behaving differentially towards 'popular' patients by treating them more favourably than 'unpopular' patients, was the first indicator for nursing care delivery practices, which may hinder access. While it may be possible to surmise that the population sample for the study did not, for example, include community nurses, one could also agree about the possibilities of generalising the findings, especially in the light of the Black Report, published eight years later. The as yet unanswered question is whether Stockwell's work was used by nurses to address issues within their practice, and, if it was, why it did not appear to have an impact on care delivery practices. Could it be that nurses were so confident that their practice was appropriate that they did not consider the need for applying the evidence to their practice? Of course, there could be other answers to this. The Black Report raised issues which were applicable to nurses as well as to the medical profession because, one could argue, nurses had had evidence much earlier than the publication of the Black Report and some kind of impact should have been observable. In order to have any impact, however, nurses must address the following questions and be clear about how to find the answers, and how to use these answers to direct their practice. The questions are:

- Who has access to the care and services that are being provided?
- What are the factors affecting people's ability to access care and services appropriately?
- How are resources allocated?
- Who determines priority?

The ethics of cost effectiveness may be considered for all the above points, and there are still conflicting views regarding the ethical implications of allowing cost to be the driving force in care and service provision. Primary care groups and trusts (PCGs/PCTs), it could be argued, have no less of a difficult task in determining cost factors than their now disbanded counterparts, the GP fundholders, or the commissioners. The removal of the internal market does not indicate any less of a focus on cost effectiveness, and it will be interesting to see how the new PCTs handle the complex issues of resource allocation to ensure maximum access to those requiring a service. District nurses have a duty to make an effective contribution to the way service provision is determined and delivered. As they have direct contact with clients on a regular basis, explicit within the political debate is the responsibility to promote access in a manner that ensures all patients receive the service they require in an equitable manner (DoH, 1999). It is the practical issues involved in this approach that will be explored here.

As you work alongside the team assessing and delivering health care in the community, you should be able to identify specific ways in which DNs work towards ensuring that the service is indeed accessible to all. This could be identifiable in a number of ways, which will include the contribution to policy decisions for the local population (their effectiveness within the PCT, or even within their own team) and the use of evidence-based practice in the direct delivery of care.

Of course, being able to identify and use the evidence in care delivery practice, and thereby influence the working of the primary health care team (PHCT) is the first step towards having the ability to be fully effective as members of the PCT. You could begin by asking the following questions:

- How does the team and/or my assessor use the evidence to inform their practice?

- How is this applied to my own learning?

For example, as you search for the evidence to study the case of a particular client or a group of clients, you may find information that district nurses may not necessarily be aware of. This could be some research-based information on a particular aspect of care assessment or delivery, possibly recently published. Would you feel confident to discuss this with your assessor and or the team? What might be their response when you raise these issues? After being in placement for a little while, you will soon have a very good idea, which you could then put to the test. This approach will give you some indication of the way the evidence is being applied, and of any direct impact it may have on the care being provided.

In terms of other applications to practice, how can you identify the ways in which access to assessment and care are equitable across client groups? Look carefully at the clients on your DN assessor's caseload and see whether you are able to spot examples of good practice in this regard. To do this effectively, you will need to consider demography (structure in terms of age/sex, employment, race, and so on) of the caseload and or community population, along with the epidemiological (disease incidence and prevalence) evidence for those populations. This should help you identify any pockets of diversity within the caseload, or the population, and ways that the service is responding to their needs.

Wilmot (1997) argues that, ethically speaking, the response of providing care in the community can be considered from varying perspectives, and possibly as a response to inequality. The idea that there will be gains and losses as a result of redistribution, and that this is determined by formal caregivers, is one concept. Formal caregivers may consider themselves as acting justly by ensuring that care delivery is accessed at the point of need. How, then, does this relate to particular groups who may have been ignored or disadvantaged in the past? Do formal caregivers see themselves as having a role in rectifying this situation? Wilmott argues that it is possible to provide formal care while accepting inequality, without necessarily understanding the possible debilitating effects on health outcomes as a result of specific disadvantage. Understanding the principle of a utilitarian approach, that is working for the greater good or happiness, based on individual judgement of what is best for an individual, may help DNs to recognise their role in making decisions about patients, and the values that may be attached to the particular judgements.

Inclusion in care planning processes

A key issue from both past and present policy initiatives, which is meant to support the concept of access, has been the need to ensure that patients and their carers (be they friends, family or neighbours) are included in assessing, planning and delivering any care that is needed (DoH, 1989 and 1996; NHS and Community Care Act 1992). To do this effectively, DNs have a responsibility to identify clearly who these participants in care might be, and to engage them in the assessment process. Being aware of assumptions which may limit the effectiveness of this process is a major aspect of care planning. For example, the fact that a patient may be supported fully by someone who is not a next of kin should be an important aspect of planning for care. Recognising that kinship ties have different connotations for individual clients will help to ensure that the package of care needed to support them will be truly sensitive to their own needs. The Carers (Recognition and Services) Act of 1995 provides details about assessment and support of carers, regardless of what their relationship to the patient might be. Understanding the need for possible respite and other types of support, and being able to include the patient and designated carers in this process, is vital if services are to fulfil the goal of being responsive to patients' needs. Could there be examples in practice when this may not occur? Consider Case Study 6.1.

Case Study 6.1

Mrs Lynton is a 70-year-old lady who lives on her own, with no next of kin in her community. She was referred to the DN following a fall, which had resulted in her being admitted to hospital with severe bruises, but no broken bones. Mrs Lynton's neighbour regularly visits to keep an eye on her. The DN did an assessment on her first visit following Mrs Lynton's discharge home, and, even though the patient identified her neighbour as her main carer, the DN informed her that she must make arrangements to move into a local home for the elderly, where she would be safe. The patient responded that she neither wanted nor intended to move into a home, as her neighbour had stated that she was quite happy to look in. The DN did not see the neighbour, but the patient was advised that it would be unfair to expect a neighbour to take on all that responsibility. The DN then recommended to the GP that Mrs Lynton should be transferred to a home. Mrs Lynton refused, and told the DN not to bother calling again.

Student Activity 6.3

◆ Thinking about the above case, would you say that this lady had been included in her care assessment and planning?

◆ What form of discrimination can you identify? Would you say that this is subtle or obvious?

◆ Identify an alternative response which could be possible and may produce different outcomes for the patient and DN.

◆ Discuss this with your DN assessor, and ask his or her views about the outcomes.

It could be argued that this DN was merely performing her role to the best of her ability, and would be quite shocked to have her actions identified as being non-inclusive and discriminatory. Yet access to care for this patient may have been jeopardised as a consequence of her behaviour. The patient does not want to see a DN again, as she does not want to be pressured into something she has no wish to do. In considering the counter argument, it could be stated that this patient's best interest was being served by the DN's recommendation. If this is the case, how could the DN have ensured that Mrs Lynton recognised this and understood it to be the best option? So, the key questions that DNs must address should help them when they encounter real clients with needs that may not necessarily equate with the professionals' perception of what is 'normal'. Older people in society may not feel that their needs are being met if their views are not heard, and DNs could end up contributing to the old stereotypes without necessarily being aware of this process. A lack of awareness is certainly not an appropriate reason to be age discriminatory. The recognition of the way that care practices may be influenced by long held beliefs about older people should help to ensure that individualised care is backed up by the application of the evidence base, in order to be able to dispel myths and break down barriers.

The following questions relate to issues in everyday district nursing practice:

- Do patients really have a say? How is this utilised and negotiated in actual care planning and delivery?
- What if patients' and clients' opinions differ from the DN's assessment?
- What methods, if any, are used to consult with diverse groups in the community?

Whether it is dealing with the larger numbers of older people in society today, working with minority ethnic or gay communities, dealing with religious or other socially and culturally diverse individuals or groups, the DN will need to identify transparent ways of working which will ensure a demonstration of awareness about the way decisions are made affecting care assessment, planning and delivery to incorporate the diversity within the community. User involvement in these processes is an integral part of the policy initiatives, and must be demonstrated, although demonstration at the clinical level could be dependent on the wider picture of available resources and examples of good practice in the commissioning processes. Cumberlege (DHSS, 1986) agrees that it is at the local level where dissemination of good practice can be used effectively to motivate and stimulate staff to address such issues. This should stimulate commitment to improved access and removal of discrimination.

Delivery of care and services

A requirement of policy initiatives is that services are delivered in such a way as to allow for sensitivity to individual wishes (DoH, 1997a). How this is translated into practice will be variable, given the range of diversity which exists. Consider the following:

- Are services delivered sensitively, and what are the practical issues affecting them?
- How is the sensitivity of the service measured or audited?
- What if patients and clients refuse to agree with the planned care to be delivered?

- How can professionals work with patients and clients to reduce non-compliance?
- What are the implications for effectiveness of the care to be delivered, and the overall goal for improvement in the patient's health outcomes?

Whether DNs are aware of the need to ensure that these questions are answered may not always be clear. We could look at an example to illustrate this point, in the form of another case study (6.2).

Case Study 6.2

Parveez Ahmed is a 54-year-old mother of three grown children. She has a self-retaining urinary catheter, which is regularly checked by the DN. On a visit to the patient's house, the DN (who had a male student out with her that day) invited the student to provide the care that Mrs Ahmed needed. The next day, there was a phone call to the DN from the patient's daughter, stating that they did not want a male student providing care for their mother. She reported that her mum had been quite distressed and that she had not been asked beforehand if she minded. The DN commented to her colleagues that she was quite surprised, as she considered Mrs Ahmed and her family to be quite Westernised, and had not anticipated that care delivery by a male student would have been a problem.

This is just one example of a service delivery problem, which, if handled differently, could have been avoided. There is also an argument that the option for patients to refuse care from particular individuals should apply to all alike, but there could be even more profound arguments in the light of resource allocations and persistent staffing difficulties, especially if this applies to trained members of staff. In this case, we are looking at a student who is being supervised by an assessor, and the need for exposure to and practice of particular clinical skills which are required to develop experience. The way this is dealt with by DNs will have a profound impact on the perception of users of the service, of its responsiveness to their needs as they perceive them.

Measuring this responsiveness may be approached in a variety of ways. Instead of knee-jerk responses to patient complaints, it may be considered more appropriate to consult them about their expectations and set achievable goals in this area, thus ensuring that patients and their significant others are aware of what is available within the remits of the resources (Wilson, 1995). It is possible that within this there could be some planning to ensure that service users have clear and appropriate information about the way services

Student Activity 6.4

♦ In considering the above case, do you agree that sensitivity was lacking in the care delivery process?

♦ What were the assumptions, if any, about the patient?

♦ How could the case have been handled to ensure a more appropriate outcome?

♦ Consider this from the student's perspective. Should clients have the right to refuse to be cared for by students?

♦ How do you think this could best be handled by workplace assessors?

are assessed and delivered, and of the realistic possibilities of what is on offer. This could have the effect of reducing the number of incidents where practice is alleged to be insensitive, thus improving users' perception of the service. It is clear then, that where users feel more involved and where sensitivity has been considered, goals for access will be enhanced. This should have a positive effect on care delivery practices and patient outcomes.

Understanding the historical and legislative basis for discrimination

If the impact of discrimination on individuals within the community is to be fully understood and recognised, the historical base must be explored so that the context can be recognised. The recent policy initiatives for *The New NHS: Modern, Dependable* (DoH, 1997a) and *Making a Difference* (DoH, 1999) identify the role of the DN as being crucial to the promotion of good practice in individual and community access to services. It is imperative therefore that the historical and legislative background is seen as providing a sound basis on which to build a foundation for the theoretical arguments underpinning the delivery of care. While some of this information may be unnecessary, a lack of understanding about the nature of society and the way structures within it shape our thinking and actions, make it difficult to promote change or fulfil the goal of improved access to care. Evidence of health inequalities from Stockwell (1972) to Acheson (1998) indicate there is much to learn. As a student on your community placement, you should be able to identify examples of practice which indicate that the issues raised are taken on board as a basis for building and improving practice. Trends set by your assessor will influence your own development and future practice. While you will encounter aspects of good, bad, and best practice, you should aim not only to differentiate between these, but also to learn to reject what is sub-standard, and use the evidence of the literature to inform the way you will practise as a fully qualified nurse. The information here should help you to identify the basis for the literature, and the relevance to your learning.

Gender perspectives

Social divisions and institutional structures have long been recognised as key reinforcers of oppressive actions, leading to unequal treatment. It is recognised that this treatment becomes embedded in institutional practices, which have tremendous impact on the lives of the individuals to whom they are applied (Thompson, 1997). Many of these are set firmly within traditional bases, which have started eroding very slowly over the past years. For example, in 1999 the government found it necessary to establish a women's unit directly answering to the Prime Minister, in order to look at the situation of women. This is an indication that gender categorisation is still responsible for a great deal of inequality within society. This is in spite of what many would consider to be great strides forward over the years. Yet it has been suggested that women themselves may be partially responsible for reinforcing some of these inequalities. The Sex Discrimination Act of 1975 had tremendous policy and practice implications, and the activities of the Equal Opportunities Commission (EOC), which was set up to enhance the working of the Act, still functions as a major aid to women, and more recently to men, who wish to challenge social or employment structures.

The differentiation process results from social stratification based on class, race, religion, disability and sexual orientation. These are still key indicators of how these groups are perceived within the society (Thompson, 1997). Legislative frameworks have been established to provide a basis from which the issues raised could be tackled. The meaning of terminology has been clearly defined in order to assist with issues such as, for example, understanding the difference between direct and indirect discrimination, and issues relating to possible victimisation as a result of challenging the status quo. It is imperative that formal nursing care providers within the community recognise and understand the issues involved. Social perceptions, which are only enforced by individual actions, may stand a better chance of changing if there is a sound level of knowledge underpinning and contributing to a wider understanding. Many of the enduring structures within society are built around the legacy of patriarchal power relations and economic interests, and these have largely contributed to the way status and opportunity are allocated within society. This is also true of ideology and use of language, which have contributed enormously to stereotypes and highlighted differences (Thompson, 1997). The need for a more enlightened view of differences that may be encountered in the community is emphasised by George (1994). The stereotypical view, that differences are automatically problematic, needs to be altered. After all, it should be possible to appreciate that not all older people are heavily dependent on care services, and diversity does not have to carry negative connotations. In order to demonstrate this awareness effectively, DNs will need to recognise and use the evidence to inform their practice. This could provide a powerful role model for influencing positive changes in social and institutional attitudes.

Race and health

The Race Relations Act 1965 (modified 1976) has been seen as the first open admission that race differentiation has a direct impact on the lives of people from minority ethnic origins. Following the Act, a Commission for Racial Equality (CRE) was set up in order to support the practical functioning of the Act. Another key issue was to clarify and define the terminology which had become part of regular use, along with the need to identify strategies to help with proof, which was a problematic issue. While there have been some strides forward in many aspects of social and institutional practice, many would argue that there are inherent problems which have had negative influences on the lives of people from minority ethnic groups. In terms of health, the Black Report (DHSS, 1980) identifies this in the way access to services has been determined, and many services structured to impede access. Within other institutional settings, for example education, police and social services, the evidence is that there are pervading perceptions which still contribute to unequal treatment (Runneymede Trust, 2000). Perhaps the best example of pervading institutional attitudes lies within the recent Stephen Lawrence incident (Macpherson Report, 1999). The findings from the report confirm the view that enduring attitudes do not simply disappear. As with other forms of differentiation, there may be possibilities of rejection and denial of the existence of a problem which, in essence, equates with a refusal to look at new ways of addressing the issues. Again, the basis for perceptions are set within enduring social stereotyping (Thompson, 1997) which must be recognised as having a direct impact on us as individuals. Only then can individuals address the issues needed to change their practice and hence positively influence institutional practices. In the case of race, the recognition of the impact on direct health outcomes must be a part of the process for DNs. For example, those race factors which have a direct influence on health outcomes will need to be recognised within appropriate assessment and care planning. The evidence is that these needs are generally not recognised by health and social care providers (Atkin and Rollins, 1993). This will make it more difficult for clinical practitioners to be . committed to changing practice when this does not appear to be supported from a policy perspective. More recently there has been a shift in policy, with the emphasis on access placing the needs of all diverse groups, and specifically minority ethnic groups, at the heart of planning (DoH, 1996).

Disability legislation – relevant issues

There has been race and gender legislation for many years, and institutions and organisations have been encouraged to adopt good practice. Disability legislation, however, has only recently been introduced (The Disability Discrimination Act 1997). The use of language, and its impact on the way marginalised groups are viewed, is equally relevant to all. This is as much an issue for people with a physical, mental or other disability as it is for others. The present emphasis, for example, on shifting the focus from a negative perception (enabling, rather than disabled) may not be considered by able-bodied people to be very significant. But for those who are having to battle daily with deeply ingrained social perceptions, the shift could mean a feeling of taking back control over aspects of their lives that have been lost. As providers of care services for the sick, DNs will come in contact with all types of patients in the community. There is a need to understand the debate and find ways of ensuring that care responses reflect that understanding. One of the major requirements is the ability to work collaboratively with other members of the PHCT. For example, where patients have mental, physical or learning disability, working closely with key workers ensures that the service being provided is as seamless as possible. The ultimate goal is to aid the improvement of the patient's health in minimum time. Issues of relevance to patients with learning or other disability, such as the need to be able to take some control of their lives, have to be a part of the way the service is delivered to clients. Case study 6.3 will illustrate the point.

Case Study 6.3

James is a 38-year-old man who has learning difficulties. He was referred to the DN for assessment regarding his insulin dependent diabetes, for which he needed daily injections. On arrival at his house, James' mother was also present, and the DN discussed James' assessment with her. James was not, however, consulted as the DN took his mother's advice that he is not very bright, and is not able to communicate well. On her return to the office, she had a call from James' key worker to say that James was upset because his mum, who had been visiting him during the day, had not allowed him any say in the care, which was agreed. The DN responded that she assumed that his mum was his main carer, and therefore had a right to be involved. However, his key worker informed her that James' mother lives out of town and just happened to be visiting that day.

Student Activity 6.5

After reading through the above case:

◆ Identify what was inappropriate about the way that the DN approached the assessment process for this patient.

◆ Discuss the case with one or more of your peers.

◆ Identify ways that you think could have helped to achieve better outcomes for the patient.

Equal opportunity initiatives: policy and practice implications

The awareness of equal opportunities focus within organisational settings is usually easily identified in advertisements, where, as a result of the legislative framework, there was a need for organisations, especially those in the public sector, to be seen to be responsive to local and national initiatives. Consequently, advertisements, for example, have long carried encouraging phrases, which are meant to identify to women, the disabled, and minority ethnic communities/individuals, the organisation's commitment to equal opportunities. Whether this written commitment is recognisable in the workforce is another issue, however. It could be argued that the key to recognising the responsiveness of any organisation could be the visible structures, which should be a feature, to support those to whom the reassurance is being given. For example, enabling those who may need wheelchair access, could require significant changes to most organisations, not just for physical access, but in terms of attitudes to the disabled, among the able-bodied workforce. It is also possible that disabled people wanting to work within a particular setting may first wish to find out how many other disabled people are successfully functioning in that organisation. The same principle applies to all other marginalised groups, especially those with visible differences, who may not want to be isolated in the workplace. It should be possible to examine an organisation's track record on these issues. However, records may not always be kept, and it is widely believed that the way equal opportunities policies are applied in practice is patchy and variable. Hence, although there are legislative frameworks, monitoring for effectiveness at organisational levels is not necessarily easy. In some instances, high profile aspects of the particular diverse group may raise issues (for example, in the recent publicity about the Armed Forces and gay people). Perhaps this is the point to remind ourselves that nursing has tended to be largely a female profession, and that there may be instances of discriminatory attitudes to men in the profession. The other side of that argument recognises that, while men may be a minority in nursing, within nursing managerial positions, they appear to maintain a monopoly, when compared to their female counterparts (Doyal, 1994).

Promoting equal access and delivery of care

For professional practice to be appropriate and effective, the allocation of resources and the delivery of health care needs to reflect the particular community to which it is being delivered. Essentially, community lifestyles and priorities will be a key feature in the organisation, assessment, planning and delivery of care services. Appropriate methods should be used to ensure that the evidence for the basis of care is sound, rather than anecdotal. As a student in the community, you should be able to identify the way that this translates into actual practice. The key issue underpinning this approach is the need for practitioners to recognise and be aware of their own differences in terms of beliefs, and how this influences their expectations of each other.

If the care delivery process is to be effective, then DNs should understand that traditional health beliefs and practices cannot be ignored or negated, simply because they do not fit in with commonly held views about health and health care. Working with patients should encourage a partnership approach, so that any planned action for the community involves wide consultation, where the views of those who will be affected will be represented.

In exploring health beliefs and practices, the application to individual practice could be helpful where, by in-depth exploration and personal observations based on the experiences of the DN, vital information can be ascertained which may impact directly on the effectiveness of certain interventions. If DNs develop regular habits of dissemination, and publish individual case reports, this will contribute to building stronger, practitioner-based research evidence. This can then be used to inform changes to practice which will benefit patients and other practitioners in the multidisciplinary team.

Working with difference and diversity – practical steps

To provide an effective service that recognises the diversity of the community, DNs will need to have the foundations of their work set within the research base. As discussed earlier, this includes recognition of the impact of social and institutional structures on our views and perceptions of diversity. Such a recognition will help to maintain awareness of the way that those perceptions may shape the delivery of care. For example, making inappropriate assumptions, not based on evidence, could actually restrict some patients' access to services, yet this may not always be recognised at a conscious level. In fact, it is in the exercise of what some patients recognise as their rights, given through initiatives such as The Patient's Charter (DoH, 1992), that DNs may first become aware that particular actions have contributed to limiting access. This could be somewhat surprising. DNs would not consider themselves to be practising in a discriminatory manner, yet the evidence from the literature identifies that discrimination is quite common across the whole spectrum of health care. In response to this, policy initiatives continue to focus on the issue of access, and the crucial role of nurses in promoting this (Acheson, 1998; DoH, 1997a, 1999). One could argue that a culture of constant awareness should be fostered if assumptions about the way practice is delivered are to be challenged by the individuals concerned. As you work alongside your clinical assessor in the community, it is useful to try and identify good practice based on the evidence, and question the way in which it is applied. The following practical steps should help to identify specific activities, which can be performed to address issues of diversity within the community and on the caseload:

- Practitioners should ensure that all patients, especially those from diverse communities understand their role and the way this relates both to the rest of the multidisciplinary team, and to the district nursing team. All explanations should be given in a way which ensures that patients understand the information and are aware of how the team works.

- When finding out about individuals, it is imperative that appropriate attempts are made to communicate directly with them. This is not necessarily always an easy process, but it should be a basic rule that we find out for sure whether direct communication is possible before making assumptions that it is not. Because of the individuality of each person, it is useful to find out, individually, how people want to be identified, what they want to be called, what their personal, religious and health beliefs are, what their main language is, and what their personal preferences are regardimg everyday experiences and lifestyle. While this is the focus for individualised care assessment and planning, it can be assumed that this cannot be always as effective as it could be if there are persistent problems with access and care delivery, as identified in the literature (DoH, 1996, 1997a, 1999). The way this information is collected will vary, and may or may not be done at once. In fact it is possible that most of this could be done on an informal basis, but it is imperative that this is used to help patients maintain their own personal identity, rather than always being defined as part of a group.

- Understanding the powerful role of language and use of terminology is an important aspect of ensuring that services are sensitive to individuals. Thompson (1997) argues that this cannot be negated or undermined where practitioners are responsive to, and committed to improving access to patients. Again, where initial steps have been taken to find out the facts about individuals, the way patients want to be identified should be clear.

- Accuracy and relevance of anecdotal information should be checked and cross referenced, using a combination of approaches, based on the evidence in the literature, what patients themselves and local communities say, personal experiences of working with clients, and through discussions with other members of the team involved in care delivery.

- Where practitioners are working in a diverse setting, it would be in their best interests to find out about the traditional healers in the community, which patients use them, and the types of problem about which they are consulted. As health care professionals, appropriate meeting and discussion with traditional healers could help to develop a measure of trust. This should be set against possible suspicion on the part of local communities, who may need to be reassured that the approaches to them are genuinely in the search for a better understanding of local health beliefs and practices.

- In order to establish a good rapport, it will be necessary to talk to individual patients about the illnesses considered to be serious in their community, and the ways that are used to handle these, for example the causes, prevention, diagnoses and treatment of these illnesses.

- Where there are variations in what is considered 'serious' within communities, talking with individuals may help to establish why this is so. Discussions can be held on an informal basis with individuals and families with whom you work. Regular team meetings to discuss caseloads should contribute to sharing and dissemination of information, fostering a better understanding of local practices in communities.

- An understanding and recognition of personal beliefs and practices does not remove the responsibility to ensure that guidelines about symptoms, which should be seen by a doctor, are provided on an individual basis.

- Patients who do not understand the way that the NHS works will need to be given guidelines which are easy to understand, in order to help them access services which may be relevant to their needs.

- The use of traditional treatments should be understood rather than discouraged, unless there is absolute evidence that this is harmful. The psychological and psychosocial effects on patients cannot be negated, but should be seen as a positive contribution to the patient's healing process.

- It is much more productive to encourage and strengthen positive approaches when working in diverse communities. Local networks and referral routes from the community could mean that health promotion work within those communities becomes much more effective. Traditional healers who are respected within the community could become powerful allies in delivering effective services if the approach used is one of searching for genuine partnership.

Conclusion

Working with, and accepting differences within health care practices in the community involves practitioners in a range of specific processes. The need for a planned and systematic approach has been strengthened by the range of policy initiatives, which identify the existence of a problem, which is persistent across health care delivery practices (Black Report, 1980; Acheson Report, 1998). Perhaps the most important is the need for a constant awareness of the way perceptions are influenced by powerful social structures, which affect the way individuals respond in the assessment and delivery of care. Past and present policy initiatives focus heavily on the crucial role of the DN in contributing to improved access of health care, ensuring better outcomes for health achievement for the whole community. In order to do this effectively, there will need to be recognition of the way certain groups have been marginalised, and specific measures taken to redress this situation. The ethical implications involved are clear. Requirements for delivering sensitive services, which are relevant to the local needs of individuals within the community, have become a key part of the DN's role. As a student in the community, the practices you observe, and in which you participate, should help to reinforce the issues discussed in this chapter. Your future role should have a sound basis from which you will be able to contribute to meeting the present policy aims for a service that is not only 'Modern and Dependable', (DoH, 1997a) but is appropriate for the demands of the new millennium. The opportunity to become major players in the way these services develop will only remain accessible if today's students recognise their own responsibilities in changing present practices by appropriate challenge to practices which may not be conducive to ensuring a widening of participation and better and more sensitive delivery of services. Clinical governance will facilitate this process, but it is up to individuals to take the initiatives forward in positive ways to benefit the whole community and ensure a cascading effect of good practice in the way care is delivered to a diverse population.

Further reading

Ahmed, W. and Atkin, K. (1996) *'Race' and Community Care*. Open University Press.
Thompson, N (1997) *Anti-discriminatory Practice*. Macmillan – now Palgrave.

References

Acheson, E.D. (1998) *Independent Inquiry into Inequalities in Health*. London, HMSO.

Ahmed, W. and Atkin, K. (1996) *'Race' and Community Care*. Buckingham, Open University Press.

Atkin, K. and Rollings, J. (1993) *Community Care in a Multiracial Britain. A Review of the Literature*. London, HMSO.

Bevan G. (1998) Taking equity seriously. *British Medical Journal*, **316**: 39–42.

Cruikshank, J.K. and Beavers, D.G. (1989) *Ethnic Factors in Health and Disease*. Oxford, Butterworth Heinemann.

Department of Health (1989) *The Children Act*. London, HMSO.

Department of Health (1990) *The NHS and Community Care Act*. London, HMSO.

Department of Health (1992) *The Patients Charter*. London, DoH.

Department of Health (1996) *Responding to Diversity. A Guide to Purchasing for Ethnic Minority Health*. London, DoH.

Department of Health (1997a) *The New NHS: Modern, Dependable*. London, HMSO.

Department of Health (1997b) *The Primary Care Act*. London, HMSO.

Department of Health (1999) *Making a Difference, the Contribution of Nursing, Midwifery and Health Visiting to Health Care*. London, HMSO.

Department of Health and Social Security (1980) *Inequalities in Health* (The Black Report). London, HMSO.

Department of Health and Social Security (1986) *Neighbourhood Nursing*. The Cumberledge Report. London, HMSO.

Doyal, L. (1994) *The Political Economy of Health*. London, Pluto.

George, M. (1994) Accepting differences. *Nursing Standard*, **8**(18): 21–3.

Gerrish, K. (1999) Inequalities in service provision: an examination of institutional influences on the provision of district nursing care to minority ethnic communities. *Journal of Advanced Nursing*, **30**(6): 1263–7.

Hopkins, A. and Bahl, V. (eds) (1993) *Access to Health Care for People from Black and Ethnic Minorities*. London, Royal College of Physicians.

Ilife, S. (1995) The retreat from equity. *Critical Public Health*, **6**: 3.

Kavanagh, K. and Kennedy, P.H. (1992) *Promoting Cultural Diversity – Strategies for Health Care Professionals*. London, Sage.

Macpherson, Sir William (1999) *The Stephen Lawrence Inquiry: Report of an Inquiry*. London, HMSO.

Mason, D. (1995) *Race and Ethnicity in Modern Britain*. New York, Oxford University Press.

Rogers, C. (1969) *Freedom to Learn: Studies of the Person*. Columbus, Ohio, Merril Publishing Co.

Stockwell, F. (1972) *The Unpopular Patient*. London, Royal College of Nursing.

Thompson, N. (1997) *Anti-discriminatory Practice*, 2nd edn. London, Macmillan – now Palgrave.

Tinker, A. (1992) *Elderly People in Modern Society*. London, Longman.

United Kingdom Central Council for Nursing, Midwifery and Health Visiting (UKCC) (1992) *Code of Professional Conduct*. London, UKCC.

Whitehead, M. (1987) *The Health Divide*. London, Health Education Council.

Wilmot, S. (1997) *The Ethics of Community Care*. London, Cassell.

Wilson, G. (1995) *Community Care; Asking the Users*. London, Chapman & Hall.

7

Effective communication in primary care

JILL BARR

Learning outcomes

By the end of this chapter you will be able to:

- Identify the need for effective communication in community nursing.
- Discuss the communication process.
- Recognise the various levels of communication of community nurses.
- Discuss the importance of quality record keeping.
- Discuss the barriers to effective communication in community.
- Discuss the variety of communication skills.

Introduction

The need for good communication awareness, knowledge and skills in nursing will be emphasised throughout your career because it is central to the therapeutic relationships that are held within nursing and patient health care. Community nursing requires effective nursing communication, maybe more so than in ward based care because there is a need for getting the *right* communication *right* first time. This is because patient or client professional contacts are more time limited, there are geographical distances between people and in terms of effectiveness and efficiency, nurses need to plan their communication activity within the allocated time span. Communication in the primary care team is also difficult when members, with different education and experiences, do not reside in the same building and where changes may be frequent. You may well find that communication in community nursing is of a different nature to ward based communication. If community nurses are to 'make a difference' to patient care, then communication skills lie at the heart of the professional care delivered. This chapter aims to explore that professional knowledge, skills and complexities within primary care.

Communication in community nursing

There are four main reasons why we communicate with other people in the community:

- To seek information
- To motivate
- To instruct
- To inform.

This may seem a rather stark way of viewing communication. As nurses, we need to be aware of the very powerful skills that exist within the activity of communicating, particularly in the therapeutic act of caring. In the community, long-term relations build up with those who live and work in an area, so professional communication should be seen in the context of providing quality community health care. Communication, therefore, is an important aspect of all care delivery. All nurses and health care workers need to be aware of the skills and knowledge needed for effective communication and the best ways of communicating with other members of the multidisciplinary and multi-agency teams. Baker and colleagues (1997, p. 54) note the value of communication in the primary health care team (PHCT) and highlight a formula to show the complexity of the communication channels:

> If n is the number of people in a primary health care team, the number of lines of communication required is expressed by the formula $(n^2 - n) \div 2$. Thus with five people in a team, there are 10 lines of communication.

Learning to be an effective and professional communicator is often a difficult journey. As a student, you are constantly trying to make sense of the various nursing areas, and the types of nursing knowledge and skills in each of those areas. The language in the different areas often changes and it takes time to integrate this new language with your own and discriminate between effective and ineffective communication. This is especially relevant where some terminology being used may not mean the same thing to all the members of the PHCT (see Chapters 1 and 6). However, poor communication can lead to substandard patient care or worse, incompetent practice leading to fatal errors with resulting disciplinary action. So it is important to recognise 'good' communication and distinguish it from 'poor' communication as early as possible in your career. The recent documents *Fitness for Practice* (UKCC, 1999) and *Making a Difference* (DoH, 1999) both identify communication as a key skill in nursing. However key skills should be underpinned with a sound knowledge base. Hinchliffe (1979) identified a skill as being either a physical or mental performance of anything that a person has learned to do with ease and precision. She feels that the learning process that leads to a high degree of performance involves the knowledge and skill becoming internalised. So while community nurses may seem to communicate easily, naturally and fluently with others, they may often have taken years to internalise the knowledge and skill. Calling at someone's door, initiating a relationship, broaching intimate questions, answering complex concerns and identifying a range of choices for individuals to meet their health needs involve a mental ability that is difficult to teach in a short time while you are out in the community. Hopefully, you will be able to observe and participate in care delivery and build up skills for the future, with the help of good assessors and supervisors and an awareness of the best care you need to deliver to your patients.

Student Activity 7.1

Think about how you communicate with others and:

◆ Make a list of your strengths in communicating with others.

◆ Give reasons why you chose these strengths.

◆ Compare these with one or two of your peers.

◆ Make notes in your portfolio.

Communication skills and knowledge

You may think that you are good at talking to other people and get on well with them. Others may feel that they are good listeners. We sometimes feel that the skill of communication is a part of our personality, which comes from our own human growth and development. Lovell (1982) suggested that all skills are learned and involve the construction of organised and co-ordinated activities. From this viewpoint, effective communication in nursing concerns more than just social communication. It is about the professional and therapeutic skill of communication.

In terms of learning, you may be able to recognise knowledge gained prior to starting your nursing course, whether it was learnt from other people or from interesting material you personally used for an assignment or for light reading. You may also have gained recent knowledge during the common foundation part of your programme.

No doubt, you will have thought about various aspects of verbal and non-verbal communication and also feel happy with the importance of listening and how to question and use 'open' questions (those requiring dialogue) and 'closed' questions (those requiring simple responses).

Student Activity 7.2

◆ Think about some of the communication knowledge you have learnt about in the past.

◆ Write down some points about communication theory that you feel are important and relevant for your placement in the community. Give reasons why you think these are important.

◆ Do this activity with one or two peers.

◆ Make notes in your portfolio.

There are many theories of communication on which you can draw. Behaviourists such as Skinner (1957) argued that operant conditioning, which emphasises the stimulus–reinforcement principle, could affect the way that people communicate with each other. Chomsky (1957), a psycho-linguist, worked on the language aspects of communication and believed that the types of language structures were generated from a set of rules, encompassing surface and deep meanings. Piaget (1955), a biologist and cognitivist, argued for a developmental view of communication and language, linking these to cognitive experiences as well as to innate factors in children. Following on from this was the later work of Rumelhart (1980) who redefined the idea of 'schemas' which were seen as the building blocks of cognition. The work of Argyle (1983) may be more familiar, as it focused on social interaction, social relationships and social behaviourism. You may wish to look at some of this material while you are in your community practice.

It may be useful here to review *how* we communicate.

The process of communication

Communication is about transferring our ideas and feelings to others. Effective communication is seen as a two-way process: a sender sends their message to a targeted person who then sends back their feedback to the original sender. If the targeted person does not receive the message, or chooses to ignore it and gives no feedback to the sender, then only partial communication takes place.

There are many models of communication that you may find interesting. One model that may prove useful in thinking about effectiveness can be seen when we think about the process of communication. The model is useful because it shows various elements of the communication process, but seeing communication as a linear process may be considered too simplistic. However, this model does highlight aspects of:

- Encoding
- Decoding, and
- Noise interference.

These are often at the heart of communication breakdown.

The Table 7.1 illustrates the variety of ways of encoding, which can be used to convey meanings.

Nurses need to be aware of the full range of ways to communicate with their patients and encourage them to communicate in return, using methods with which they are familiar.

Table 7.1 Various forms of communication encoding

Verbal codes	Non-verbal codes
These include the sounds we send to each other, aided by our sophisticated human neurolinguistic anatomy and physiology. This ability is said to place us apart from other animals.	These may be considered to be partially innate and partially culturally defined.
	Body language:
	These are body actions, which are partly learnt through the socialisation process and are partly innate. They may reinforce verbal messages but they may also show contradictions. Examples include eye contact, touch, facial expressions.
	Other communication forms:
	These have developed throughout civilisation and have required the manufacture of tools such as chisels, paper, pens, computers and so on, which provide alternative channels to convey messages. Examples include writing, Braille, art, music.

Language as a form of encoding

Any language can be seen in terms of its symbols. As children, we learn to speak and write our own language through the socialisation process. The written form of language is seen as more formal and permanent. We often take literacy for granted in this country but many people in the world are unable to read and write in the formal language of their own country. It is also true that there are people in Britain who have not got the skills to read and write. Written symbols are associated with a developed educational system and access to that system. There is a need to learn about these symbols; the rules of their ordering and the meanings attached to the sequences of these symbols.

Language may be conveyed immediately from our voices through sound wave channels to recipients' ears, from words on paper, paper substitute channels, recording sounds on video or tape for more permanence.

Spoken language/accents

The spoken word is learned informally through the socialisation process and there are variations noted in various geographical areas. For example, there are distinct dialects in Scotland, Newcastle, the Black Country and Cornwall. These are due to the historical migration of different peoples globally.

It has also been noted that there are now distinct variations of language between young people and older people, between various ethnic groups in the same geographical area and also between social classes. The same is true for the wide range of accents, which you may be aware are used regionally, and which may serve to reinforce assumptions about patients. This richness in diversity could be seen as a sign of global development and maturity. However it could also be seen as a means for social exclusion from the resources within a community or a country and thus will affect access to health care.

Student Activity 7.3

♦ Think back to the model of communication described in Table 7.1 and the text immediately preceding it.

♦ Make a list what you think may affect the *encoding and decoding* of language symbols when nursing patients in the community.

♦ Discuss your list with your assessor.

You may well have thought about patients or clients whose first language is not English and how they may find difficulty expressing themselves in their efforts to get their messages or information through to a nurse. This is also true for nurses who wish to give information to patients who do not speak their language. This may pose difficulties for nurses who may see this difficulty as a patient problem and end up 'blaming' them for not being able to speak English *rather* than questioning their professional ability to communicate creatively and effectively. Discriminatory behaviour must always be questioned. So what can nurses do? Many nurses take on the challenge of learning new languages (and dialects) such as Hindi or Gujerati in order to communicate better with their patients. Chapter 6 highlights the importance of self-awareness for all nurses working within our culturally diverse society and is linked to the UKCC's *Code of Professional Conduct* (1992) which makes clear the responsibility of the nurse to respect the individualism of patients and clients.

Nurses can use other symbolic channels besides spoken English. They can also refer to available translating services as soon as possible if there are real communication barriers. Time and limited resources within the community often deter nurses from attempting this approach. However, if there is enough demand, more resources may be brought in.

When nurses assess the needs of their patients, they need to recognise the wider issues affecting communication. These could include:

● Infants or children who may not have a developed language.

● People with learning disabilities who have delayed language development.

- People who are challenged in reading and writing
- Cultural differences in dialects, accents, class and ethnic background.
- Disabilities such as deafness, strokes and neuro-muscular problems, diseases affecting speech structures (that is, mouth, throat and respiratory tract) as well as mental health problems.

Unspoken language

The issues just discussed relate to the language as a symbol for encoding. However, we also use unspoken or non-verbal communication to convey extra meanings. The main channels for communication come through our:

- Appearance
- Facial expressions
- Eye contact and use of eyes
- Use of body space near others
- Use of body gestures
- Use of hands in gestures
- Gait
- Use of space and territory.

Non-verbal communication issues may pose difficulties for those attempting to communicate because of:

- Developmental immaturity
- Cultural differences in non-verbal behaviour
- Visual problems, blindness
- Neuro-muscular problems affecting mobility of the body, facial or limb movements
- Cerebral trauma, infection or disease
- Social problems
- Mental health problems.

These difficulties may be assumed to lie with the patient or client, but they could well be issues affecting the nurse as well. Nurses, as individuals, will have their own personal issues, socially or medically. For example, patients may find it difficult to understand the nurse whose concentration is impaired by a raging toothache and who does not feel able to respond very easily.

Student Activity 7.4

◆ Think about some examples of effective communication by a community nurse that you have seen in practice.

◆ Make notes on why you think these were effective.

◆ Write down what you learned from this.

◆ Discuss these with one or more of your peers.

Other non-verbal codes used to convey messages

The ability to encode and decode as an alternative for speech is also a sign of human development. The need for messages and meanings to have some relative permanence has been a challenge for many centuries.

The changing social conditions, such as an increase in mobility, role changes within a family or small community, the availability of natural resources and a need for a sense of identity as the world becomes more complex, may well be seen as important in bringing in alternatives to speech and language.

From the cave pictures in the history books to sculpture, architecture and photography, as well as the development of musical notation, numeracy and Braille systems, through to the digital age of television, photography and now the Internet, communication has developed in a wide variety of ways outside language. These ways of encoding can also convey thoughts and meanings through time and space.

The use of art may be a creative way to help patients express themselves when they have a physical or mental illness that inhibits speech. Children or adults who have underdeveloped speech may be encouraged to identify their

Student Activity 7.5

◆ Identify from your experience as a student the ways that nurses use to convey non-verbal symbolic codes when working with patients.

◆ Ask one or more of your peers to do the same.

◆ Compare and contrast your list.

◆ Make notes for your portfolio.

worries or concerns through drawing. Computer technology has also allowed some patients with deteriorating neuro-muscular conditions to communicate with the world via Possum machines. People with learning disability may well enjoy the use of 'stimulation rooms' which are a form of textural art to stimulate the senses and allow self-expression. Photographic representations are important aids for remembering individualism and family experiences for all those who may not be in control of their own health. Some nursing and residential homes actively encourage relatives to bring in photographs and memorabilia for their kin who are unable to look after themselves.

The *written word* is considered to be an advanced system of symbols and when patients are unable to speak, the use of the written word may be a useful alternative if the nurse uses the same language as the patient. Nurses may often use health education leaflets to reinforce a verbal message. The idea that literacy has affected health overall and provided opportunities for improvement in life chances and choices goes without saying. The ability to disseminate knowledge about healthy living and different health services, through health education in the form of posters, literature and books has expanded the general public's view of health and ill health. Health education material using written messages is a useful resource for nursing care. However, it is not suitable for all situations.

It was Neil Postman, in 1983, who argued that the advent of the printing press in the 15th century gave rise to the discrimination between childhood and adulthood. Prior to this, virtually all human communication was through word of mouth, stories, ballads and wise sayings. Even the reading that was available was done out loud. The use of the spoken word as narrative for research purposes may be an issue for exploration, in order to preserve its importance especially in varied cultural environments. The printing press revolutionised the availability of 'ideas' but as a consequence, children were separated from the adult world. This process is continuing with the advent of the home computer, giving children the opportunity to explore alternative realities.

Written documentation for record keeping in nursing is also important and you will get an opportunity to notice the various forms of records when you are out in community practice. This topic will be returned to later.

Communication as a form of social control

Communication, as it is, cannot be just seen as a neutral aspect of nursing... 'that comes with the job'. Communication represents some stance in the social world. The way nurses choose and use their communication and language is a powerful source of social control. It has to be remembered that nurses are dealing with very vulnerable individuals and the ethical consideration of 'doing no harm' often requires a deeper understanding of communication.

The Marxist view sees communication as contributing to the domination of some groups or individuals over others (Crawford et al., 1998) This can be illustrated by the use of medical jargon within the context of the social construction of illness. Nurses view 'patient compliance' in a positive light and 'non compliance' as a negative response and may well approach patients based on these responses. They may sometimes give more communication time to those with less need than those with more need as identified by the inverse care law (Stockwell, 1972). Indeed Crawford and colleagues (1998) highlight institutionalised discrimination of cultural and racial biases that are made via language in nursing, for example by pathologising the black family (p. 177) and by limiting the communication time for patients from ethnic minorities to express themselves (p. 203). They also note that communication with elderly patients is often in a patronising tone (see also Chapters 6 and 13 in this book).

Edwards and Noller (1993, p. 207) argue that, 'Inappropriate or mismanaged communication can contribute to the psychological and physical decline among the elderly.' In addition, the work by Crawford et al. (1998, p. 182) highlights the frequent assumption that older patients will be suffering from hearing and comprehension impairment. Communication using high pitched and slow intonations with childish expressions is often used. Written nursing records can also illustrate ethical problems. These authors coin the phrase 'firing paper bullets', referring to the fact that communication in writing may actually work against the patient:

> overdosing client records with judgmental terms may be just as toxic as overdosing with medication.

The fact that patient-held records are now a feature of care in the community should alert those working with patients of the need to be aware of the way that records are written. Remember that patients have direct access to these notes, and will often take them out to read as soon as the district nurse or other health care worker has left.

From a feminist perspective, the various forms of language and knowledge often distinguish the world of women and men in health care. Traditionally, men as doctors and women as nurses has meant that the latter have been more hesitant to offer opinions or question medical expertise. Gendered records towards *masculine* ideologies may also have been favoured in the past at the expense of feminine perspectives. Binnie (2000) identifies 'new nursing' in health care and argues for nurses to become aware of their role in health care. For example, during a medical consultation, a nurse could sit beside the patient's bed, encouraging consultants to come down to the same level, making the situation less intimidating for the patient, rather than the nurse standing behind the doctors and, like the patient, becoming invisible.

Levels of communication

It could be said that nurses communicate on different levels. There are four main levels of communication for community nurses:

- Therapeutic communication
- Interprofessional communication
- Administrative communication
- Political communication.

Therapeutic communication

Nursing patients, whether sick or well, is said to involve the therapeutic *use of self* (Peplau, 1987). The level of communication you use when nursing will depend very much on your own self-awareness and interpersonal skills that have developed during your life and since you commenced your programme. Benner (1984) identified stages in nursing development, where there is a growth in skills and knowledge from a novice stage to an expert stage. Despite this being a useful incremental model, it does not always take into account any changes in situations that occur regularly, which may affect the knowledge and skills an individual nurse may require. For instance, moving into a new clinical area or a change in what is seen as acceptable practice. So, in the past, nurses focused on educating people by passing information to clients and patients, for them to absorb. Research questioning the value of this then moved the goalposts and a more participative style of communication was required. This meant that those who were more expert in *lecturing* skills needed to learn the skills of *facilitation* on an individual or group work basis.

Milburn and colleagues (1995) identified that it was patients who really valued nursing communication:

> The bother that nurses go to ... when you are low they're there holding your hand ... It's a gentle sweetness; They show they care by sitting and talking ... spending time.

> I want them to listen to me when I need them ... When I get bad news (about this cancer) I need someone to sit and listen and to know they don't leave you when you get bad news. (Milburn et al., p. 1096)

McLeod (1998) supports the importance of *listening*, in a professional sense, within the context of 'the Narrative Approach'. He identifies the real need of patients to 'tell their story'. Sometimes patients depict their story *as* a hero/heroine with the use of language in terms of 'fights and battles' against diseases and problems but there were some who find it difficult to express their feelings of 'fear and fright' which is described as the lesser of the 'dominant narratives'. McLeod goes on to identify that there is a real therapeutic value in storytelling, which can have a direct influence on health status. The importance of listening and promoting 'listening communication' is therefore vitally important as a therapeutic skill. Therapeutic communication is therefore *deep* in nature as opposed to social communication which is *superficial*.

However, communication difficulties in health care are often at the root of dissatisfaction on the part of patients and families, despite the advances made in research and the introduction of training and development programmes for nurses. Patients often make complaints about poor communication and the lack of information they receive.

Quite often, students and some nurses feel unable to cope with the enquiries about illness and treatment and often use a range of techniques to avoid answering. These include:

- *Evasion* – moving quickly on to another topic of little significance.

- *Diversion* – moving quickly on to another topic of significance.

- *Blocking* – responding by asking another question, stating a point of issue or even abruptly cutting short the conversation which stops the progression of the patient's enquiry.

It might come as quite a shock to hear these negative criticisms about communication in nursing. However research has shown that nurses learn in their training not to become personally involved with patients' problems (Altschul, 1972; Wells, 1980). So we need to be aware of ineffective as well as effective communication between nurse and patient.

Student Activity 7.6

Have you ever been in a position in the community where a patient asked you a question and you truly did not know the answer?

- ◆ Write down how you responded.

- ◆ Discuss your response with your assessor/supervisor.

- ◆ Keep a record in your portfolio.

Non-verbal communication

A patient often senses non-verbal messages from a nurse first. So it is important to look at these in order to aid effective communication.

1. *Warmth* can be conveyed by smiling and by maintaining an 'open' posture, that is, keeping arms and legs uncrossed. Touching the patient appropriately and sensitively may also help.

2. *Appropriate positioning of the body can convey attention to the patient.* Leaning forward, being at the same (or lower) eye level as the patient and maintaining eye contact without staring, shows the patient that you have an interest in what they have to say. Occasional nodding of the head signals to the patient that you understand them and wish them to continue on with their communication.

3. *Unconditional positive regard* involves a positive frame of mind, which demonstrates a total acceptance of and feeling for the patient's unique position which requires an attentive purpose, regardless of one's personal views about them or their illness (see Chapter 6).

Verbal communication

Language: tone, pace. When we talk to patients, it is important that we think about the tone and pace of our expression. When we are rushed, driving from one home to another in bad traffic conditions and with lots of things on our mind, it would be easy to give the impression of being frustrated, angry or even disinterested by the tone of our voice. We also need to take care that we are not speaking too quickly.

Questioning allows nurses to gather information and data for assessment by encouraging a response from a patient. It also allows patients an opportunity to explore their own feelings on an issue. The nurse should therefore use questioning with the aim of giving patients an opportunity to express themselves. There are two types of questions that can be asked:

- 'Closed' questions
- 'Open' questions.

'Closed' questions are necessary sometimes to elicit information quickly mainly for the nurse's benefit. They often usually elicit a 'yes', 'no' or factual information such as a name or an address.

> *Nurse:*   Do you sleep well?
> *Patient:* Yes, usually.

However, it may be necessary for nurses to ask patients to give non-verbal responses if communication difficulties are severe and answers are needed quickly. For example, a patient may be asked to blink once for 'yes' and twice for 'no'. Closed questions have their value when patients may find difficulty breathing or expressing themselves for a number of reasons.

'*Open*' *questions* invite patients to describe their answer in more detail.

> *Staff Nurse:* What kinds of things help you to settle to sleep at night?
>
> *Patient:* Well, I usually like a cup of cocoa about ten o'clock and then I like to have a wash, brush my teeth and settle into bed by reading a chapter of my novel.

There is also a range of professional communication techniques, some of which give patients an opportunity to be able to 'tell their story'.

- *Maintaining silence* is a purposeful activity in order for patients or their relatives to process their own information before expressing it.

- *Reflecting* helps patients to think about expanding on an area of thought. Nurses use reflection to help patients to expand or 'open up', as it avoids the use of direct questions. Too many questions can make the patient feel intimidated. Saying a key word back to a patient invites them to explore their thoughts and feelings. However, they can also choose to 'block' further dialogue.

> *Patient:* I feel so lost without Michael.
> *District nurse:* 'lost?'

Student Activity 7.7

- ◆ Observe a nurse–patient contact in the community and estimate the ratio of open to closed questions. Was there a rationale for the type of questioning?

- ◆ Discuss your observations with your assessor/supervisor.

- ◆ Make notes in your portfolio.

- *Echoing* uses a similar technique but the last few words of the patient's sentence are echoed back to the patient, for example:

> *Patient:* I have had such trouble with the pain in the wrist.
> *Community nurse:* Pain in the wrist?

- *Paraphrasing* is a similar technique in which the nurse uses his or her own words to restate the patient's ideas or feelings. This may be useful to help a patient expand or clarify their thoughts, or indeed it may help to summarise an issue in order to move on to another issue. For example:

> *Patient:*   I sometimes get so angry that I cannot move as quickly as I want and then I can just dissolve into tears at the thought of it all.
>
> *District nurse:* It sounds as if you feel a mixture of frustration and despair?

- *Advising* is communication, which offers the patient some advice relating to health.

> *Patient:*   When do you think I should take these tablets, nurse?
>
> *District Nurse:* Well, the Medicine Formulary recommends that Ibuprofen should be taken after meals to avoid the drug reacting with strong gastric juices and affecting the lining of the stomach. I would suggest taking them about half an hour after breakfast, lunch and dinner. What do you think?

- *Reinforcing* patients' understanding of health-enhancing activities is a useful method of encouraging partnership.

> *Patient:*   Should I try to keep my legs supported under a footstool until my leg is better?
>
> *Nurse:*   Well, yes, that is one of the best things you can do while you are sitting here in your chair watching the television. If you haven't got a footstool, a few cushions may help to raise your legs up to allow the blood to return more easily to your heart.

Student Activity 7.8

- ◆ While out visiting, listen carefully to your community nurses and identify the use of any of the techniques described above.

- ◆ Try, consciously, using any of these techniques with your patients.

- ◆ Make notes of the outcome of the interaction.

Dealing with patients who are dying

This is always challenging for student nurses, but it is also a difficult area for professional community nurses. Tschudin (1988) identified three important needs of patients in this situation:

- Physical symptom control
- Psychological support of the patient
- Psychological support of the family.

Holistic nursing involves addressing all these issues simultaneously. Doyle (1990) highlights the skill of nurses in making sure patients do not feel that their symptoms are trivial. It is important that patients are involved in as many decisions as possible regarding their care, particularly as their control in other areas of their life has been removed from them. Guild (1995) identifies the importance of:

- Effective listening to what is said *and* what is not said
- Use of eye contact and 'open' body language
- Appropriate touch
- Avoidance of false reassurances (see Chapter 14).

Dealing with patients who are aggressive

There is a growing awareness that nurses are facing difficult situations, which are threatening in a personal way. This is a challenge to community nurses in terms of developing appropriate skills and knowledge, and dealing effectively with such situations. Aggression can be seen as a normal human behaviour, which helps individuals express particular difficulties facing them, and which may be caused by intrinsic or extrinsic factors.

Expert skilled observation is very important in order to note specific changes in patients. Violence rarely occurs out of the blue. Some of those changes may be:

- Restlessness
- Inability to sleep
- Preoccupation
- Abruptness
- Reluctance to becoming involved in social interactions
- Uncharacteristic rudeness
- Mood changes.

Vanderslott (1992) suggests the value of counselling patients in aggressive situations. Counselling is *not* about advising, *but* about helping through listening. Appropriate support and reassurance should always be offered to patients who become aggressive.

Inter and intraprofessional communication

Inter and intraprofessional communication involves conveying messages across primary, secondary and tertiary health care areas for the benefit of patient care. Interprofessional and intraprofessional communication occurs within primary health care, the wider community and between staff in the hospital and the community through formal and informal meetings, the use of patient records, telephone systems and communication books. In this context, nurses and other health care professionals hope to work together effectively. Multi-agency working has been the focus of much health policy. The Health Act 1999 highlights the need for collaboration instead of competition, which resulted from the NHS and Community Care Act 1990.

However, the effectiveness of communication in the community has often been seen as problematic. Collaboration between doctors and nurses is still an issue (Allendale, 1999; Reeves and Freeth, 2000). This may be due to the different and separated training of the professions. It could, however, also be linked to society's high expectations of their roles which leave little opportunity for quality time together. Community relationships are probably much better than those in the acute sector because nurses and doctors often have a more settled relationship. Davies (2000) argues that transformational leadership may be the answer, especially when there is a focus on welcoming challenge and working confidently within teams with a respectful and trusting culture. Affirmations, acknowledgements and recognition are important.

Collaboration between nurses in different environments, however, causes communication problems. Saville and Bartholomew (1994) highlight the particular communication problems of planned discharges from hospitals and their impact on district nursing. From their research in two geographical locations in London, they found that almost three-quarters of all district referrals appeared to have caused problems, lack of communication being given as the most important factor. Most of the problems affected the over 75 age group, comprising the most vulnerable patients.

In this age of technology, the most important information may fail to reach the primary health care team (PHCT), which is often only a few miles away from the general hospital. However, advances in technology mean that community nurses have now become more contactable, and this may ultimately lead to greater access to health care (Haggard, 1997). District nurses now carry mobile phones, have access to facsimile machines, computers, answerphones and the Internet. However, now that communication is more complex it is also more burdensome, requiring new skills and management expertise for community nurses. Some patients in the community find change difficult and dislike using new technology that dehumanises the interaction and so limits their access.

Student Activity 7.9

◆ Ask your district nurses what types of communication problems they have with hospital discharges that are referred to their team.

◆ Make a list of the most serious to the least serious.

◆ Record in your portfolio.

There has been much research into how students learn in the community (Ferguson et al., 2000). The value of these settings has been identified for pre-registration students as making allowances to be more involved, with knowledge, skill and expertise being shared through discussion, reflection and narrative. They highlight the value of community experience for student nurses, along with the one-to-one relationships. They identify the role of the nurse within the PHCT as facilitating learning of these essential skills:

● Communication

● Collaboration

● Team working.

All of these are required for practice.

As students in a new setting of 'community nursing', you may find that certain 'community' jargon and language is used that you are unfamiliar with until you have been working there for a while. Chapter 1 highlights some of this language.

What kind of words do you remember hearing that were new to you? You may have heard lots of conversations about 'daily diary sheets' and wondered if they were a certain kind of linen used for diarrhoea if the words were

Student Activity 7.10

◆ Think about some jargon words or abbreviations you have encountered for the first time on your community placement.

◆ Write down what you think these terms mean.

◆ Discuss them with your assessor/supervisor.

spoken quickly, only to find that these were part of the administration paper work. Other jargon such as ECRs, ECGs or TLC, explained below, may also be seen as quite confusing to newcomers.

- *ECRs:* Extra contractual referrals, that is, patients who live outside the local health authority (HA) area but have requirements within another health authority.
- *ECGs:* Electrocardiograms.
- *TLC:* Tender loving care.

Trained professionals need to make sure that students, unqualified staff and importantly patients and their carers do not get confused with the many jargon terms that set up barriers to effective communication. You have a responsibility, however, as a student, to ensure that you check the meanings of terminology, so that you can be aware of the meanings that are being applied at the time of use.

Professional community nurses are responsible for passing on their communication skills and knowledge of the professional discipline to you as students and to new members of staff. For example, practitioners and nurse lecturers work together to support and train student nurses to the competence levels required at registration, and communication is always part of your learning.

Student Activity 7.11

♦ Think about your community experience and jot down some of the important aspects of the way the practice staff have communicated their knowledge and skills to you.

♦ Keep notes in your portfolio.

Record keeping

Records in nursing should be seen as part of any of the levels of professional communication. In reality, they are more often seen and used to enhance interprofessional communication than being used with patients to communicate health enhancing activities. The inclusion of record keeping at this point reflects this but could have been included in any of the sections.

Nursing communication is rooted in oral tradition. This has meant that nursing and health care *knowledge* was not recognised or even regarded as credible in the past, because it lacked permanence. Lumby (1991) has pointed out that this tradition has meant that it has not even been possible to publish nursing and health care practice knowledge books as it was doctors who always published medical and care books. Nursing and midwifery knowledge was seen as having lesser value than medical knowledge, of which it was merely a part. O'Brien and Pearson (1993) suggest that one of the reasons why the real knowledge of nursing practice is seldom documented is precisely because nursing information is central to practice. It is taken for granted and accepted by expert nurses almost 'without thinking'. Such forms of knowledge fall outside what is deemed to be real science. It is interesting to recall that Florence Nightingale (1859) believed writing down one's observations about patients to be a mental crutch that would diminish the nurse's capacity to observe and remember. She permitted it reluctantly but with the focus on patient assessment:

> if you cannot get the habit of observation one way or another, you had better give up being a nurse, for it is not your calling, however kind and anxious you may be. (cited in Eggland and Heinemann, 1994, p. 4)

Written channels have in recent years been required in order to pass information on to different staff as a legal and professional requirement. Eggland and Heinemann (1994, p. 1) define a clinical record as:

> The comprehensive collection of data that describes a patient's condition, health care needs, health care services received and responses to care.

Clinical records, therefore, are used to inform others about the needs and progress of patients, clients and families in respect of their overall health. However they are also used to instruct others of what is expected of them in continuing care. When used with patients, clinical records aim to motivate and help in the learning process. They are also useful learning and motivational aids for students and learners, aiming to keep them focused on 'best practice'.

Student Activity 7.12

- Reflect on a good example of record keeping you have seen in the community.
- Why did you feel it was an example of best practice?
- Think about confusing or badly kept records seen in the community.
- Why were they so poor?
- Write some notes about your observations.

There are various types of patient records that may be seen in the community. The following types may be seen while you are on your placement.

- Handwritten records
- Patient-held records
- Critical pathways
- Computerised care records
- Multi-agency records.

You may not have seen all these examples but look out for them in the future.

Student Activity 7.13

- ◆ Write down a list of the advantages and disadvantages of computerised care records.

- ◆ Ask your assessor/supervisor about other forms of records that you may not have seen in use.

You may have felt that they could be more efficient in saving time for documenting usual and expected aspects of care. They may also be used to remember aspects of practice expected in certain care situations. The use of computerised records can also save space in GP surgeries where storage over many years is a problem.

Some disadvantages of nursing records could be that individuality of care is not reflected in the documentation, or that there is an inability or difficulty in highlighting specific issues for individuals. Doctors sometimes complain that some of their computerised records do not allow them to *document* certain areas that they have checked to be normal when performing a clinical examination. It will only allow them to register a problem. There are also fears that computerised records may be 'lost' if the hardware is stolen or breaks down for a period of time. So in many areas both manual and computerised records are often kept simultaneously.

Record keeping and the law

Record keeping is seen in the context of professional standards of practice and within a legal framework. This is a very important aspect. There are ethical issues concerning:

- Integrity
- Truth

Table 7.2 Retention of records (may be affected by local policies)

Maternity records	25 years
Children	Up to the age of 25 years/10 years after death
Patients under Mental Health Act 1983	20 years/10 years after death
Prisoners and Armed Forces	Not destroyed
Others	10 years

- Respect
- Confidentiality
- Consent, and
- Informed decision making.

The Access to Health Records Act 1990 and the Data Protection Act 1984 give patients and clients specific rights, concerning their records. There are general rules about the length of time clinical records may be kept (Table 7.2).

Value of record keeping

Record keeping is not only used as a form of communication but can be used for the following

- Legal protection
- Reimbursement
- Patient education
- Quality assurance
- Research.

Records and documentation are the primary communication tool that reflects nursing and care philosophies, models, structure, processes and outcomes.

Student Activity 7.14

- ◆ Discuss with your assessor/supervisor the models of nursing, which are reflected in the records used in your community.
- ◆ Is there any way of checking on their effectiveness with individual patients?
- ◆ Make notes on your thoughts in your portfolio.

Table 7.3 Points for inclusion on clinical records

- The collection of data to identify needs
- Problems and concerns
- Reactions and responses to existing or potential health needs
- Goals set and planned interventions
- The review and goal evaluation, which should highlight the effectiveness of the professional input by examining the outcomes or responses

---

It is usual to see a range of conceptual care models within community nursing. Roper et al. (1983), and Orem (1980, 1995) feature predominantly within district nursing. However practice nurses, health visitors, psychiatric nurses and child health nurses will relate to different models, because of the type of work they do and their different perspectives.

Nurses can communicate, in writing, with each other and other agencies through nursing records and through the Lloyd George records (named after the Lloyd George National Insurance Act 1911) which are kept in the GP surgery. Indeed, Baker and colleagues (1997, p. 57) note that:

> the key clinical communication tool in the UK general practice is the patient record and most practices have at least twenty people requiring access to clinical records.

Ideally, clinical records should show a range of issues, as shown in Table 7.3.

How realistically do you think these issues are documented in practice? Which issues are the most important?

Practice nurses may find that they have very little space and time to record all these items for each individual contact they see. However, it would certainly be helpful for patients who are visiting the surgery on a regular basis, so that the service delivered can be monitored.

Student Activity 7.15

◆ Now, have a look at some examples of a district nurse's 'care plan' in practice. This would be kept in the patient's home.

◆ Check to see whether it meets the requirements noted above.

Guidelines on record keeping are useful tools to help us reflect on the skill of record keeping. Sometimes we do not always show *the choices* we offer patients, so it is also useful to note what health care services have been offered even though they may have been refused, through choice.

The UKCC (1998) provides guidelines for professional record keeping. The updated version should clarify issues and stress the importance of professional practice. It sets out the need for all entries to be:

- Factual, consistent and accurate.
- Up-to-date, and informative about the care and condition of the patient or client.
- Written clearly in a manner that the text can not be erased.
- Dated, timed and signed.
- Free from abbreviations, jargon, meaningless phrases, irrelevant speculation and offensive subjective statements.
- Readable on any photocopies.
- Wherever possible, written with the involvement of the patient or client and their carer.

Nursing and health care record keeping has been criticised (Castledine, 1998; Tingle, 1998). The deterioration in record keeping is thought to be due to various factors:

- It is not considered to be a skill that needs to be taught or corrected when poor.
- A considerable number of personnel are giving care and recording it in the nursing records.
- Health care interventions and communication channels are complex.

Improving clinical communications

Tingle drew attention to a report prepared in 1998 by the Clinical Systems Group (CGS) of the Department of Health, on *Improving Clinical Communications*.

The report's findings showed that *few records* are made:

- Of *decisions*
- Of *who is responsible* for carrying out tasks
- Where care is shared there is *rarely a full record* of all events even in GP records
- Specific advice or information is rarely recorded and there is *inaccurate information and widespread duplication.*

Why do you think there are these weaknesses?

Record keeping is considered to be a *formal channel of communication*. It would be too easy to say that there is never enough time for good record keeping but the main problem lies in poor clinical management, poor training and poor monitoring of records. Documentation for care, therefore, needs to be constantly monitored and audited. Standards must be measured so that the skills of professional staff in record writing are improved, thus giving value to the professional care on offer.

Informal communication is considered to be the type of regular communication which is not recorded, and which goes on daily between health care staff. Informal communication involves non-verbal and verbal communication. The 'handover' or case discussion forums may include a mixture of formal and informal communication. The informal channels of communication have an important role to play here in terms of culture, induction of new staff, team building and support, as well as an educational role.

Student Activity 7.16

Observe the allocation process in the DN team and make notes on how the DN sister/charge nurse:

◆ Communicates with the team in order to distribute the workload.

◆ Receives feedback from the team.

◆ Responds to various suggestions or issues raised about patient care.

Lally's (1999) research into nurse communication found that, in the process of 'handover', goals and *values* relating to nursing practice were passed on to the team members. This had the effect of facilitating cohesiveness and a sense of 'belonging' within the team.

Professional research

It is important that nurses try to share their knowledge and 'best' practice with others. One way may be to give a presentation, hold a workshop or contribute to a conference. A wider audience can be reached by publishing your research and ideas. Specific pieces of research or articles that start to stimulate research can be communicated to professional groups through journal articles and books. These are powerful methods of reflecting the amount and quality of activity that goes on in search of truth and theory within the professional groups.

There is a wide range of journals, each with a particular market. Some journals contain little more than a range of opinions but keep people in touch. At the other end of the continuum, others have research articles that must pass several review panels before being accepted.

Student Activity 7.17

Review and make notes on the following:

♦ The type of research /evidence for practice that is kept at your base.

♦ The use of this research by qualified nurses.

♦ Keep a record in your portfolio, for possible use when writing assignments or care studies.

Presentations

In health care, presentations are used frequently as a means of cascading information verbally to a number of people. The advantage may be that this gets information quickly to a large number of people. It may be used as a forum for changing attitudes and values more easily. It may also be seen as more participative management of information sharing, depending on the involvement of those attending. Preparing a presentation on a topic is a good way of reinforcing your own learning. Many of you will recognise the amount of knowledge you acquire when you have to present in a classroom.

The disadvantage is that making a presentation involves public speaking skills, and many staff feel they lack confidence or skills in this area. It also involves releasing staff from their normal day-to-day role and is time consuming and therefore expensive.

Administrative communication

Other types of communication are required in community nursing. These may involve top down (management) information or bottom up information. Such flows of information are part of the organisational requirements that enable the trust or practice to operate.

Policies and procedures

Policies are written forms of internal communication to show employees *how* the organisation will achieve its objectives. A policy document is a way of representing 'the way things are done here.' Policies provide the broad framework for decision making in an organisation as well as clarifying roles and responsibilities.

Mullins (1993, p. 281) describes policy as, 'a guideline for organizational action and the implementation of goals and objectives'. However, some policies are directly influenced by government legislation. The ones that first spring to mind may well be the *equal opportunity* policies and the *health and safety* policies. These are policies which are meant to protect all staff in terms of their human, physical and employment rights. Ultimately such policies should have a positive effect on patient care.

On the other hand, policies could be seen as a way of *controlling* staff (Huczynski and Buchanon, 1991, p. 587), by illustrating acceptable behaviour within the organisation.

Procedures are now even more specific, with written communication about how certain tasks will be carried out. You may have seen procedures about what to do in case of a fire. After reading them, you should then have the knowledge about your responsibility in terms of alerting the fire brigade, making patients safe and evacuating buildings.

Student Activity 7.18

- ◆ Find some of the Trust's policies and procedures that are kept at your base.
- ◆ Identify which policies are directly linked to national government policy.
- ◆ Jot down how they affect direct patient care.

Administrative computer work

You will no doubt notice that community nurses are involved in completing daily diary sheets, which give the following information to their managers:

- The patient's name, details and identification number
- Objective for contact
- Care or treatment given
- Time taken

- Possible outcome
- Date of next contact.

This information is then keyed into a computer programme either by the nurses themselves or by clerical staff. This is a large part of the expectation of the role in community nursing. The information forms part of the financial planning required by Trusts in order to identify trends of health needs and the use of resources in meeting those needs. There have been various systems that have been taken on to monitor the large amount of data. The Financial Information Planning (FIP) system was one of the first used when information was required. Community Information Systems (CIS) is another information system that might be used in your community, but systems are changing regularly.

Community nurses are expected to be involved in Patient's Charter monitoring, caseload analysis and audit. This information is required for the purposes of reviewing performance and activity. You should become aware of these activities while on your placement, and use the opportunity to talk with the DN team about the value of this information.

Political communication

In political communication, power and influence play a major part in the communication process, and the health of the community or population underpins practice. It involves inter-agency working and the build up of communication channels between a variety of agencies, based on the principle that health is multi-faceted. Nursing as a discipline becomes visible, often when medical involvement is weak. The skills and knowledge of nurses can be used to highlight the health expertise of a group of professions as lobbyists or advocates for the rights and needs of a variety of subgroups, such as those in poverty, ethnic minorities, the homeless, the lone elderly, the mentally and learning ability challenged. Community nurses will be involved with inter-agency working through formal and informal routes, to support patients and clients in gaining extra resources and benefits for their specific needs.

Case conferences

These are meetings which require a range of individuals from the many agencies involved in a single patient case to meet together to offer their opinions of the patient and family with complex needs. Case conferences may occur in the patient's own home setting, in hospital prior to discharge or, occasionally, at another venue. They are an important part of good collaboration, and you should take the opportunity, if you are able to, to attend a conference so that you can observe the process in action.

Student Activity 7.19

Negotiate with your assessor to attend a case conference if possible during your placement.
Make notes of the following:

♦ Which professionals attended.

♦ Their power and influence in contributing to the conference.

♦ Was the patient, and their carer(s), given a 'voice'?

♦ The outcome of the conference.

Reports

Reports are more commonly required in nursing, midwifery and health visiting than in medicine, for example. A report is a document that may:

● State facts

● Analyse issues

● Give professional opinions

● Report progress

● Draw conclusions

● Make proposals.

They are commonly used instead of conference attendance. They may also be written to inform or even persuade others as well as to initiate a change. A report may be part of a bid for more resources in a ward or within a team, or it may be needed to evaluate a new service.

Reports are often requested to provide part of a multi-agency picture of a patient or client from a health perspective. It is usual for a senior member of the team to produce the report but they may gather information from any member of a nursing or primary health care team.

Writing reports about patients has implications for patient confidentiality, and therefore needs to be done with patient collaboration. It is necessary to get patients and their relatives to agree what you have written before a report is sent off to a third party.

Letters

Letters are used in a wide variety of uses in health care. There are various reasons for letter writing:

- Letters of referral
- Letters for influencing decisions
- Letters to influence quicker action taking.

In terms of formality, it is useful to keep copies of letters sent as well as those received to reflect the total correspondence. Nurses, midwives and health visitors are an influential professional grouping, and their letters make an impact on decisions that are based on health grounds.

Barriers to effective communication

Student Activity 7.20

♦ During your experience in the community, think about the real barriers to effective communication.

♦ Make notes of these ideas and discuss them with your assessor, identifying which of these are the most important.

The communication problems that occur within the community are an ongoing issue. During your placement you may make your own minds up about the reasons for this. However, communication is a complex professional skill which depends on the various people involved in the interactions. The main barriers to effective communication relate to:

- Skills
- Attitudes
- Experience
- Knowledge
- Values
- Social and cultural factors.

We must try to recognise these barriers within ourselves but also help others to become aware of them for the overall benefit of patient care.

Conclusion

The ability to communicate effectively is an essential component of nursing practice and the delivery of total health care. It is a complex process that involves the transmission of *mutually understood meanings and symbols* among individuals. In the community, communication establishes the nurse–patient relationship and is a means to effect change. Multi-agency communication is also vital and requires constant collaborative attempts.

Community nurses engage in communication at a variety of levels during their daily work. Nurses need to exercise their communication skills, using all available channels, if they are to benefit patient care in all its diversity. Effectiveness involves clear, concise, organised messages that are acceptable and familiar to recipients of those messages. Finally, allowing the patient or client to 'tell their story' should be of paramount importance to any community nurse.

Further reading

Ellis, R., Gates, R. and Kenworthy, N. (1995) *Interpersonal Communication in Nursing*. London, Churchill Livingstone.

Kagan, C. and Evans, J. (1995) *Professional Interpersonal Skills for Nurses*. London, Chapman & Hall.

Morrison, P. and Burnard, P. (1997) *Caring and Communicating: The Interpersonal Relationship in Nursing*, 2nd edn. Basingstoke, Macmillan – now Palgrave.

Robinson, L. (1998) *'Race', Communication and the Caring Professions*. Buckingham, Open University Press. Especially Chapter 7: Facilitation and the development of rapport; and Chapter 15: Constraints on using effective interpersonal skills.

References

Allendale, E. (1999) Interprofessional working: an ethnographic case study of emergency health care. *Journal of Interprofessional Care*, **13**: 139–50.

Altshul, A.T. (1972) *Patient–Nurse Interaction – A Study of Interaction Patterns in Acute Psychiatric Wards*. Edinburgh, Churchill Livingstone.

Argyle, M. (1983) *The Psychology of Interpersonal Behaviour*, 4th edn. Harmondsworth, Penguin.

Baker, M., Maskrey, N. and Kirk, S. (1997) *Clinical Effectiveness and Primary Care*. Oxford, Radcliffe Medical Press.

Benner, P. (1984) *From Novice to Expert: Excellence and Power in Clinical Nursing Practice*. Menlo Park, Addison-Wesley.

Binnie, A. (2000) Freedom to practise: the doctor–nurse relationship. *Nursing Times*, **96**(9): 44–6.

Castledine, G. (1994) The standard of nursing records should be raised. *British Journal of Nursing*, 7(3): 172.

Castledine, G. (1998) The blunders found in nursing documentation. *British Journal of Nursing*, 7(19): 1218.

Chomsky, N. (1957) *Syntatic Structures*. The Hague, Mouton.

Clinical Systems Group (1998) *Improving Clinical Communications.* Wetherby, Two Ten Communications.

Crawford, P., Brown, B. and Nolan, P. (1998) *Communicating Care: The Language of Nursing.* Cheltenham, Stanley Thornes.

Davies, C. (2000) 'Vive la difference'. That's what will make collaboration work. *Nursing Times,* **96**(15): 27.

Department of Health (1990) *The NHS and Community Care Act.* London, HMSO.

Department of Health (1997) *The New NHS: Modern, Dependable.* London, HMSO.

Department of Health (1999) *Making a Difference, the Contribution of Nursing, Midwifery and Health Visiting.* London, The Stationery Office.

Doyle, D. (1990) *Symptom Control in Terminal Care.* North Berwick, Tantallon Press.

Edwards, H. and Noller, P. (1993) Perceptions of overaccommodation used by nurses in communication with the elderly. *Journal of Language and Social Psychology,* **12**(3): 207–23.

Eggland, E. and Heinemann, D. (1994) *Nursing Documentation: Charting, Recording and Reporting.* Philadelphia, JB Lippincott.

Ferguson, C., Whyte, D. and Anderson, C. (2000) Learning in the home care setting. *Journal of Community Nursing,* **14**(2): 13–19.

Guild, R. (1995) Effective communication. *Journal of Community Nursing,* **9**(7): 10–14.

Haggard, L. (1997) Commissioning services to meet identified needs. In Hennessy, D. (ed.) *Community Health Development.* Basingstoke, Macmillan – now Palgrave, pp. 62–85.

Haynes, W. and Shilman, B. (1998) *Communication Development: Foundations, Processes and Clinical Applications.* Philadelphia, Williams and Wilkins.

Hinchliffe, S. (1979) *Teaching Clinical Nursing.* London, Churchill Livingstone.

Huczynski, A. and Buchanon, D. (1991) *Organizational Behaviour,* 2nd edn. Hertfordshire, Prentice Hall.

Lally, S. (1999) An investigation into the functions of nurses' communication at the intershift handover. *Journal of Nursing Management,* 7: 29–36.

Lovell, B. (1982) *Adult Learning.* London, Croom Helm.

Lumby, J. (1991) Threads of an emerging discipline. In Gray, G. and Pratt, R. (eds) *Towards a Discipline of Nursing.* Melbourne, Churchill Livingstone, pp. 461–83.

McLeod, J. (1998) Listening to stories about illness and health: applying the lessons of narrative psychology. In Bayne, R., Nicolson, P. and Horton, I. (eds) *Counselling and Communication Skills for Medical and Health Practitioners.* Leicester, The British Psychological Society.

Milburn, M., Baker, M.J., Garner, P., Hornsby, R. and Rogers, L. (1995) Nursing care that patients value. *British Journal of Nursing,* **4**(18): 1094–8.

Mullins, L. (1993) *Management and Organizational Behaviour,* 3rd edn. London, Pitman Publishing.

Nightingale, F. (1859) *Notes on Nursing.* London, Duckworth.

O'Brien, B. and Pearson, A. (1993) Unwritten knowledge in nursing: consider the spoken as well as the written word. *Scholarly Inquiry for Nursing Practice,* **7**(2): 111–24.

Open Tech/Manpower Services Commission (1992) *Interpersonel Skills, Open Learning for Nurses.* Continuing Nurse Education Programme, Barnet College, London.

Orem, D.E. (1980 *Nursing Concepts for Practice,* 2nd edn. New York, McGraw-Hill.

Orem, D.E. (1995) *Nursing Concepts for Practice,* 5th edn. St Louis, Mosby.

Peplau, H.E. (1987) Nursing science; a historical perspective. In Parse, R.R. (ed.) *Nursing Paradigms, Theories and Critiques*. Philadelphia, WB Saunders, pp. 13–29.

Piaget, J. (1955) *The Language and Thought of a Child*. New York, Meridan Books.

Postman, N. (1983) *The Disappearance of Childhood*. London, W. H. Allen.

Reeves, S. and Freeth, D. (2000) Learning to collaborate, *Nursing Times*, **96**(15): 40–1.

Roper, N., Logan, W.W. and Tierney, A. (1983) *The Elements of Nursing*, 2nd edn. Edinburgh, Churchill Livingstone.

Rumelhart, D. (1980) Schemata: the building blocks of cognition. In Haynes, W. and Shilman, B. (eds) *Communication Development*. Philadelphia, Williams and Wilkins, p. 110.

Saville, R. and Bartholomew, J. (1994) Planning better discharges. *Journal of Community Nursing*, **8**(3): 10–14.

Skinner, B.F. (1957) *Verbal Behavior*. New York, Appleton Century Crofts.

Stockwell, F. (1972) *The Unpopular Patient*. London, Royal College of Nursing.

Tingle, J. (1998) Nurses must improve their record keeping skills. *British Journal of Nursing*, **7**(5): 245.

Townsend, P. and Davidson, N. (1990) *Inequalities in Health*. London, Penguin.

Tschudin, V. (1988) *The Patient with Cancer*. London, Prentice Hall.

United Kingdom Central Council for Nursing, Midwifery and Health Visiting (1992) *Code of Professional Conduct*. London, UKCC.

United Kingdom Central Council for Nursing, Midwifery and Health Visiting (1998) *Guidelines for Records and Record Keeping*. London, UKCC.

United Kingdom Central Council for Nursing, Midwifery and Health Visiting (1999) *Fitness for Practice*. London, UKCC.

Vanderslott, J. (1992) A supportive therapy that undermines violence. *Professional Nurse*, April: 427–30.

Wells, T. (1980) *Problems in Geriatric Nursing*. Edinburgh, Churchill Livingstone.

8 Assessing the needs of individuals and communities

NAOMI A. WATSON

> **Learning outcomes**
>
> By the end of this chapter you will be able to:
>
> ■ Define needs assessment and care planning within the context of the relevant legislation.
>
> ■ Explain the concept of needs, and assessment processes within theoretical frameworks.
>
> ■ Consider the major factors influencing community and individual needs.
>
> ■ Discuss the role of the community nurse (adult branch) in the recognition, and assessment of needs, and in ensuring appropriate care planning and delivery.

Introduction

Needs assessment processes in the community are an important part of the role of community nurses. The recognition of individual and community needs, and the ability to prioritise for effective health outcomes, now form key features of care delivery practices for all community nurses, including district nurses (DNs) (DoH, 1991a). The ever problematic issue of resource allocation and the requirement that available resources are used not only effectively, but efficiently and economically, places on DNs the responsibility of ensuring that a clear understanding of local and national initiatives underpins their approach to assessing, planning and delivering care to individuals and to the community (Gilman et al., 1994). As a student in the community, you will very soon become aware of the different meanings, which may apply to the use of some terms. This is a problem applicable to some commonly used terminology within nursing and health care practices. 'Needs' is one such term. Individual clients in a community may have views about their needs, which may be similar to, or different from professional perspectives. The same could apply to national and local community initiatives, as there may not necessarily be agreement by all concerned about the priorities, and how the available resources should be allocated. When this is combined with the requirement for community personnel to work collaboratively at all times, in order to provide optimal benefits for patients and clients, the possibilities for tension within the relationships become more marked.

This chapter will explore the concept of needs assessment and care planning by considering the frameworks from the individual and professional perspectives. It will discuss possible ways in which effective collaboration may ensure that outcomes for individual patients and clients will reflect both national and local priorities, with benefits for all. It aims to provide an overall

Student Activity 8.1

- ◆ As you reflect on what you have read so far, make a list of what you think the general needs of the public may be.

- ◆ Place these needs in order of priority.

- ◆ Make a list of the reasons why you have prioritised these needs in the way you have done.

- ◆ Compare your list with those of some of your peers.

- ◆ Is there anything on your list which could be classed as a 'want' rather than a need?

- ◆ Discuss what you think the differences may be.

- ◆ Make notes in your journal/portfolio.

understanding of the background and concepts of the processes involved, so that these can be applied to the nursing care of adult patients. This should facilitate awareness of community and individual needs within the context of limited resource availability and national and local priorities.

Service provision: underpinning requirements

The main purpose of assessing needs is to ensure that the service to be provided will be relevant and appropriate, the ultimate goal being to ensure positive health outcomes for patients and their communities. Some would argue that health gain should be recognised as the greatest need of individuals and communities, as this focus would help to remind clinical practitioners that simply delivering health care is no longer an option. All formal caregivers must now consider the wider implications of limited resources set against increasing demands in a climate of rapid changes in policy processes (Trent Health, 1993).

Vetter (1997) states that in order for service provision to be appropriate, it should be:

- Accessible
- Relevant to the whole community
- Individually effective
- Equitable
- Socially acceptable
- Efficient and effective.

In order to be able to apply the above criteria, community nurses must be able to recognise not only the theoretical basis of the discussion, but the political impact of diminishing resources, set against the ever increasing cost of health care with equally increasing demand and expectations from individuals within the community. Whether or not the issue of demand for health care exceeding the supply is a reasonable and valid argument for rationing services, this could still be an issue which community nurses may have to grapple with. What is certain is that limited resources demand new ways of working, which should place all community nurses in a key position, not only as possible advocates for their clients, but as important contributors to innovation and effective caseload management (Armitage, 1997).

From an epidemiological perspective, the health needs debate includes not only the incidence and prevalence of disease, but the cost effectiveness of care delivery and health service availability. This is considered by some to be biased towards a medical model of assessment and delivery (Blackie and Appleby, 1998). Others would argue that there have been competing perspectives between the purchaser, the provider and the consumer. Purchasers have been concerned with the commissioning issues of the internal market, prior to it being abolished. Top of the provider's agenda are issues about whether the service is being prioritised or rationed, and how this may differ. Meanwhile the key issues, as Vetter (1997) sees them, for consumers relate to equity and accessibility.

Understanding theoretical frameworks

It is possible to conceptualise the theory of health needs into the following perspectives:

- Individual
- Community
- Professional
- Political.

From an individual perspective, humanist theories of needs have provided a basis for community nurses to understand how patients may respond or perceive those issues which directly affect them. Maslow (1943) identified a hierarchy of needs, which recognised basic physiological needs as having priority over higher order needs, and gives the individual few choices in terms of how these needs are met. While the hierarchy is an appropriate tool for considering individual needs, this must be set against the ability of the individual to exercise personal choice, regardless of risk. The possibility of conflict in the relationship is therefore an important issue, which should be considered and managed effectively.

Bradshaw (1972) also identified a 'taxonomy of needs' which recognises differences in perceptions, applicable individually in the community, professionally, and politically. The fact that felt needs (as perceived by an individual) may not necessarily reflect expressed need (the demand for a service), also illustrates the powerful choice factor, which individual patients and clients can use, and which must be handled with a high level of awareness by community nurses. Normative needs, as perceived by any professional in the multidisciplinary team, may or may not have any bearing on felt or expressed need. Comparative need, which underpins access and equity, has to be clearly understood if the community nurse is to be effective at ensuring that the political/professional/community and individual interfaces are able to fit appropriately for maximum effect. Within the individual aspect, there is also the perception of the carer, which the DN must also consider in order to show recognition of the legislative requirements in ensuring that both patients and carers are able to benefit from appropriate positive health outcomes (DoH, 1995; Nocon, 1996). Within this professional perspective, one has to ask whether the commissioning process, which formed the basis of the purchaser/provider debate, was legitimately and fairly able to identify and meet needs either on an individual or a community focused basis. The argument for prioritising for care delivery could be that demand inevitably exceeds supply, with rationing of health care being considered an acceptable way of limiting access. This is not without its controversies, however, as the waiting lists for the acute sector have shown (Vetter, 1997). Vetter also argues that demands for health care do not necessarily equate with actual need, which is why more articulate and persistent patients are able to have their unnecessary demands met. This is set against the backdrop of patients who have been thrown off general practitioners' (GPs) lists because of 'expensive' needs. The abolishing of this internal market by the Labour government has been seen by some as the first step in resolving these issues. However, the role of the community nurse in the new structures, the primary care groups and trusts (PCGs/PCTs) may have to be seen as it evolves. It will be interesting to observe how the role of the DN will develop within the PCT, and whether opinions about priorities for the needs of individuals and communities will be synchronised. Active participation in the decision making process for resource allocation is now a real possibility for DNs. It is likely, however, that their level of participation will depend on a combination of factors, among which will be their ability to demonstrate with credibility, by the application of evidence based practice, the extent of their understanding about the importance of the individual, and the community as client. As you participate with your assessor and members of the DN team in assessment processes in the community, you should be able to recognise, in practice, the interrelationships which should be evident from the particular approach to the patient's needs assessment process. For example, are there any tensions between the individual and professionals' perception of what their needs are? If so, how are these managed? What are the similarities

Student Activity 8.2

Once you have started your community placement, in order to get an early overview of the needs assessment process, you need to get a feel of the neighbourhood in which you are working.
Negotiate an afternoon with your assessor to do the following:

♦ Visit local shops, on foot preferably. Try using local cafés, go to the library and visit the leisure centre and post office. Make sure it is safe to wander around.

♦ Observe carefully the people you meet as you wander around.

♦ Who are they? Older people, or young mothers? Younger people on the streets?

♦ What is access like to the places you have visited? Did you see any disabled persons using local facilities?

♦ What are people like in the area? Are they friendly? Find out by asking for some directions, if possible. Or talk to people to find out how they feel about living in that community, in terms of the benefits and disadvantages.

♦ Write down your observations and discuss them with a) your assessor, and b) your peers in other placements, to compare and contrast the information.

♦ Keep notes of your discussions in your diary or portfolio.

and/or differences between individual, community, professional and political concepts of needs, and what are the underpinning factors that make for a productive working relationship between them?

An understanding of the community response to the perception of health needs can be enriched by looking at self-help action groups. These provide clear evidence of the ability of the community to organise itself, with or without the help of health care professionals, in order both to generate funding, and to lobby the political and professional sectors as necessary, if they feel that the focus of resource allocation is inappropriate, uneven or unfair. The importance of the voluntary sector is now well recognised. It has a key role to play in the collaborative processes which are essential to effective care delivery (Billis and Harris, 1995) However, even with a well established sector, new groups are continually emerging, and are contributing in tangible ways to the debate on the best ways to use diminishing resources. The extent to which community nurses recognise their role in supporting such groups may be a contributing factor to the way their services are perceived in the community.

Robinson and Elkan (1996) agree that understanding the theoretical base is an important determinant of successful caseload management for effective and innovative care planning and delivery.

Student Activity 8.3

◆ Is it possible to plan for, and deliver, care based on individual perceptions of need in the community?

◆ How can individual needs be appropriately considered in the light of diminishing resources?

◆ Discuss your ideas with one or more of your peers.

◆ Make notes on your discussion in your journal/portfolio.

Searching for health needs may not have always been recognised as an important indicator for the nursing care of sick adults, the process having had a longer history in health visiting (Luker, 1987). However, the urgency of this factor in the light of diminishing resource and changing focus of care, is now an important issue for district nurses.

The political perspective and process have always been major contributors and possibly triggers to the 'needs' debate in health care. Indeed, they could be seen also as a major contributor to the persistent medical model (DoH, 1991a). For example, *The Health of the Nation* (DoH, 1991b) identified diseases and conditions for which targets were set. The extent to which the promotion of health is considered within the medical model may be marginal, but the move to focus on health gain as the major need may help to shift the balance to a model which takes a more holistic view.

Factors influencing individual and community health needs

As shown in Table 8.1, the health both of individuals and of communities may be affected by many different factors. This is particularly relevant to DNs, concerned as they are about the health status and health care of sick adults in the community (Turton and Orr, 1993; Blackie and Appleby, 1998).

Community nurses are usually well aware of the impact of an unhealthy environment on health outcomes for individuals and communities. Whether it is in the workplace, the environment generally or in the type of housing, the impact on health status can be quite profound. The problems of multiple

Table 8.1 Factors influencing health status of individuals and communities

Housing	Race/ethnicity – access issues
The environment – pollution, workplace issues	Gender issues, male and female
Deprivation (poverty), socioeconomic status	Unemployment
Leisure facilities	Resource allocation

deprivation as a consequence of interrelated factors may occur where there is poor or inadequate housing, unpleasant polluted environments, limited facilities for leisure or education, and poor job prospects. Within the workplace, the high levels of workplace stress due to factors such as bullying and harassment, is now an emerging issue (Wilkinson, 1997). The impact of poverty is also widely discussed (see Chapter 5), and the need to recognise the links to poor health outcomes is essential. The lack of availability of affordable leisure facilities and parks, especially in dense urban areas could be key contributors to high levels of accidents, for example (Turton and Orr, 1993). As far back as 1980, the Black Report identified that limited access to services for minority ethnic patients had a negative effect on health outcomes. The same is true of the failure to take into consideration those factors, which may be of particular relevance to the health of minority communities. For example, sickle cell disease, Thalassaemia, hypertension and diabetes for Asian and African Caribbean communities (Cruikshank and Beavers, 1989). The health of men and women may be directly influenced by a number of factors producing negative health outcomes. The present emphasis on the health of men, especially regarding prostate cancer in older men, and testicular cancer in younger men, is emerging as one of great importance, given the view that men do not appear to access health services unless they are forced to do so by their women folk, usually when a crisis has occurred. Although women have been considered always to have access to health care by virtue of their role as carers, the level of isolation experienced by certain groups of women may have adverse effects on mental health. High levels of unemployment and/or expectations have been said to be the key indicators for the present increase in the suicide rates of young men.

The resource allocation issue has a long-standing controversy. Whitehead (1987) found that more resources tended to be concentrated in the south rather than the north ('the north/south divide'). This discussion still takes place today, with controversies about the uneven allocation of lottery funds. It is easy to recognise the effects such issues could have on individuals and communities.

The government initiative on 'healthy cities' recognises the impact of such factors on health outcomes, and frameworks have now been set up to ensure that the issues are addressed. The establishment of primary care groups (PCGs) was seen as a major landmark in the development of community health care. Following on from this has been the establishment of health action zones (HAZs) to deal with the problem of deprivation and its devastating effects on health. Perhaps the main emphasis is the involvement of local providers of health care, together with the business community, to ensure that a comprehensive effort is used to tackle the existing problems. Such schemes have only recently been introduced, and have yet to be evaluated for effectiveness.

The establishment of primary care trusts (PCTs) in the community moves these processes further towards providing a service that is as comprehensive as possible, originating at the start of a patient's encounter with formal health care systems. The structures are aimed at ensuring appropriate co-ordination at all levels, with primary care finally receiving the kind of emphasis that has always been reserved for the acute sector (see Chapter 15).

As you work in the community, you will no doubt be exposed to information which will help you to form your own opinions about how well the initiatives appear to be shaping up. It is possible to determine the extent to which they are working for the benefit of patients and their communities. Applying the processes to individual patient experiences can be compared and contrasted with the experiences of other patients in the same community, or in neighbouring areas. Your peers and assessor will also provide help with information that will help you to have an informed opinion.

Student Activity 8.4

♦ Ask your assessor to arrange for you to spend some time in another placement.

♦ If you are able to negotiate for more than a day, spend some time, not just with a DN team, but with another member of the PHCT, such as the health visitor.

♦ Find out what their views are about that particular community, and its health needs.

♦ Identify what they have said in common, and what the differences are.

♦ Discuss these with your peers who are normally in the placement you are visiting.

♦ Make notes on your discussion in your journal/portfolio.

Determining health needs

Decisions about health needs may be made by a variety of individuals who may be formal or informal carers. The patient, his or her carer, relative, friend, teacher, community worker, or any member of the primary health care team (PHCT) may each have their own personal ideas about the priorities of someone in their care who is sick, or about the situation in a particular community. Sometimes, this makes for conflicting situations, which may not be in the best interests of the patient (Armitage, 1997). A particular problem area is cross-communication dilemmas, and professionals may need to make themselves responsible for preventing these. In spite of the potential problems, it is still important that those who are closest to the patient, and directly involved in providing health care, should be able to contribute to the assessment and care planning processes. The Carers (Recognition and Services) Act 1995 ensures that the voice of carers is explicit within the process, with the entitlement to an individual assessment as a carer, subject to set criteria. DNs, by virtue of their traditional roles, may be more in tune with the needs of individuals and their carers. In understanding the community as a client, a wider construct becomes necessary, as the role and function of public health concepts become more functional. Blackie and Appleby (1998) state that this involves a mixture of knowledge and skills, which combine nursing and public health to provide breadth and depth for practising effectively within the context of primary care. Determining health needs becomes an activity which is informed by the influences of the individual, the community, and those public health issues, as identified from the relevant local searches. Public health is understood, from Blackie and Appleby's (1998) perspective to indicate that the needs of the wider community are considered for the greater good of all, in that community. The available data provides information on individuals, families, and the wider community, essentially meaning that the approach provides a holistic view which could serve to empower local communities to take action on local health issues. Traditionally, this is not a role that DNs have assumed, but new community nurses, regardless of specialism, must now use this approach to inform their practice.

Student Activity 8.5

♦ During your time with your assessor, find out from him or her the extent to which the needs of the wider community are used to inform the assessment process of individuals.

♦ Discuss the same point with a DN from another team in the same placement, and look for similarities and differences.

♦ Identify what you think possible public health issues may be for differing groups of clients on your assessor's caseload.

♦ Check with your assessor to see if there is agreement.

♦ Make notes in your journal/portfolio.

The Health of the Nation (DoH, 1991b) and, more recently, *Our Healthier Nation* (DoH, 1998) use information from the public health domain to look at trends and set targets for improvements. But it should be remembered that the information used is based on normative and comparative needs, while disregarding felt and expressed needs, effectively silencing individuals and communities. Geographical areas are also used, which are usually different from practice population areas (Blackie and Appleby, 1998). The other important issue to be aware of here is that this approach encourages a medical model of identifying and planning for health needs, thus limiting the possibilities of using a holistic approach. This sometimes tends to present a confusing picture of the true status of a community. The need to become organised through the establishment of pressure groups can perhaps be put into perspective. Note the extensive numbers of voluntary groups in the community, some large and well established, some very small, all working to draw attention to the local situation with a view to attracting more funds from a variety of sources, usually beginning with individual beneficiaries.

Joint assessments, the health/social care interface

As far back as 1980, the Black Report identified the possible influences of social factors on health. More recently, Sir Donald Acheson (1998) has confirmed that this is a perpetual problem, which still needs to be addressed by all professionals. The impact of poverty has been covered in this text (Chapter 5). Joint assessments, as identified by the legislation (NHS and CCA, 1990) were meant to recognise the need for a combined approach, which would recognise the interface. This would ensure that DNs and social care professionals work together where appropriate, undertaking joint assessments on a needs led rather than a service led basis, for the benefit of the patient. The aim was to ensure that a flexible approach was used to maintain patients' independence as far as is possible. Social services are able to offer such support as home help services, transport for day care attendance, meals on wheels services, and respite care to enable carers to have a break. You should find out from your assessor the criteria which are used to determine the need for a joint assessment, and, where possible, try to be in attendance at one of these.

Care planning and care delivery frameworks

The assessment process is the start of what should be a systematic approach to dealing with the needs of the patient. Planning the care is done on the basis of a conceptual framework, which should be determined from the assessment. The care plan should have a clear statement of how the needs of the patient will be met, following full discussions and agreement with the patient, the carer, and any other relevant member of the PHCT. There is a possibility that most DN teams will be using one or more frameworks, based on the types of patients they usually have on their caseload. As a student, you should be able to assess the suitability of the framework in use, to determine if this is the most appropriate. The Roper, Logan and Tierney model (1983), with its Activities of Daily Living is widely used, as is the Orem (1980) model, which concentrates on self-care issues. It is possible however to identify other frameworks which may be appropriate, and it is useful to try and apply one or more of other conceptual frameworks, or to use an eclectic approach in the application of a framework (Fraser, 1996).

If you have the opportunity to follow a patient through a study in your placement, you may wish to consider drawing up your own framework for planning and delivering care. It is important to ensure that the use of a model of care is directly applicable to the patient's personal circumstances, rather than because it is the one used by all practitioners in the team. However, where the types of patients on a caseload are similar, one can understand the decision of DN teams to focus on the use of one or two models only. The model should include a regular review and evaluation process and outcomes of care, integral to the plan, and the dates for this should be stated. In most districts, a Community Charter has been drawn up which, along with the Patient's Charter (DoH, 1993), provides the patient and community with specific plans for particular outcomes. These may be used as a measure of the type of care being delivered. A copy of the care plan is also held by the patient, who has access to its contents. It may be worthwhile to agree the contents with the patient, and explain these. This will ensure that there is transparency, enabling both patient and carer to feel that they are fully included in the process.

Student Activity 8.6

♦ Identify the conceptual frameworks which are in use at your placement.

♦ Ask your assessor how the decision is made over which framework is used to plan and deliver health care.

♦ Do you think the frameworks in use are the most effective? Say why or why not.

♦ Look carefully at one or more care plans of patients on your DN's caseload.

♦ Have they used a holistic approach to the patient's assessment and care planning? Identify how this is observed.

♦ Compare the frameworks in use in your placement, with one or more of your peers from another placement.

♦ Check the web site of another health district and see if there is any information about conceptual frameworks in practice.

♦ Keep notes in your journal/portfolio.

The role of screening in the assessment process

DNs use a number of screening tools, either on an individual basis or to screen groups within a community. Tissue viability is the subject of regular screening for older people who may be vulnerable to skin deterioration. The use of the Waterlow score is widely encountered by students. The same is true of the Doppler test for identifying leg ulcers. Make sure that you are aware of the way these screening tests are applied, and how they are used to plan for effective care.

From a community perspective, the use of indicators to assess the community's social deprivation scale helps to ensure that the wider issues of deprivation are understood and are used to inform the way care is assessed, planned and delivered. The Jarman index is used to identify the population status, and includes the following variables: single parent households, children under five years old, older people living alone, unemployed people, mobility of the population, overcrowded housing, unskilled people, and minority ethnic peoples. The Townsend score looks at variables based on mortality and morbidity rates, considering percentage of unemployed people, percentage of households without a car, percentage of households living in overcrowded conditions, percentage of households not owner occupied. The ACORN classification looks at socioeconomic status and health within the general practice population. This is a classification of residential neighbourhoods and uses census data, which gives sociodemographic information, for units of 300 in the population. Local public health departments and departments of general practice usually have this information (Blackie and Appleby, 1998).

Student Activity 8.7

♦ Find out from your DN assessor, or a member of the team, about the types of screening tools that are used in your place-ment, and how they are administered.

♦ How is this incorporated into plans for the care of patients?

♦ Compare the information with one or more of your peers in a different type of placement.

♦ Make notes on your findings in your journal/portfolio.

Health promotion in care delivery practice

The role of health promotion in the care of sick adults was emphasised as a major requirement of the legislation, yet it has not always been clear whether DNs see this as part of their remit for meeting the needs of sick patients in their care. Perhaps the reason for this has been in the way traditional health promotion concepts in the community have developed over the years, with the health visitor and school nurse being seen as the professionals directly linked to promoting the health of individuals and communities. By virtue of the systematic process of assessing the needs of individuals and their commu-nities, the DN's role as a health promoter becomes clearly recognisable. Pike and Forster (1994) state that, in considering the concepts of health promotion, the 'health story' includes the following aspects: cure, care and quality of life, people's own views about their health, preventive measures and education. DNs should be, and usually are, involved in all of these processes with individuals and groups of patients in their care. For example, a group of patients who regularly attend a clinic for diabetes, leg ulcers or other clinical problem, will give the DN an opportunity to actively engage in each of the aspects described above. Whether it is related to dietary and other lifestyle factors, or teaching particular skills such as appropriate self-administration of insulin, the importance of the DN's health promoting role is obvious. Of course, all formal caregivers should recognise this as an important feature of the care that they provide, and be responsible for contributing to promoting the health of individual patients and their communities (see Chapter 9 for further discussion and application).

Student Activity 8.8

♦ Identify specific health promotion activities carried out by your assessor and other members of the team, with individuals and groups on the caseload.

♦ Make a list of these activities.

♦ Find out from your assessor about his or her understanding of the health promoter role.

♦ Ask your peers in another setting to do the same, and compare your findings.

♦ Make notes in your journal/portfolio.

Confidentiality and inter-agency collaboration

The emphasis on the need for greater inter-agency collaboration is one of the major issues within the legislative frameworks (NHS and CCA, 1990). While it is acknowledged that this has many advantages (Øvretveit, 1993), it is also recognised, as discussed earlier, that there could also be difficulties, due to the traditional approaches of professionals who have tended to work independently. Another issue which could become problematic is that of confidentiality. Blackie and Appleby (1998) identify confidentiality as a major principle of primary health care, with patients who are on the receiving end needing to be reassured that their problems remain private. The same emphasis is also made within the UKCC *Code of Professional Conduct* (1992), which requires patient confidentiality to be foremost in the assessment and delivery of care. But how can this be maintained when a wide range of professionals may have access to information about the patient? In many areas, local arrangements are made to overcome this problem. For example, some other members of the team may be asked to sign confidentiality clauses, or access to certain records is restricted or denied.

In any event, the rights of the patient are paramount and the DN has a responsibility to ensure they are not jeopardised in any way. Perhaps a safe principle on which to practise is to ensure patients' involvement in any decisions, so that their voices can be heard (Billings, 2000). Where this is possible, patients and their carers should be consulted about information held on records, and asked their views about other members of the PHCT having access. This should always be treated as a matter of great importance, and it should never be assumed that patients are happy for everyone, including even their nearest and dearest carers, to know about information relating to themselves. The only way to be sure is to ask the patient, and this should be done in such a way that patients feel empowered to decline access to information about themselves if they so choose.

As a student, you can find out from your DN if there is a locally agreed policy on what is to be done about confidentiality when there is involvement by multiple members of the PHCT.

Identifying the role of the community nurse: sick adults

Within the legislation, the role of the nurse is clearly stated. In summary, the nurse's responsibilities are as follows:

- To develop a profile of the patient as an individual and of the patient's community.

- To identify any potential and actual nursing needs that patients may have, through a structured assessment, which may be in collaboration with social services if necessary.

- To ensure that the DN caseload is appropriately analysed, and to consider whether there is a pattern in the type of patients. This could help in identifying whether there are others on the caseload with similar conditions, who may be able to offer support to the patient.

- To plan the care by outlining the patient's and community's needs, with clear statements of how these will be met, and in direct consultation with the patient and any informal carers involved.

- To deliver the planned care in a sensitive manner. To ensure it is acceptable, and thereby maximise the chances for effectiveness, which will lead to the most positive health outcomes.

Developing a profile of the patient and the patient's community

Profiling lies at the heart of the assessment process, and is imperative for an effective assessment. The DN will need to establish a rapport with individual patients, thereby encouraging trust and co-operation, as well as sharing of information about themselves. A patient profile is essentially a history taking, but unfortunately this term may be too reminiscent of the medical model which is not fully inclusive of the patient. But while the development of a profile needs to be fully interactive, the DN is collecting information and making observations that will inform the way needs will be assessed and care delivered. Because of the relative ease with which assumptions may be made about patients (Thompson, 1997), it is imperative that the personal profile is seen as providing information about the patient, by the patient, fully inclusive of how he or she wishes to be known, and including the patient's own views about the illness and the care required. This is an explicit requirement of the legislation (NHS and CCA, 1990). While the personal profile may include contributions from significant others who may be involved in the care, it is good practice to ensure that, as far as possible, it is the patient who provides the information, and who gives permission for information to be taken from carers.

In developing the patient's profile, some of the information may come from other professional sources. It is important to have the patient's views and perceptions about these. For example, information may need to be checked and confirmed as correct and relevant. Basic information needed in the profile includes personal details such as name, address, age, marital status, significant others, nursing and medical history, history of present illness, treatment and medications, among others. The extended list in Table 8.2 is not exhaustive, but helps to remind DNs of the need to use a comprehensive approach so that individuality and uniqueness of the patient can be maintained.

Table 8.2 Individual profiling of patients

Age, date of birth	How individuals identify themselves, for example black, gay, working class and so on
Sex	Education
Place of birth	Employment, past and present
Family history	Hobbies and interests
Sexual orientation	Personal aspirations
Racial background	Preferred food
Religious beliefs	Political beliefs
Disability	Preferred newspapers, radio, TV and so on
Languages spoken	Preferred music

The patient's community: demography and epidemiology

Equally relevant to effective assessment is a sound knowledge about the patient's community. We have already discussed the importance of social and community influences on health outcomes. This information is crucial to the process of making an appropriate assessment. Not only does it help with ensuring that a holistic view is maintained, it should also provide an accurate indication of the range and quality of services on offer. This would go some way towards highlighting any gaps in the service provision, so that they can be addressed in the strategic planning processes (Moon and Gould, 2000). This is the opportunity for DNs to become key contributors to the policy processes which inform the way the services they provide and deliver are organised and funded. Turton and Orr (1993) stress the importance of spending time to get to know the community. DNs, by virtue of working in a community, usually have a good grasp of the major issues within that community, particularly if they affect health outcomes. Table 8.3 gives an overview of demographic and epidemiological information.

Understanding of community processes is enhanced if the information can be compared with other local areas and with the national situation. This helps to make a stronger argument for resources to be made available if needed, and where possible. It may also help to put the situation into an appropriate

Table 8.3 Community profiling

Factors	Issues of relevance
Environment	Type of area: inner city/urban, rural. General state of tidiness. Facilities: leisure centres, parks. Range of shops: pharmacist, post office and so on. Transport: public, private and community. Obvious health hazards: motorways, canals, factories and so on
Housing	Types of housing: private, council, and so on. Relationship of housing to shops and facilities: play areas for children, library, community centre
Health care facilities	Health centre, GP surgery, nearest hospital and emergency centres. Residential homes for older people
Social services and voluntary services	Local social services office, Benefits office, sheltered housing/hostels, local job centre, Day centres for elderly, mental illness, people with learning disability, Age Concern, Red Cross
Employment opportunities	Major industries, level of unemployment. Travelling to work outside of area, numbers. Types of jobs advertised locally
Population structure	Breakdown of area by age and sex. Groups in the community with special health needs, for example minority ethnic groups, older people, and so on. Disease profile: incidence and prevalence of disease. Patterns of disease. Morbidity and mortality data

perspective, demonstrating which needs do not require immediate intervention. Armitage (1997) agrees that effective intervention will depend on the severity of the problem, the feasibility or acceptability of the planned intervention, the level of community involvement and the resource implications. Until a full community profile has been compiled, it will not be possible to determine what may be an appropriate intervention. The challenge of this task is perhaps an issue for DNs, given that this is not necessarily a role which they have traditionally carried (Appleton and Cowley, 2000). Collating the community profile will involve compiling information based on available data, which will need to be analysed by summarising the information, making sure there is emphasis on the relevant issues or problem, and setting targets for achievement (Burton, 1993). DNs may need to identify support for these activities to help them become more effective in these roles. Essentially then, the demographic information about the community should provide information which will help you determine how that community is able to support patients who have particular needs. The epidemiological information will give statistical data on the incidence and prevalence of disease in the community, to help you draw on comparisons and possible contrasts locally, nationally and internationally, if necessary (Moon and Gould, 2000).

Student Activity 8.9

◆ Read Chapter 2 of Moon and Gould (2000).

◆ Using the information provided, start collecting epidemiological information about your locality.

◆ Discuss with your assessor how you plan to do this, and what possible sources might be available.

◆ Make sure you are able to compare the information with other localities and with the national data.

◆ Keep notes in your portfolio.

Potential and actual needs

Potential needs are those that may develop as a consequence of present deficits. For example, a patient with an abnormal screening score for skin integrity may be considered as having a potential need for action to prevent actual skin breakdown. This could be the need for a certain type of mattress, and/or particular focus on health promotion activities to encourage dietary changes, which may help to prevent skin deterioration and breakdown. Actual needs are those which may be specific to the clinical manifestation of a particular illness, combined with the social, psychological, emotional and other external demographic, epidemiological and political factors which impact on patients' experiences of their illness. The same is true of the process for the community needs.

A community with a high deprivation score could have potential needs which should be identified and planned for. For example, if there are high levels of unemployment, and large numbers of single parents or young people, these factors would need to be considered in planning for services, as they could be the precursors to actual and/or potential needs in the community. These services do not necessarily have to be provided by the DNs; however, the referral to other agencies may have to be made by them. Effective referral systems indicate good inter-agency collaboration among members of the PHCT.

Student Activity 8.10

Look at the documentation of assessments done by your clinical assessor, and list the actual and potential needs that have been identified. Were these based on an individual assessment, or was the patient's community considered?

♦ Identify the screening tools which were used to identify these needs.

♦ Compare and contrast your findings with those of your peers from another placement.

Caseload analysis

A caseload is the designated population within a practice, for which the DN or other community nurse is responsible. Within this remit, the DN in this instance, is responsible for ensuring that the needs of patients on the caseload are being met (DoH, 1991b). To do this effectively, issues in identifying actual and potential nursing needs must be identified. The DN will need to monitor the types of intervention on the caseload, and their appropriateness. Local and national policy responses to the need for improving local services should be identified. The DN also has a responsibility to ensure that the health needs of the patient are compared and balanced with those of the wider community. He or she should also be able to prioritise these needs and contribute to local community health profiles (Hawkins et al., 1994).

Planning and delivering care to patients

All of these factors will have an impact on the way care is planned and delivered. The legislation states that care planned and delivered should be clearly documented and only carried out in close consultation with, and with the agreement of, the patient and his or her carer. The framework used for the documentation should clearly identify specific steps that will be taken in the planning and implementation stages, and dates for the actual review and evaluation of progress. Challis (1994) believes that managing patient care will involve tremendous co-ordination, with the consideration of the effective use of the available resources. The extent to which DNs are able to apply this will depend on the perceptions of the local team and the way resources within that team have been allocated. Certainly, the need to ensure that the basis for care is firmly placed within the evidence, will strengthen the DN's contribution and ensure that it is valuable. Clinical governance will provide the opportunities for the DN, as an autonomous practitioner, to effectively contribute to the process by advocating for, and empowering patients and carers in the community to improve outcomes for health (Armitage, 1997).

Student Activity 8.11

Practice application for student nurses:

♦ Ask your assessor for blank copies of the documentation which is used in the assessment process in your placement. This should include skin integrity assessment tools, community deprivation assessment tools and so on.

♦ Check that these are the same for the rest of that locality.

♦ Negotiate some time with your assessor to take you through the actual process, from referral to evaluation of the care delivered.

♦ In identifying the conceptual frameworks that are used, be able to comment on their effectiveness or ineffectiveness. To do this, you will need to look at patients' records. Negotiate this with your assessor.

♦ Make notes in your journal/portfolio.

Conclusion

Needs assessment and care planning are integral to the delivery of care and services, and to ensuring positive outcomes for health. This is as true for individuals as it is for communities. The many factors that influence health and health outcomes must be considered if effective assessment is to take place. The evidence in the literature suggests that individual and community influences are equally important in terms of the effects on health outcomes. Social, demographic, epidemiological and political factors need to be considered in the light of changing emphasis on the care of patients in the community, and the new focus on primary care as a major consideration for the future of health care delivery.

The development of PCGs and PCTs (see Chapter 15) demonstrates the political commitment to ensure a radical shift in emphasis, so that patients are supported as far as possible as close to their primary source of access to health care. DNs have a major role to play in this process, as the key professional and member of the PHCT with responsibility for providing nursing care to sick adults. A clear understanding of the interface between the many factors which impact on the patient's health, and the ability to translate this understanding into appropriate action for patients, is crucial if the DN is to be effective in this role. Using the evidence from available research will help to strengthen this focus, and will provide benefits both to patients and to DNs who, rightfully, will be able to become key contributors to the policy processes which influence resource allocation and changes to the practice of nursing in the community. This chapter has tried to identify the key issues to be considered, and should help you as students to become critically aware of how practice is being informed by the processes, and the way that this is identifiable in the actual roles of the practitioners.

Further reading

Armitage, L. (1997) Identifying health needs. In Hennessey, D. (ed.) *Community Health Care Development*. Basingstoke, Macmillan – now Palgrave.

Blackie, C. and Appleby, F. (eds) (1998) *Community Health Care Nursing*. London, Churchill Livingstone. Chapters 8 and 9.

USEFUL WEB SITES

Department of Health http://www.open.gov.uk/doh/nhs.htm

Public Health Laboratory Service http://www.open.gov.uk/cdsc

UK Clearing House on Health Outcomes http://www.leeds.ac.uk/nuffield/infoservices/UKCH/home.html

References

Acheson, E.D. (1998) *Independent Inquiry into Inequalities in Health*. London, HMSO.

Appleton, J. and Cowley, S. (2000) *The Search for Health Needs*. Basingstoke, Macmillan – now Palgrave.

Armitage, L. (1997) Identifying health needs. In Hennessey, D. (ed.) *Community Health Care Development*. Basingstoke, Macmillan – now Palgrave.

Billings, J. (2000) Lay perspectives on health needs. In Appleton, J. and Cowley, S. (2000) *The Search for Health Needs*. Basingstoke, Macmillan – now Palgrave.

Billis, J. and Harris, T. (1995) *Voluntary Agencies*. London, Macmillan – now Palgrave.

Blackie, C. and Appleby, F. (1998) *Community Health Care Nursing*. London, Churchill Livingstone.

Bradshaw, J. (1972) The concept of need. *New Society*, **30**: 640–3.

Burton, P. (1993) *Community Profiling – a Guide to Identifying Local Needs*. Bristol, SAUS Publications.

Challis, D. (1994) Care management. In Malin, N. (ed.) (1994) *Implementing Community Care*. Buckingham, Open University Press.

Cruickshank, J.K. and Beavers, D.G. (1989) *Ethnic Factors in Health and Disease*. London, John Wright.

Department of Health (1990) *The NHS and Community Care Act*. London, HMSO.

Department of Health (1991a) *Care Management and Assessment, a Practitioner's Guide*. London, HMSO.

Department of Health (1991b) *The Health of the Nation*. London, HMSO.

Department of Health (1993) *The Patient's Charter*. London, HMSO.

Department of Health (1998) *Our Healthier Nation*. London, HMSO.

Department of Health and Social Security (1980) *Inequalities in Health* (The Black Report). London, HMSO.

Fraser, M. (1996) *Conceptual Nursing Practice. A Research Based Approach*, 2nd edn. London, Chapman & Hall.

Gilman, E., Munday, S., Somervaile, L. and Strachan, R. (eds) (1994) *Resource Allocation and Health Needs. From Research to Policy*. London, HMSO.

Hawkins, M., Hughes, G. and Smith P. (1994) *Community Profiling – Auditing Social Needs*. Open University Press.

Hennessy, D. (1997) *Community Health Care Development*. Basingstoke, Macmillan – now Palgrave.

Luker, K. (1987) *Health Visiting*. London, Blackwell Science.

Maslow, A. (1943) A theory of human motivation. *Psychological Review*, **50**: 370–96.

Moon, G. and Gould, M. (2000) *Epidemiology: An Introduction*. Buckingham, Open University Press.

Nocon, A. (1996) *Outcomes of Community Care for Users and Carers*. Buckingham, Open University Press.

Orem, D. (1980) *Nursing: Concepts of Practice*, 2nd edn. New York, McGraw-Hill.

Øvretveit, J. (1993) *Outcomes of Community Care for Users and Carers: A Social Services Perspective*. Buckinghamshire, Open University Press.

Pearson, P. and Spencer, J. (1997) *Promoting Teamwork in Primary Care*. London, Edward Arnold.

Pike, J. and Forster, K. (1994) *Health Promotion*. London, Heinemann.

Robinson, J. and Elkan, R. (1996) *Health Needs Assessment – Theory and Practice*. London, Churchill Livingstone.

Roper, N., Logan, W.W. and Tierney, A.J. (1983) *Using a Model for Nursing*. Edinburgh, Churchill Livingstone.

Thompson, N. (1997) *Anti-discriminatory Practice*. Basingstoke, Macmillan – now Palgrave.

Trent Health (1993) Every Nurse's Business. The Nursing, Midwifery and Health Visiting Contribution to the Achievement of the Trent Strategy for the Health of the Nation's Targets. Staffordshire, Trent Health.

Turton, P. and Orr, J. (1993) *Learning to Care in the Community*, 2nd edn. London, Edward Arnold.

United Kingdom Central Council for Nursing Midwifery and Health Visiting (1992). *Code of Professional Conduct*. London, UKCC.

Vetter, N. (1997) *Purchasing and Providing Health Care. A Practical Guide*. Cheltenham, Stanley Thornes.

Whitehead, M. (1987) *The Health Divide*. London, Health Education Authority.

Wilkinson, C. (1997) *Workplace Health*. London, Blackwell Science.

Wright, J. (1998) *Health Needs Assessment in Practice*. London, BMJ Books.

9

Promoting the health of the client and the community

CAROL WILKINSON

Learning outcomes

By the end of this chapter you will be able to:

- Assess the relevant health initiatives within national and international contexts and identify their implications for nursing.
- Analyse the political, social and ethical implications for health promotion.
- Recognise the practical implications of health promotion work by nurses in the community.

Introduction

The aim of this chapter is to help you to understand and outline the issues affecting health promotion for nurses in the community setting. You will also have the opportunity to review developments in health promotion since the Ottawa Charter, and in doing so be able to identify the alliances that nurses can make to promote health in the community.

Examples from current practice will be cited, with a view to helping you find your role as a student, and as a future community nurse, in the continued development and evaluation of health promotion to benefit everyone in the community.

The new millennium has encouraged everyone to take stock of developments in the field of health promotion. Since the Ottawa Charter (WHO, 1986), health promotion activity has made strides in terms of alerting individuals to lifestyles and behaviour issues and their impact on health, identifying the health needs of populations, formed new models and approaches to health promotion and, now the development of tools for the evaluation of interventions.

Inequalities continue to persist in terms of socioeconomic status, and access to health services. Indeed, Richard Wilkinson's (1996) analysis of industrialised societies has alerted us to the adverse effects upon health of relative inequalities in income where differing levels coupled with social circumstances, produce stress, low self-esteem and poor social relations. These in turn carve out the health outcomes experienced by people in the community.

Community, or the sense of community has altered in the British context over a thirty year period. The nuclear family and lone parent families are now common features of the society. Increased social mobility and dispersal of populations has given rise to new communities with alterations in common culture and sets of beliefs. This has given rise to a multiplicity of values and diversity in needs and expectations (see Chapter 6).

Nurses and other health professionals working in the heart of the community, are in an ideal position to influence and improve the health of the population. Indeed, making use of the social capital that a community has to offer encourages partnership and builds alliances. Everyone has a part to play. As a student, you should not only be able to identify examples of good practice, but also to participate in a range of activities with your assessor/supervisor and other members of the primary health care team (PHCT).

A worldwide review of community based alliances for health promotion undertaken by the Health Education Authority (HEA) for the International Conference on Health Promotion based in Jakarta 1997, has provided some interesting developments in this growing field. The most current leading example in community health promotion is located in Costa Rica. Health promotion interventions formed the catalyst for cross-governmental working. Local participation at all levels has become the norm and has included needs assessment; community development projects, improved educational opportunities for women and children and investment in programmes for the poorest in communities. This has provided measurable benefits in service provision, access to health care, reduction in infant mortality, improvement in social relationships, norms, values and new policy development.

Student Activity 9.1

◆ Make a list of activities you have been able to identify in your practice placement as specific activities for promoting the health of patients on your assessor's caseload.

◆ Discuss these with one or more of your peers to see how the list compares and contrasts with a list from another caseload.

◆ Keep a record of these in your portfolio.

Vienna Declaration on Nursing in Support of the European 'Health for All' Targets, 21–24 June 1988

This European Conference drew together nurses from 32 countries in the region, to examine their role and functions in light of the Health for All (HFA) strategy. The main aim was to bring health to the attention of ministries of health, trades unions of health professions and regulatory bodies of the regions. The declaration intended that, as a requisite for developing their role as health promoters, nurses should act as partners in decision making at not only local, but regional and national levels. They should have a greater role in empowering individuals, families and communities to become more self-reliant and to take charge of their health developments. The Vienna Declaration paved the way for nurses to take the lead in providing clear and valid information to patients on the positive and negative consequences of different types of behaviour, and on the merits and costs of different options for care.

What did this mean in reality for UK nurses?

Initially, this extended the process of *decision making* in the health services. It brought nurses into the debate about health promotion matters, which related to their patients and themselves as a profession (Butterworth, 1988; Thomas and Wainwright, 1996). The how, the why, the strategies and the consequences were thought about and developed especially in relation to the nursing curriculum and subsequent practice.

As far as health promotion activity is concerned, in the primary care setting a considerable amount of what is perceived to be health promotion is undertaken on a group basis by nurses and health visitors (Sourtzi et al., 1996). There were some problems to overcome. It has been argued that traditional nurse training gave little or no preparation for such a role (Thomas and Wainwright, 1996). Subjects such as ethics, health promotion and social policy were subsequently introduced into the curriculum to develop the political awareness of nurses. This was strengthened with the Community Care Act 1992 and the Calman–Hine Report (1995) which shifted the focus of care and demands for early intervention, acute stage treatments, continuity of care and role extension. Health promotion was a part of this process underpinning an ideological shift set in train by the move towards market forces and closely linked to issues assuming prominence in the new climate of care within community nursing. Health promotion was set to extend beyond traditional boundaries with a greater focus on collaborative health promotion. This of course, meant that all nurses had to recognise their unique role in the process, rather than make assumptions that health promotion activity was the specific role of particular nurses in the community. Student Activity 9.1 should have helped you to identify some of the ways in which DNs, as a part of their role, for example promote the health of patients who may be chronically sick.

In terms of the practicalities of fostering *empowerment* of patients, the issue in relation to health care was engendered in the philosophy of nursing in acute as well as primary care services. However, it was brought into sharp focus when it was discovered that a greater examination of the role of community nurses was necessary. Preliminary studies such as that by Thomas and Wainwright (1996) found nurses lacked knowledge, training and expertise. This was coupled with the issue of definition. What is health promotion, and how did it differ from health education, which straddled alongside the nursing ethos for many generations?

It must be noted that this early study into nurses' perception on their new role in health promotion was problematic. In fact, the narrowness in perception of health promotion that the researchers posited to their fellow nurses was quite marked. For instance, Thomas and Wainwright (1996) discussed *role modelling and tactics* in health promotion, which presented an outmoded 1970s' image of health promotion:

> Some issues featured more in one group than the other. For example, the use of fear tactics was highly prioritised as an issue by the district nurses, but scarcely featured for the health visitors. The health visitor, however, included immunization issues, which were not addressed by district nurses. (Thomas and Wainwright, 1996: p.102)

The provision of *information* on health and health care has also been brought under closer scrutiny. For example, nurses' approaches to health promotion, the introduction of The Patient's Charter (1993) and the co-operation in information provision. There is a long way to go in pushing the boundaries forward. Currently, the concept of health promotion based on the primary health care team seems to be limited to the activities of the GP and practice nurse, with small scale collaboration with other health authority staff. The development of skills in communication with different client groups, getting to grips with new computerised technology and the dissemination of information by those other than the doctor and manager will need to be more closely examined.

Student Activity 9.2

♦ Look again at the list of health promotion activities that your assessor undertakes.

♦ Are you able to identify their effectiveness?

♦ What methods, if any, are used by the DN to evaluate these activities?

♦ Make notes in your portfolio.

The nurse education curriculum and health promotion

One of the main potentials in health promotion is to bridge the theory/practice gap and to have solid evidence of what works and the limitations of specific undertakings. The debate in the field of health promotion generally continues although the employment of specific research techniques continues to bring evidence forward from the field. Evaluation is still poor as the combination of techniques is only gradually being employed (Oakley, 1998).

To bridge the gap, the nurse needs to observe what is going on in practice, record it, reflect upon it, consider whether it is the best technique for her patient, or how best her patient's needs can be served within each situation. Is it best to suggest nicotine patches without counselling in order to stop smoking? Is it more favourable to suggest dieting to a patient without providing them with information on the impact on their metabolism, or on the importance of combining diet with a sensible exercise regime?

Nursing skills

Nursing skills are important if health promotion is to be meaningful, and have a greater guarantee of success. As you work alongside your DN assessor, you should be observing these skills in action, and learning to recognise their effectiveness in your own development on your placement, and in your work with patients. The skills are as follows:

- Observation
- Communication
- Listening
- Reflection
- Prioritising
- Knowledge
- Monitoring
- Awareness of limitations.

Knowledge too is important but there are limitations and often providing the client with too much may hinder their perception and progress in development. Striking a balance between prior knowledge, acquiring new knowledge and the client's personal circumstances must be gauged carefully for success. Questions that need to be asked are:

- What are the innovative ways that exist in working with patients and are these in their personal interests?
- Is there a general awareness of factors affecting health and self and how these can be brought to bear on the execution of health improvement work?

Student Activity 9.3

Do this activity with two or three of your peers.

♦ Discuss your own values in relation to health and health care.

♦ In what ways can your values impinge on your work with patients?

♦ Give examples of how the health values of patients can be mobilised to meet their needs.

♦ What action can clients take within their communities to improve and enhance their health status?

♦ Make notes on this discussion in your portfolio.

These are all considerations for the nurse. (Chapter 8 provides further information about factors affecting the health of individuals and communities.)

In relation to their own interests, principles and practices outlined by the WHO (1985) for nursing and health promotion include the following:

1. Opportunities for students to enhance their own health through relaxation training, stress management, complementary therapies, sports facilities and communication.

2. Holistic and diverse approaches for promoting health and well-being.

3. Knowledge and skills to facilitate community participation such as assertiveness skills, networking with voluntary and statutory agencies.

4. Evidence of knowledge in the social and behavioural sciences.

5. Evidence of health education and advocacy skills.

During the 1980s, Meyer (1986, 1988) developed a consensus view based on expert opinion of what health promotion within nursing education should be. This view suggested that health should be threaded through the curriculum, integrated with other subjects, should explore wider social and political aspects, emphasise the community, explore learners' own values and attitudes and be taught using formal methods. As mentioned earlier, the necessary skills for health promotion include communication, advocacy, collaboration, mediation and negotiation. Awareness and development of these skills need to begin within the curriculum if we are to overcome the problem identified by Thomas and Wainwright (1996) of problematic focus in terms of the role of community nurses in health promotion activities.

The important aspects in terms of curriculum design and development required prioritising specific elements. For example, policy makers and educa-

Student Activity 9.4

♦ Find out whether there is a health promotion specialist practitioner in your locality.

♦ If there is, negotiate with your assessor to spend some time with this person.

♦ Find out what is involved in their role, and how this relates to the role of the DN.

♦ Make notes in your portfolio.

tionalists had to make explicit the body of knowledge which comprised health and health promotion, and acknowledge the time and staff development required to integrate these concepts into the curriculum (Smith et al., 1995).

Practitioners, educationalists and managers were required to review and critique the concept of health promotion currently in use and to redefine it in a theoretically meaningful way for nursing, midwifery and health visiting. Changes in health policy mean this requires periodic revision. In some areas, a specialist lecturer-practitioner/facilitator role was developed, the principal aim being to guide and support students and qualified staff in enhancing and promoting the health of patients and clients (Smith et al., 1995).

Values and approaches to health promotion must be embedded within the curriculum and become a part of the culture of nursing. New paradigms in health, which originally emanated from Alma Ata and the HFA philosophy, should also be incorporated into the curriculum. These include the notions of equity, empowerment, multisectoral activity and the psychosocial element.

Perhaps it is best at this stage to define these specific notions then develop their meaning in light of advancing healthy communities.

Psychosocial

There is a distinct recognition that psychosocial aspects of life influence the health of people within society. For example, it is acknowledged in the early 21st century that stress, or at least the ill effects of the condition, are precipitated by a multiplicity of factors. These may include working conditions, family relationships where there is no single causative factor to ill health. Also what makes young women smoke is not only peer pressure, but a combined association with level of education, family conditions, vulnerability, and the link to prevention of weight gain. Wilkinson emphasises the psychosocial:

You can be happy eating chips. But sources of social stress, poor social networks, low self-esteem, high rates of depression, anxiety, insecurity, the loss of sense of control, all have such a fundamental impact on our experience of life that it is reasonable to wonder whether the effects on the quality of life are not more important than the effects on the length of life. (Wilkinson 1996: pp. 5–6)

Equity

One of the key concepts originally identified under the HFA strategy was the notion of equity. It is about ensuring an equal opportunity for all citizens of obtaining and maintaining good health so that inequalities in health and health status no longer exist between and within countries/societies (Rathwell, 1992).

The term, however, is considered on a broader set of assumptions especially in relation to health planning and development. Equity incorporates the notion of social justice. A variety of possible definitions of equity exists, including the following:

- Equal health
- Equal access to health care
- Equal utilisation of health care
- Equal access to health care according to need, and
- Equal utilisation of health care according to need.

To take these notions further, there have been greater distinctions within the vertical and horizontal contexts. Horizontal equity implies equal treatment for equal need. For example, all pregnant women without complications would receive similar care. Vertical equity implies the unequal treatment of unequal need. It suggests that differing levels of health provision be made available for pregnant women expecting no complications from those with likely complications. It also suggests different levels of care for pregnancy as compared to other health needs, such as coronary patients. In planning services it is relatively easy to understand the concept of horizontal equity, although it may be difficult to achieve. However, the concept of vertical equity is far harder to apply, requiring a working definition of need, and value judgements about how to react and how to prioritise services for relative needs (Green, 1994).

With reference to the community, access to primary care may be equitable, however, it does not always follow that equity will be achieved especially in referral to specialist care. It is acknowledged that there is wide variation in the behaviour of GPs and nurses in their referral practices, which are independent of patient conditions and social situations (Blaxter, 1984; Noone, 1989; Ham and Mitchell, 1990; Hoskins and Maxwell, 1990). For example, in areas of high unemployment or in the inner city, there are higher rates of utilisation of primary care but this is not borne out in the same number of referrals (Blane et al., 1997). (Chapter 6 provides more discussion on working in a diverse community.)

Empowerment

Empowerment is one of the main philosophical components in health promotion. It implies a relationship between the individuals and their environment. It is intended to facilitate healthy decision making as well as attempts to achieve the best for the individual through fostering sufficient skills and knowledge to enable participation in the decision-making process. The relationship is intended to be nurturing and reciprocal (Tones, 1997). You may find it useful to consider the extent to which your DN assessor is able to empower the patients with whom she or he works.

Student Activity 9.5

If you have had an opportunity to observe and/or discuss empowerment strategies with your DN assessor, negotiate some time with a health visitor to see whether you are able to compare and contrast the methods used to empower patients.

◆ Discuss these with one of your peers and with your assessor and the health visitor concerned. What do you think may be responsible for the differences/similarities?

◆ Make notes in your portfolio.

Multi-sectorial planning

The attainment of good health requires a concerted approach by all sectors of society. The health sector alone cannot manage schemes or achieve health improvement for all (Rathwell, 1992). To this end, you should be aware of a variety of approaches from all public sector services, as well as the private sector, in dealing with the issues under discussion. The legislation outlined the need for all sectors to participate in the processes. Healthy cities initiatives bring together all these groups in order to ensure that the approach to dealing with problems of health promotion is as seamless as possible.

'Our Healthier Nation'

The Green Paper *Our Healthier Nation* was introduced by the Labour government in February 1998. Its intention was to provide a platform to debate and develop new strategies for health improvement in England and Wales. One of the ways it differed from its predecessor *The Health of the Nation* (DoH, 1991) was in concentrating on four rather than six targets: Cardiovascular disease and strokes, cancers, accidents and mental health. And for the first time in almost 20 years, the social agenda was reintroduced into health. This is not to say that health professionals were unconcerned with such matters. On the contrary, it is the case that the health promoting philosophy harnessed in Alma Ata had that very intention. But its interpretation in Britain and parts of Europe has been very localised.

The issue of promoting health in specific settings has made its return. Drawn into this social health ethos is a great sense of community development and participation as being necessary ingredients to drive initiatives forward. *Our Healthier Nation*'s two key aims of improving health of the population are:

1. To improve the health of the population as a whole by increasing the length of people's lives and the number of years people spend free from illness.

2. To improve the health of the worst off in society and to narrow the health gap.

Although targets are beneficial for the obvious reason for accounting for change, achieving improvement in health and reduction in inequalities will require more than balancing accounts. It will need a cultural shift to focus on structural changes such as better housing, employment, access to health care services for all, investment in communities, bringing back pride in the family and family life, whatever its constituents, finding not only ways of dealing with poverty as a result of circumstances of birth or lack of employment, but also providing support for families that break down as a result of separation, divorce and bereavement. Health is only one part of the equation. Approaches that foster health development and improvement within and between communities need to be found.

An example of ongoing initiatives is the establishment of health action zones (HAZs). The concept here aims to use an inclusive approach in dealing with the problems, by recognising the contribution of a multiplicity of factors to the health outcomes of individuals and communities. This recognition ensures that a focus is given to all the possible factors influencing health status. Both public and private providers of services, including the business community, employers, schools and other educational settings, are encouraged to participate in improving this status.

Student Activity 9.6

♦ Find out whether your locality is part of a health action zone (HAZ).

♦ If it is, discuss with your assessor what this means for people in the community.

♦ Find out if DNs contribute in any way to this process.

♦ If your locality does not include a HAZ, spend some time either searching the Internet or do a library search to find out what the prerequisites are for the establishment of a HAZ, and the possible benefits for the community from this approach.

♦ Keep notes of your findings in your portfolio.

The Ottawa Charter: developments

The Ottawa Charter was established in 1986 following in the spirit of Alma Ata nine years earlier. The Alma Ata Declaration of 1977 committed all member countries to the principles of Health for All by the year 2000. The main direction advocated a shift in focus towards primary health care but, at the same time, drove commitment to community participation and intersectoral action which became the primary elements of all serious health promotion programmes. The WHO in Europe launched its own programme on health promotion in 1984. This subsequently gave rise to the first international conference on health promotion in Ottawa, Canada in November 1986.

The Charter set a new challenge for a move towards a new public health, which attempted to reaffirm the values of social justice and equity as prerequisites for health, advocacy and mediation intended to be the processes by which such aims could be realised. The Charter was intended to achieve Health For All by the Year 2000 and beyond.

The Charter also identified specific actions for the achievement of health improvement for all nations around the world. Its ideals were established in a definition, which identified health promotion as a process enabling people to increase control over, and improve, their health. The aim is to reach a state of complete physical, mental and social well-being by being able to identify and realise their aspirations, satisfy their needs, and change or cope with their environment. Health is therefore considered as a resource for everyday life, not the objective of living. The concept is meant to be a positive one, emphasising social and personal resources as well as physical capacities. Hence, health promotion is seen as not just being the responsibility of the health sector, but as going beyond healthy lifestyles to well-being.

Student Activity 9.7

◆ With two or three of your peers, discuss the above description of health promotion.

◆ Identify the extent to which the ideas represented in this description are achievable in your locality.

◆ Compare and contrast the information with that of your peers.

◆ Are you able to identify examples of participation in the health outcomes of your locality by providers other than the health sector?

◆ Make a list of these, and state their involvement.

◆ Keep records for your portfolio.

Prerequisites for health

The Charter underlined specific prerequisites for health which are fundamental. Conditions and resources for health are peace, shelter, education, food, income, a stable ecosystem, sustainable resources, social justice and equity. Improvement in health requires a secure foundation in these basic prerequisites, as well as in the processes of advocacy, mediation and enabling.

Advocacy

Within these prerequisites, positive health is generally seen as a substantial resource for economic, personal and social development. It is a necessary dimension in maintaining quality of life. Health promotion action through advocacy can make a contribution to the factors such as biology, culture and behaviour that can be equally harmful or favourable to health. Nurses' role in this process is a key factor in the contribution to health outcomes for individuals and communities.

Mediation

The prerequisites and prospects for health cannot be ensured by the health sector as sole provider. Professional and social groups and health personnel have a major responsibility to mediate between differing interests in society for the pursuit of health. Health promotion strategies and programmes should be adapted to the local needs and possibilities of individual countries and regions to take into account differing social, cultural and economic systems. The establishment of HAZs in the UK can be seen here as important for this process.

Enabling

Health promotion focuses on achieving equity in health. Health promotion action intends to reduce differences in health status and ensure equal opportunities, especially in terms of resources, to enable all people to achieve their fullest health potential. The process of enabling people to take control is seen as crucial for health. A secure foundation includes the provision of a supportive environment, access to information, life skills and opportunities for making healthy choices.

'Health Promotion Action'

As well as the specific prerequisites identified above, specific action was identified to mobilise the 'Health Promotion Action'. This includes five key elements:

- Building healthy public policies
- Creating supportive environments
- Strengthening community action
- Developing personal skills, and
- Reorienting health services.

The following sections from the Ottawa Charter demonstrate this:

1. *Building healthy public policies*

Health promotion extends beyond health care. It places health on the agenda of policy-makers in all sectors and at all levels, directing them to be aware of the health consequences of their decisions and to accept their responsibility for health. Health promotion policy combines diverse but complementary approaches including legislation, fiscal measures, taxation and organizational change. It is co-ordinated action that leads to health, income and social policies that foster equity. Joint association contributes to ensuring safer and healthier goods and services, healthier public services, and cleaner, more enjoyable environments. Health promotion policy requires identification of obstacles to the adoption of healthy public policies in non-health sectors, and ways of removing them. The aim must be to make healthier choice the easier choice for policy-makers as well as individuals and communities.

2. *Creating supportive environments*

Our societies are complex and interrelated. Health cannot be separated from other goals. The inextricable links between people and their environment constitute the basis for a socio ecological approach to health. The overall guiding principle for the world, nations, regions and communities alike is the need to encourage reciprocal maintenance – to take care of each other, our communities and our natural resources throughout the world should be emphasised as a global responsibility.

Changing patterns of life, work and leisure have a significant impact on health. Work and leisure should be a source of health for everyone. The way society organises work should help to create a healthy society. Health promotion should generate living and working conditions that are safe, stimulating, satisfying and enjoyable.

Systematic assessment of the health impact of a rapidly changing environment – particularly in areas of technology, work, energy production and urbanization is essential and must be followed by action to ensure positive benefit to the health of the public. The protection of the natural and built environments and the conservation of natural resources must be addressed in any health promotion strategy.

3. *Strengthening community action*

Health promotion works through concrete and effective community action in setting priorities, making decisions, planning strategies and implementing them to achieve better health. At the heart of this process is the empowerment of communities, their ownership and control of their own endeavours and destinies. Community development draws on existing human and material resources in the community to enhance self-help and social support, and to develop flexible systems for strengthening public participation and direction of health matters. This requires full and continuous access to information, learning opportunities for health, as well as funding support.

4. *Developing personal skills*

Health promotion supports personal and social development through providing information, education for health and enhancing life skills. By so doing, it increases the options available to exercise more control over their own health and over their environments, and to make choices conducive to health. Enabling people to learn throughout life, to prepare themselves for all of its stages and to cope with chronic illness and injuries is essential. This has to be facilitated in school, home, work and community settings. Action is required through educational, professional, commercial and voluntary bodies, and within the institutions themselves.

5. *Reorienting health services*

The responsibility for health promotion in health services is shared among individuals, community groups, health professionals, health service institutions and

governments. They must work together towards a health care system, which
contributes to the pursuit of health.

The role of the health sector must move increasingly in a health promotion direction, beyond its responsibility for providing clinical and curative services. Health
services need to embrace an expanded mandate, which is sensitive and respects
cultural needs. This mandate should support the needs of individuals and communities for a healthier life, and open channels between the health sector and broader
social, political, economic and physical environmental components.

Reorienting health services also requires stronger attention to health research as
well as changes in professional education and training. This must lead to a change
of attitude and organization of health services, which refocuses on the total needs
of the individual as a whole person.

(Ottawa Charter, WHO Regional Office for Europe,
August 1986, pp. 1 and 2)

Student Activity 9.8

♦ With a group of your peers, consider the five areas discussed
   above.

♦ Discuss the extent to which your DN assessor is able to
   contribute to the processes required for each.

♦ Make notes on specific activities, which you have seen or
   participated in, that have supported the concepts discussed.

The Ottawa Charter: issues

For the first time, an agenda with underpinning political and social principles
was set for achieving health for all peoples of all nations. It prioritised and
structured health development, which differed from single issue
programmes, for example reduction of malaria, or oral rehydration in developing countries, as in the 1960s and 70s, and defined the issue of health
promotion, a much broader concept than the old notion of health education.

The Charter also took on the WHO definition of health and made the
notion more people focused within a broader social context. The concept of
health, an abstract term was strengthened by the *notions* which included:

● The recognition and satisfaction of need
● Adaptability to one's environment

- Making use of social and personal resources
- Well-being.

The Charter formed the foundation for other initiatives and development of strategies to promote health. For example, the Healthy Cities campaign, Local Agenda 21 and Sustainable Development, as well as local strategies for health improvement in a variety of countries. It focused attention on processes and methodologies to promote health, thereby extending the definition of health improvement beyond education. It created a new language that continues to be debated and extended. For example the buzz words lifestyle, health promotion, empowerment were being hotly pursued and contested in the late 1980s and through the 1990s. There was also the impetus for health improvement on a grand scale. The approach was intended to be vertical, horizontal and diagonal, so that by the end of the 20th century, health improvement and involvement in promoting health had become the domain of many sectors of society. The ideology of health promotion as expressed in the Charter placed emphasis on prevention, despite the fact that much of the driving force came from the public health movement, which was medically orientated. The Charter provided an international and national arena for debating issues in health promotion. It also assisted in strengthening the resolve of parties concerned in health to reduce inequalities in the health of populations. Further, the Charter encapsulated the spirit of primary health care and the strategy for achieving Health for All.

Criticisms

The Charter and the issues emanating from it, which included the spirit of new policies and strategies for health, experienced much criticism.

First, many advanced countries including Britain devised their strategies to improve health alongside the underpinning notions of the Charter. However, while the social and other environmental factors influencing health may be recognised in the policies of health promotion, many of the targets set relate to disease or to biological or behavioural risk factors, parallelling the rapid shift from comprehensive to selective health care (Baum and Saunders, 1995). This was very apparent in the policy document *Health of the Nation* (DoH, 1991).

Second, the Healthy Cities campaign, seen as spearheading community action to promote health, has been criticised for being too bureaucratic. It advocated the language of radical social movements on change through conflict. However, despite its success in places like Sheffield and Toronto, it fell short of its radical ideals and instead translated into consensual and incremental change (Baum and Saunders, 1993).

Third, the term 'healthy public policy' refers to all general governmental policy that has an impact on health. Healthy public policy may be seen as part of the health promotion policies as defined in the Ottawa Charter (WHO, 1986). At the 1988 WHO Adelaide Conference on Health Promotion – Healthy Public Policies, four key areas were defined as priorities for healthy public policy for immediate action. These were support for women's health, food and nutrition, tobacco and alcohol, and creating supportive environments. Specific emphasis was put on healthy public policy in the developing world (Hetzel, 1989). While building on the same background as the initiatives on health promotion, the healthy public policy approach may reveal a greater orientation towards public health, social justice and social policies, and avoid the victim-blaming more prone to emerge in strategies focusing on individuals and lifestyles. However, in the UK much attention was paid to lifestyle issues alone – for example, reducing obesity among women under the age of 40, reducing teenage pregnancies, heavy focus on HIV/AIDS campaigns as an individual problem. It is only recently that the new Labour government is seen to be making some headway in healthy public policy. Rathwell (1992) also saw the issues in Europe lacking the appropriate resources and infrastructure.

The Charter encapsulated the spirit of the primary health care movement through health promotion and HFA 2000. However the resources to support these movements in any substantial way were considerably lacking. Indeed, it has been observed that, on a global scale, the primary health care movement has been dependent almost exclusively on goodwill. The proposal of establishing a Global Advisory Council as a means of exerting pressure on various health for all partners to comply with their commitments has not been successful and the need for such a mechanism has yet to be devised (Tarimo and Webster, 1995).

For a time, there was a considerable gap between theory and practice (Bryant, 1988), although it must be emphasised that research and development in this field is being generated, but resources are rather limited. The strategy was dismissed as unrealistic and the WHO should be called to account in the light of something so unworkable in terms of achieving its realistic aims. De Kadt (1982) underlined the doctrinaire nature of the HFA strategy and its offshoots and its nebulous phraseology, which acted as a blanket substitute for real practical solutions. The goals were seen as unrealistic (Peabody, 1995) and there was also insufficient support on an international level to implement particular aspects of the policy in its entirety (WHO, 1987, 1993).

Finally, the age-old problems of class and professions ensued. The role of the medical profession's conservatism coincided with the interests of the elite which ensured the failure of Health for All and supported the choice of selective strategies with a framework better suited to the medical profession's interests (Green, 1994). The interests and class background of the medical profession do not coincide with the aims of primary health care, equity and public health in many countries (Zaidi, 1986; Mangelsdorf et al., 1988; Mburu, 1989; Sherraden and Wallace, 1992; Woelk, 1994).

A number of issues converge. Emerging developments are the ideas that emanate from the concept of *social capital* and *healthy living centres*. Although from different perspectives, they bring together development and participation in communities for health improvement. To develop this further, we will consider the issue of social capital.

The concept of social capital

There are social relationships which come into existence when individuals attempt to make best use of their individual resources, but are not necessarily seen as components of social structures. Loury (1977) introduced the term *social capital* to describe these resources. For Loury, social capital is inherent in family relationships and community organisation, and is useful for the cognitive or social development of a child or young person. These resources differ for different persons and can constitute an important advantage for children and adolescents in the development of their human capital. Similar ideas were introduced by Loury in the field of economics to identify the social resources considered beneficial for the development of human capital.

Student Activity 9.9

◆ Consider the extent to which the individuals in your locality are able to benefit from an understanding, and application, of the concept of social capital.

◆ How can they be helped in this process by the DN?

◆ Share your ideas with one or two of your peers, and discuss these with your assessor.

Social capital is defined by its function. It is not a single entity but a variety of different entities with two distinct features. They consist of some aspect of a social structure and they facilitate certain actions of individuals who are within the structure. Like other forms of capital, social capital is productive, making possible the achievement of certain ends. It is created when the relations among persons change in ways that facilitate action. Putnam (1993) takes this further in the expression of social capital as features of social organisation such as networks, norms and trust that facilitate co-ordination and co-operation for mutual benefit. Social capital enhances the benefits of investment in physical and human capital. Social capital espouses collective action, partnership and social solidarity. In line with notions identified in

healthy policies mentioned in this chapter, it involves making use of collective resources without necessarily incurring high economic costs.

A good example of social capital in action is discussed by Putnam (1993)
relating to the Italian communities of Tuscany and Emilia-Romagna, where
citizens are engaged in public issues, not merely through patronage, but in a
spirit of trust and abiding law. Leaders in these communities are relatively
honest and committed to equality. Social and political networks are organised
horizontally rather than hierarchically. Democracy flourishes through solidarity and participation.

He also sees similar action in the black churches of African American
peoples. The church provided the organisational infrastructure for political
mobilisation during the Civil Rights Movement. As far as health is
concerned, community participation and solidarity can best be seen in Costa
Rica where health policies were specifically devised by the communities. Solutions for health improvement were also created and executed by them.

Issues relating to social capital for health

The concept is as yet untested in Britain, although there are moves to incorporate the notion of social capital into health policy and action to improve
health at community level. Summoning the resources of churches and voluntary agencies is only slowly being seen as having workable potential, perhaps
more so for the voluntary sector than for churches. Perhaps society has come
to expect more from the demands created jointly by policies, increasing
knowledge and its statutory services. For social capital to mean something,
the ability to command resources through social networks must be separate
from the level or the quality of such resources. This is important for poor
communities when social capital and the benefits derived from it may be
confused, the term merely relegates the notion to the already successful
continuing to succeed (Portes and Landolt, 1996).

Community membership brings with it the demand for conformity. Those
who do not conform run the risk of being ostracised. This kills creativity and
individual expression. In sectors where the notion of social capital has been
tested, the fact still remains that inequality of opportunity exists. For
example, in American society where industries with strong social ties exist,
newcomers often find themselves unable to compete, no matter how accomplished their qualifications and skills. African American contractors
attempting to carve a niche in white and immigrant dominated construction
industries find themselves unable to do so (Portes and Landolt, 1996). In
fact it increases discrimination rather than acquisition of human capital.

Many communities in Britain are fragmented by their inability to access
sufficient resources and health services (Ahmad and Atkin, 1996). Caution is
needed in order to mobilise social capital into practical solutions.

Healthy living centres

One of the policy pronouncements indicated in *The New NHS: Modern, Dependable* (DoH, 1997), is the introduction of healthy living centres. Its aim is to provide greater access to primary health care services to communities in Britain. Whether it bridges the gap between health improvement and summoning social capital is as yet an unknown quantity.

The Life Project: Wirral

During the early 1990s, an alliance was formed between Wirral Health Authority, Wirral Borough Council and the University of Liverpool to improve health of the community. The alliance was embedded in a philosophy of empowerment, and committed to raising self-esteem and developing opportunities for its people. The focus was on the development of a coronary heart disease (CHD) risk prevention strategy.

Strategic aims:
1. To improve the health, quality of life and general well-being of residents of the target area of Wirral.

2. To promote a number of key behavioural changes related to the risk factors associated with CHD.

3. To assess scientifically the state of health and fitness of residents of the target area.

4. To improve the long-term survival prospects and quality of life of coronary patients by introducing an exercise-based rehabilitation programme.

5. To improve self-esteem within the community.

6. To encourage and support community responsibility as one of the major methods of improving health and fitness.

7. To encourage collaboration between the agencies involved in order to provide the necessary leadership, human and physical resources and information.

8. To assess savings on health resources as a result of the project.

9. To provide training in health-related leadership with corresponding employment opportunities.

The initial aim during 1993 was to establish a network of contacts in three parts of the district. A mobile trailer was used for screening and networking in community centres, public houses, nightclubs, car parks and other public places. Once the links were established, information and guidance were developed and provided relating to local opportunities, services, therapies, referral points for health and leisure services. Recipients of the service were encouraged to negotiate a lifestyle action plan, which gave them access to a

The Life Project: Wirral continued

range of rehabilitation courses. These featured, for example, exercise on prescription, and help with smoking cessation. Opportunities for health improvement were offered at community centres, GP surgeries, leisure centres, community colleges and working men's clubs.

To support the initiative, a number of volunteers and tutors were recruited. A training programme, which included nationally recognised qualifications, attracted approximately 80 candidates per year and provided professional training, ongoing support, job creation and increased opportunities in the local community.

The initiative was positive in the sense that it brought people together to achieve specific aims, which it did with very positive spin-offs for the local communities. Much of it rested on goodwill of the people, an example of investing in social capital. Whether it is sustainable with limited financial resource is as yet unknown, and the extent of participation and the engendering of a community spirit which is sustainable and moves beyond the specific project remains to be seen.

Student Activity 9.10

◆ What do you think healthy living means?

◆ Are you able to identify any examples depicted in the locality of your placement?

◆ Describe the role that DNs and the voluntary sector could play in assisting older patients to survive the winter months.

◆ Make notes for your portfolio.

The current intention is to give communities free rein to set up their own centres through mobilising their creative resources in ways specific to their own community's needs. The intention is not to pursue a single centre or building as such, but for the community to offer a range of services and facilities from various sectors within itself. There is an emphasis on partnership, for example voluntary agencies joining forces with the NHS or the local council with public health departments. The intention is to provide complementary facility to the government's public health action on reduction in inequalities in health. Some economic resources will be provided through the New Opportunities Fund.

Emerging issues for 2001 and beyond

Although the nursing curriculum has developed to incorporate health promotion, albeit on an incremental scale, the practice within community settings still requires considerable development. This can only come about through continuous observation and research of community nursing around the world. This, however, begins with all nurses, including students, at the clinical level. They need to engage themselves in activities which show that they are aware of the implications of this requirement, and their role within it. At the beginning of a new century, nurses need to find new ways of supporting their clients in the community. It will require collaborative efforts as the nurse's role and skills are finite. Collaboration with other agencies will be necessary to deal with continuing health related problems including the following:

- *Literacy* and the educational status of women. These are known to be core long-term determinants of health. In many countries women's education remains far below the levels necessary for sustained improvements in health status.

- *Ageing*, which is now a major demographic factor of change in many developing countries, and in all Western countries. The rate of growth in the population over 60 years of age in countries as diverse as China, Indonesia, Brazil and South Africa is higher than more developed countries. A rapidly growing challenge for health and social welfare policies is to provide assistance for these people on a par with their European and North American counterparts (Ebrahim and Kalache, 1996).

- *The widening gap* between rich and poor, and widening inequalities in health present a formidable obstacle for attempts to reduce health inequalities.

The Jakarta Declaration (WHO,1997)

The Fourth International Conference on Health Promotion was the first of its kind to be held in a developing country and to involve the private sector in supporting health promotion. Since the Ottawa Charter, evidence has emerged that:

1. Comprehensive approaches to health development are the most effective. Those which employed combinations of the five strategies are more effective than single track approaches.

2. Settings offer practical opportunities for the implementation of comprehensive strategies. These included local communities, cities and municipalities with their schools, markets, workplaces and health care facilities.

3. Participation is essential to sustain efforts. People have to be at the centre of health promotion action and decision-making processes for them to be effective.

4. Learning about health fosters participation. Access to education and information is essential for achieving effective participation and the empowerment of people and communities.

New priorities in health promotion for the 21st century

Under the Jakarta Declaration specific priorities have now become prominent to take forward the vision of health improvement for communities around the world. The main aims are:

- To promote *social responsibility* for health
- To increase *investment* for health development
- To consolidate and expand *partnerships* for health
- To increase *community capacity* and *empower* the individual
- To secure an *infrastructure* for health promotion.

Social responsibility

Both the private and public sectors should conjoin to pursue policies and practices that:

- Avoid harming the health of other individuals
- Protect the environment and ensure sustainable use of resources
- Restrict production and trade in inherently harmful goods and substances, such as tobacco and armaments as well as unhealthy marketing practices
- Safeguard both the citizen in the marketplace and the individual in the workplace
- Include equity focused health impact assessments as an integral part of policy development.

Investment

The current investment in many countries in health is insufficient, and could be utilised more effectively. Increasing investment for health development requires a positive and multi-sectoral approach. This should include housing and education policy. Greater focus is to be placed on marginalised populations, older people, women and children.

Partnerships

In accordance with WHO guidelines, partnerships are being encouraged to improve health along health and social boundaries. Health is a feature of society and hence its promotion and improvement is being encouraged and developed within this context.

Community capacity and empowerment

Training, education, leadership and greater access to resources is encouraged within groups, communities and organisations. Empowering people is likely to bring them greater access to the decision-making process. The harnessing of information and social capital is seen as an integral part of this process.

Infrastructure

New sources of funding are required to assist in building global, national and local structures. A concerted effort will need to be harnessed by governmental, non-governmental, educational institutions and the private sector. Greater emphasis is now being placed on settings for health.

Conclusion

Healthy communities need a concerted effort on the part of policy advisers, planners, health professionals and voluntary groups. Investing in social capital requires an understanding of empowering people. This requires practical application to realise health improvement and ambitions. It also requires a contribution from governments in terms of economic resources, and building an infrastructure to mobilise opportunity for its communities.

The contribution of community nurses towards shaping healthy communities is now being recognised by policy frameworks. The development of knowledge, skills and further research into the needs of clients, from a variety of backgrounds and circumstances, is now an ongoing aspect of the work of nurses. Many now recognise the need to become more proactive in ensuring that actions are firmly based within the available evidence, which they may have to seek.

As a student, your role is an equally important one, as you prepare to become a practitioner for the future. The need to stimulate discussion and debate while gaining your experience in the community will help to generate a healthy approach to understanding theoretical concepts, and applying these to practice.

Further reading

Heritage, Z. (1994) *Community Participation in Primary Care*. Occasional Paper 64, January. London, Royal College of General Practitioners.

Sourtzi, P., Nolan, P. and Andrews, R. (1996) Evaluation of health promotion activities in community nursing practice, *Journal of Advanced Nursing*, 24: 1214–23.

Thomas, J. and Wainwright, P. (1996) Community nurses and health promotion: ethical and political perspectives, *Nursing Ethics*, 3(2): 97–107.

Wilkinson, R. (1996) *Unhealthy Societies*. London, Routledge.

USEFUL WEB SITES

European Network of Health Promotion Agencies (ENHPA) www.nigz.nl/enhpa.html

European Public Health Alliance www.epha.org

World Health Organization (WHO) www.who.int/regions/weu.html

Healthy Cities Project www.who.dk/healthy-cities/

Department of Health UK www.doh.gov.uk

Our Healthier Nation and other government health reports can be located at: www.official-documents.co.uk/document/cm43/4386/4386.htm

Health Development Agency Enquiries www.hea.org.uk

References

Ahmad, W. and Atkin, K. (1996) *'Race' and Community Care*. Buckingham, Open University Press.

Baum, F.E. and Saunders, D. (1993) Healthy cities and change: social movement or bureaucratic tool? *Health Promotion International*, 8: 31–41.

Baum, F.E. and Saunders, D. (1995) Can health promotion and primary health care achieve Health for All without a return to the more radical agenda? *Health Promotion International*, 10: 149–60.

Blane, D., Brunner, E. and Wilkinson, R. (1997) *Health and Social Organization: Towards A Health Policy for the 21st Century*. London, Routledge.

Blaxter, M. (1984) Equity and consultation rates in general practice. *British Medical Journal*, 288: 1963–7.

Bryant, J.H. (1988) Health for All: the dream and the reality. *World Health Forum*, 9: 291–302.

Butterworth, C.A. (1988) Breaking the boundaries: new endeavours in community nursing (inaugural lecture). Manchester: University of Manchester Department of Nursing.

Calman, K. and Hine, D. (1995) *A Policy Framework for Commissioning Cancer Services*. London, DoH/Welsh Office.

De Kadt, E. (1982) Ideology, social policy, health and health services: a field of complex interactions. *Social Science and Medicine*, 16: 741–52.

Department of Health (1991) *Health of the Nation*. London, HMSO.

Department of Health (1997) *The New NHS: Modern, Dependable*. London, HMSO.

Department of Health (1998) *Our Healthier Nation*. London, HMSO.

Ebrahim, S. and Kalache, A. (1996) *Epidemiology in Old Age*. London, BMJ Publishing/WHO.

Green, A. (1994) Decisions about health servies should not be made purely on the basis of achieving efficient allocation and utilisation of resources. *World Health Forum*, **15**: 30–1.

Ham, C. and Mitchell, J. (1990) A force to reckon with. *Health Service Journal*, **100**: 164–5.

Hetzel, B.S. (1989) Healthy public policy in the Third World. *Health Promotion*, **4**: 57–61.

Hoskins, A. and Maxwell, R. (1990) Contracts and quality of care. *British Medical Journal*, **300**: 919–22.

Loury, G. (1977) A dynamic theory of racial income differences. In Wallace, P.A. and Le Mund, A. (eds) *Women, Minorities and Employment Discrimination*. Massachusetts, Lexington Books.

Mangelsdorf, K.L., Luna, J. and Smith, H.L. (1988) Primary health care and public policy. *World Health Forum*, **3**: 509–13.

Mburu, F.M. (1989) Non-governmental organisations in the health field: collaboration, integration and contrasting aims in Africa. *Social Science and Medicine*, **29**: 591–7.

Meyer, J.E. (1986) Exploratory study to describe the process and impact of introducing a new health education component into the basic nursing training curriculum. MSc Dissertation. London, King's College.

Meyer, J.E. (1988) Health promotion in basic nurse training conference paper. In Weare, K. (ed.) *Developing Health Promotion in Undergraduate Medical Education*. London, BMJ Publishing.

Noone, A. (1989) Do referral rates differ widely between practices and does supply of services affect demand? *Journal of the Royal College of General Practitioners*, **39**: 404–7.

Oakley, A. (1998) *Welfare Research: A Critique of Theory and Method*. London, Routledge.

Peabody, J.W. (1995) An organizational analysis of the World Health Organization: narrowing the gap between promise and performance. *Social Science and Medicine*, **40**: 731–42.

Portes, A. and Landolt, P. (1996) The downside of social capital. *The American Prospect*, May–June, **94**(26): 18–21.

Putnam, R.D. (1993) The prosperous community: social capital and public life. *The American Prospect*, **13**(Spring): 1–13.

Rathwell, T. (1992) The reality of Health For All 2000. *Social Science and Medicine*, **25**: 731–42.

Sherraden, M.S. and Wallace, S.P. (1992) Innovation in primary health care community health services in Mexico and the United States, *Social Science and Medicine*, **35**: 1433–43.

Smith, P., Masterson, A. and Lask, S. (1995) Health and the curriculum: an illuminative evaluation – Part 1: methodology, *Nurse Education Today*, **15**: 245–9.

Sourtzi, P., Nolan, P. and Andrews, R. (1996) Evaluation of health promotion activities in community nursing practice, *Journal of Advanced Nursing*, **24**: 1214–23.

Tarimo, E. and Webster, E.G. (1995) Primary Health Care Concepts and Challenges in a Changing World. Division of Strengthening of Health Services. Current Concerns. SHS Paper No. 7, Geneva, WHO.

Thomas, J. and Wainwright, P. (1996) Community nurses and health promotion: ethical and political perspectives, *Nursing Ethics*, 3(2): 97–107.

Tones, K. (1997) Health education as empowerment. In Sidell, M., Jones, L., Katz, J. and Peberdy, A. (eds) *Debates and Dilemmas in Promoting Health: A Reader*. Basingstoke, The Open University/Macmillan – now Palgrave. pp. 33–42.

Wilkinson, R. (1996) *Unhealthy Societies*. London, Routledge.

Woelk, G.B. (1994) Primary health care in Zimbabwe: can it survive? *Social Science and Medicine*, 39: 1027–35.

World Health Organization (1981) *Global Strategy for Health for All by the Year 2000*. Geneva, WHO.

World Health Organization (1985) *Targets for Health for All by the Year 2000*. Copenhagen, WHO.

World Health Organization (1986) *Ottawa Charter*. WHO Regional Office for Europe, Geneva, WHO.

World Health Organization (1987) Economic Support for National Health for All Strategies. A40/Technical Discussions No.2, Geneva, WHO.

World Health Organization (1993) Report of the Executive Board Working Group on the WHO Response to Global Change. Paper EB/92/4. Geneva, WHO.

World Health Organization (1997) The Fourth International Conference on Health Promotion: New Players for a new Era. The Jakarta Declaration. Geneva, WHO.

Zaidi, S.A. (1986) Why medical students will not practise in rural areas: evidence from a survey, *Social Science and Medicine*, 22: 527–33.

10

Coping with chronic illness in primary care settings

NAOMI A. WATSON

Learning outcomes

By the end of this chapter you will be able to:

- Define pathology in relation to chronic illnesses which may be encountered in the community.

- Identify a range of common pathological conditions that have been observed in the community, and understand their impact on patients and families.

- Discuss the provision of care for the chronically sick.

- Discuss the role of informal care in the support of patients who are chronically ill.

- Identify government initiatives, past and present, which support carers.

- Reflect on the role of the voluntary sector as seen while on placement in the community.

Introduction

This chapter will look at common chronic pathological conditions and the way they are managed in the community. The aim is to help you identify the features of chronic illnesses on your assessor's caseload, the impact on individuals and carers, and the support networks that exist within the legislative framework, to help patients and their families cope with chronic illness.

The present focus on shifting the balance of care for sick adults to the community could be seen by some as a mere continuation of a trend which has existed for some time. Indeed, it could be argued that the community has always been the focus of care for the chronically sick, and the role of the district nurse (DN) has, in the main, provided support for the chronically sick in the community. Working with other carers, especially informal networks, to ensure that the usual side effects from chronic conditions are appropriately cared for, is a key part of the DN's role. Additional support, for those who need it, is usually available from statutory, voluntary and informal service networks.

Murray and Lopez's (1996) Disability Adjusted Life Years (DALYs) scale, is a useful way of measuring the effect of chronic diseases on the life of individuals in the community. Among the range of chronic illnesses to be encountered in the community, the prevalence of conditions such as cancers, cardiovascular related illnesses, including strokes, heart disease, hypertension, diabetes, and other conditions such as Alzheimer's disease, are all a regular feature of the DN's caseload. Dealing with the side effects from these illnesses, however, could arguably be the major focus of the DN's work. Community health care should aim to promote good health, prevent ill health and enable people in the community to cope with illness or impairment (DHSS, 1986). These are activities that are central to the work of DNs. Patients with a chronic illness needing support, and having interventions from the DN should be able to receive this with the DN acting as co-ordinator for any other services that may be required.

The increasing number of older people in the community means that the caseload of the DN is likely to reflect this trend. While the majority of older people lead busy, active lives (Donnellan, 1995), those seen on the DN caseload may reflect resultant effects of a sedentary lifestyle, possibly brought on by a chronic illness. Butler (1997) argues that growing numbers of older people could mean an increasing burden in terms of disability for society, and hence for services in future. Warner and colleagues (1998) remind us that the bulk of care for older people is not provided by statutory services, but by families and other carer support networks who, by virtue of the demographic changes, will also be growing older.

Student Activity 10.1

♦ What would you say are the features of a chronic illness?

♦ How does this differ from an acute illness?

♦ Discuss your views with one or more of your peers.

♦ Keep notes in your portfolio.

Defining and understanding chronic illness

The use of the term 'chronic' to describe an illness indicates a persistent condition of long-term duration, where the disease progression is slow, or there may be little change generally. This differentiates it from an acute illness, which is usually resolved quite quickly (Thorne, 1993). The range of diseases involved is far reaching, with the common problem usually being that the condition remains with the affected person for the rest of the lifespan. The actual illness may not necessarily be as problematic as the side effects it causes.

These effects may or may not be observable, depending on the type of illness. For example, in the case of a problem such as a venous or arterial leg ulcer the physical effects will be quite marked, and may be disfiguring for the legs of the suffering patient.

'Silent' illnesses, such as hypertension and diabetes, where the outward physical effects may not always be seen, could become life threatening unless careful regular screening occurs.

Chronic illnesses are common to large numbers of people in the community. Their onset varies, and may be triggered by an acute episode, although it is possible for a disease to progressively develop over many years. Degenerative conditions are a good example here. The way individuals respond to their particular disease will vary according to the type of illness, their own perceptions of illness, and the social and cultural constructs within which they have

Student Activity 10.2

◆ Make a list of chronic conditions that you have encountered while on your placement, on your supervisor's caseload.

◆ Ask your supervisor how this compares to the caseloads of others in the team.

◆ Compare your list with those of your peers in another area.

◆ Are you able to notice any trends?

◆ Make a note of any trends, which you and your peers have been able to identify.

to live. Thorne (1993) agrees that people may not always be able to explain their personal experiences and feelings about a longstanding illness. However where side effects are obvious, this may help patients to articulate the problem. Unfortunately, in some instances, long-term conditions which require some kind of nursing intervention over a long period may tend to blur professional perspectives on the seriousness of the effects on patients. There may be a tendency to think that patients have assumed passive sick roles, rather than wishing to co-operate to get well (King, 1985). This may be because the general focus of care tends to be towards a more acute, curative approach, and hence the expectation of improvement in a chronic condition may still be a dominant feature of the care delivery process. The extent to which this is possible may not always be realistic (Thorne, 1993), although present policy in the UK discusses the need for health improvement programmes, intended to move individuals towards more positive health outcomes (DoH, 1997).

The chronic illness experience is heavily individualised and it is difficult (if not impossible) to be prescriptive about possible outcomes. One has to surmise, however, that a combination of approaches to care is as applicable here as in other situations. For example, an assessment of needs for an individual with a chronic illness will follow similar patterns to others. Identifying the demographic and epidemiological factors influencing the patient's condition, and looking at possible frameworks within which to plan and deliver care, will be important features of the process (see Chapter 8 for information on needs assessment).

Screening programmes and health promotion for these individuals may help to identify ways of alleviating and/or improving the actual effects of the illness, rather than curing the illness itself.

Some common conditions which may be chronic: effects on individuals and families

It is imperative that you remember that the side effects from these conditions may be more problematic for patients than the conditions themselves. Nonetheless, having a good understanding of the original reasons for a problem will help in the recognition and care of the physical effects on patients. Identifying the possible problems of patients who may be suffering from a particular condition may help you to better understand the patient's perspective on the effects of the illness. For example, the patient suffering from an AIDS-related illness may perhaps be dealing with social isolation, or family rejection, depending on the community in which they live, and the involvement and knowledge of their family. The level of isolation may also be dependent on what is known about the cause of the disease.

Patients who are suffering from problems related to haemoglobinopathies (for example sickle cell anaemia, thalassaemia) may have no outward signs of a problem, but may suffer varying levels of severe pain which may not always be understood by formal carers (Anionwu and At, 2000). The patient who has problems with circulation, and has a resultant arterial or leg ulcer, will have obvious disfigurement of affected leg(s), and will suffer from the effects of altered body image. The same will be true for patients who suffer from a neurological condition, such as a degenerative motor neurone disease where physical changes are obvious even if they have been slow to develop.

While the obvious physical effects can be quite marked, the social and emotional effects can also be devastating, as much for family members as for patients themselves. If we remember that the family usually bears the main burden of care for chronically sick members, it is easy to understand that this will affect them. This does not apply only to the many adjustments that will be needed in the family to provide care, but also to the impact on family relationships which can be quite marked.

King (1985) found that chronic illness within a family is usually characterised by chronic grief, which may follow a staged process involving a reaction to loss (Chapter 14 provides an overview of the grieving process). This is understandable, given the fact that family members may remember a once active patient, who has been slowly reduced to dependence, and the resultant pain that this brings to the individual concerned. Loss, in these circumstances, is related to loss of function of an organ, strength, independence, sexual function, ability to pursue previous leisure activities, body image, self-worth, feeling of well-being, and role related losses such as loss of the ability to function in family, work or social roles. The grieving process may be experienced by patients themselves, and by significant family members. Community nurses caring for patients need to be aware of this, so that stages in the process can be recognised for what they are, and appropriate support provided when needed.

Challenges to patients and families

Patients with a chronic illness have to live their lives, dealing with the personal, family and illness problems that each day brings. Patterns of dealing with this will vary, as individuals will have different personal skills, different support networks, and different social and cultural perspectives on what is happening to them. For most patients, however, dealing with the daily issues of a chronic illness may include efforts to prevent any acute crisis, or managing one when it occurs. This involves being able to recognise and deal with these events. Patients will also perhaps have to make sure that medical treatment regimes are being followed. This could include having to deal with debilitating side effects from such regimes. Living with a chronic illness involves immense adjustment. Lifestyles will have to be modified and social interactions re-negotiated, with priorities being changed and the environment adapted to accommodate possible physical symptoms of the illness.

Where treatment regimes (for example regular dialysis) are time consuming and frequent, family routines may be disrupted, and the patient easily fatigued. Adjusting family patterns to cope with this is going to be essential. Where the outcome of an illness is unpredictable, this could put strains on family relationships and make management difficult. Troublesome symptoms may cause major social disruption resulting in isolation of the patient, and the process of adjustment should perhaps be focused on living life as normally as possible, in order to make the illness and its effects as acceptable as possible. Patients will usually be helped in the process by significant others within the family, who will assist, protect, control and generally cover for the sick person, acting as their agent (Strauss et al., 1984; Corbin and Strauss, 1991).

Loeb and colleagues (1992) identify a list of conditions, which may be chronic and have visible, physical and/or non-visible effects on patients and families, that community nurses should be aware of. It is of course imperative to remember that many patients cope with a multiplicity of complex problems, all of which may contribute to the chronic state of their ill health. The problems may be interrelated, hence the need for knowledge about the conditions, combined with an awareness that the personal effects on individuals could be very different. When set within an appropriate conceptual framework, the holistic approach to identifying the patient's needs should ensure that the actual disease does not become the focus of the search. Rather, this should be the impact of the disease on the person's life. This does not, however, negate the need to be aware of what these conditions are. Understanding the aetiology and likely outcomes will ensure that you are better informed when discussing these issues with patients, their carers and members of the multidisciplinary team. The list does not include the myriad of social situations which may contribute to chronic illnesses, including violence and family problems, alcohol and related addictions or other social and environmental problems such as homelessness and workplace health problems (Smith et al., 2000).

- *Cardiovascular/circulatory conditions:* for example venous/arterial leg ulcers, coronary artery disease, hypertension, congestive heart failure, valvular heart disease, chronic arterial occlusive disease.

- *Respiratory conditions:* for example asthma, cystic fibrosis, occupational respiratory diseases, chronic obstructive pulmonary disease.

- *Neurological conditions:* for example Parkinson's disease, Alzheimer's disease, multiple sclerosis.

- *Immune and haematological conditions:* for example AIDS, haemophilia, sickle cell disease, thalassaemia, rheumatoid arthritis, systemic lupus erythomatosus (SLE), iron deficiency anaemia.

- *Cancers:* for example lung cancer, colorectal cancer, laryngeal cancer, leukemia, breast cancer, cervical cancer, bladder cancer, testicular cancer.

- *Gastrointestinal conditions:* for example irritable bowel syndrome, inflammatory bowel disease, cirrhosis, chronic pancreatitis, hiatus hernia, constipation, faecal incontinence.

- *Endocrine conditions:* for example diabetes mellitus, hyperthyroidism, hypothyroidism.

- *Renal and urological conditions:* for example chronic renal failure, neurogenic bladder, urinary incontinence.

- *Gynaecological conditions:* for example endometriosis, infertility.

- *Musculoskeletal conditions:* for example osteoporosis, osteoarthritis, chronic low back pain, scoliosis.

Student Activity 10.3

- From the list of chronic conditions, choose one or two, and identify specific effects from which patients are likely to suffer.

- Negotiate with your assessor for an opportunity to talk to some of the patients on his or her caseload, to see whether your list corresponds with what patients actually say about the effects of the condition on their lives, and on their families.

- Keep a record in your portfolio.

Provision of care for the chronically sick: the district nurse

The community provides care for individuals who are chronically sick in a variety of ways. The range of care providers varies depending on the type if care that is required (see Chapter 1). Statutory providers of care include health services and social services and, where appropriate, you should experience joint assessments between these two major providers taking place in the community (see Chapter 8 for more information about needs assessment). The role of the DN as a key worker in this provision has been identified by all the policy documents since 1990 (DoH, 1990, 1997, 1999). However, Nolan and Nolan (1995) argue that some types of care strategies reflect treatment for acute illnesses. Corbin and Strauss (1991) have developed a trajectory scale as a model for delivery of care to chronically sick patients. While there is a requirement for increased collaboration across all providers, it could be argued that this is more important for DNs and social services providers, given their roles as key participants in care for the chronically sick. Other providers include the voluntary sector, now a major force in care delivery, supporting patients and families. Groups with interest in particular diseases, such as diabetes, asthma, AIDS, and Alzheimer's disease, have long participated in providing care within a specific focus. The private sector, providing nursing homes, and agencies enabling patients to access care for a fee, are also recognised as being key players in terms of what is available in the community. DNs are required to work closely with them to ensure that patients gain the most appropriate service. Informal carers, however, form the majority of caregivers in the community, and have now been recognised within legislation as requiring particular support from DNs.

Student Activity 10.4

♦ Choose one case from the list of pathological conditions which you made earlier.

♦ Reflect on the person who is suffering from this chronic condition, and ask your supervisor about the individual.

♦ Find out how this person is supported with the illness.

♦ Who are the informal carers involved?

♦ Are there any voluntary services in use?

♦ Find out who the voluntary providers are, and whether the provision is free.

♦ Look up the article by Corbin and Strauss (1991), cited in the reference list.

♦ After reading this, make sure you understand how a trajectory model may be applied in the community.

♦ Discuss this with your assessor.

♦ Make notes in your portfolio.

The role of informal care in the support of patients: policy initiatives

Family caregivers play a key role in supporting and caring for patients who are chronically sick. From as far back as 1982, the Equal Opportunities

Commission (EOC, 1982) supported the voice of carers, recognising the majority of them as being women. Informal care is usually unpaid care. Family members provide this out of a feeling of duty, and the member of the family providing the most care is usually female. The care provided is said to save the government billions of pounds each year, hence the continued emphasis on ensuring that the role of informal care is recognised. Family caregivers undergo tremendous changes in response to the chronic illness of their relative. Major adjustments in lifestyle take place not just for the affected individual, but for the carers as well. The loss of normal function has an impact physically, socially, psychologically and economically (King, 1985). The accompanying grief will also have an impact on formal caregivers, in both negative and positive ways. In line with the staged process of grieving (see Chapter 14 for more information on death and dying), feelings of denial, anger, sadness and withdrawal may all precede coming to terms with the condition and attempting to live life as normally as possible. Family members often feel powerless at being unable to do much, if anything, to reverse the situation (Miller, 1992). The responses experienced will vary depending on the type of illness, and the visibility or outward effects of the condition.

Changes in family composition over the years have altered the structure, and in part, the function of the family (Dimond and Jones, 1983). However, even where there are major adjustments, it is still recognised that this unit still accounts for most of the care needed.

The work of the DN with family caregivers is now set firmly within the policy, requiring that all regular carers of the chronically sick be recognised, and action taken to ensure that their needs are met (DoH, 1995). This entitles regular carers to their own assessment of their care needs, with the requirement that plans are set in place to ensure that these needs are being addressed. The need to work in partnership is also a requirement within this context, especially relevant to local authority providers of social care services and DNs. Those caring for individuals as part of a voluntary organisation are not included in this provision, neither is it clear how the role of close friends and neighbours will be perceived, and whether an assessment will be possible in those circumstances.

Family carers are involved in a range of activities, which aim to support the sick member. These activities range from administering treatments, applying certain dressings, collecting prescriptions, accompanying the patient to attend hospitals or other community centres, providing transport, escorting and being there when needed. They are involved in handling any crisis that may occur as a result of the condition, and are usually there to help following the event. Lubkin (1990) describes the role of family caregivers as being either care providers or care managers. The role in use will depend on the economic situation of the family. Lubkin argues that where there is appropriate funding, care managers will arrange for caring tasks to be done by others, and pay for this facility. She also argues that where providers immerse themselves in physically meeting all the needs of the patient, psychosocial needs (described by her as transporting, for shopping and so on) may not be met. The evidence for this in the UK is still unclear, although the nature of the illness will dictate the amount of intervention from family carers. But the major strength is that they are usually on call 24 hours a day if and when needed.

Because the majority of carers are women, the way the care is provided may be dependent on the amount of information known about diet, medication, and available health and social services. This may be especially difficult to manage effectively following discharge from a period in hospital. In a grounded study of strategies used by mothers and daughters, Bull and Jervis (1997) concluded that difficulties in care management post discharge were because of lack of relevant information. Nonetheless, carers do the very best they can, even without appropriate support from statutory services. The new Carers (Recognition and Services) Act 1995 now ensures that the voice of carers can be heard, and their views listened to, and used in assessment, planning and delivery of care.

The role of the voluntary sector in supporting carers

Patients in the community have a long history of self-support, usually initiated by a concerned carer, or patient who has been dissatisfied with the level of statutory response in terms of service availability. As a result they have mobilised themselves, with or without the support of community nurses, and formed pressure groups, to lobby locally and/or nationally for more funds. Consequently, a wide range of voluntary organisations has grown out of these groups, many of which have become quite powerful national lobby groups. The voluntary sector is well established, and past and present governments have recognised the key role that they play in the provision of a range of services, reflecting both health and social care, to the community. There is a requirement that, when forging partnerships, the voluntary sector must also

Student Activity 10.5

♦ Find out from your assessor if there is a carers' support network in your locality.

♦ If there is, make arrangements to visit the group, to find out how support is organised.

♦ If there isn't one, ask your assessor why.

♦ Find out from your peers in a neighbouring locality if there is one.

♦ Make notes in your portfolio.

be considered as part of the equation, and should be consulted in the decision-making processes preceding planning and delivering care (DoH, 1990, 1997). The examples are numerous, but mention of cancer services is one area where the voluntary sector has made great contributions. The hospice movement was borne out of voluntary services, as were Macmillan Cancer Relief and the Marie Curie Foundation.

In this area, funding is usually from private individuals who may use a variety of sources, such as local or national fundraising events and donations from members of the public. Other major voluntary organisations, also involved in research and education, include Age Concern, the British Red Cross, and MIND (the Foundation for Mental Health). Support for older people is extensive, providing care or assistance with caring in a variety of ways. This could be with helping individuals to remain as independent as possible, or supporting them when they need help with an illness.

Many new voluntary organisations are equally successful in supporting individuals locally and nationally. For the majority of illnesses, a voluntary group is usually able to provide support, information and guidance to people in the community.

The voluntary sector is still growing. As a student, you should ensure that you spend some time finding out about the work of the voluntary sector in your locality, and the specific ways in which they help people in the community. Within the process of needs assessment (see Chapter 8), the requirement that you spend time finding out about facilities, include all services provided by the voluntary sector.

Student Activity 10.6

◆ Choose a patient from your DN's caseload, with an unusual illness, if possible.

◆ Find out if there are any voluntary groups specific to that problem, locally or nationally.

◆ Ask your DN to help you decide how you are going to search for the information nationally.

◆ If there is no support group or voluntary body, make notes about how you think one could be established in that locality. What do you think would be the requirements for setting up such a group?

◆ Keep a record of your notes in your portfolio.

Health promotion in chronic illness

Promoting the health of people with a chronic illness may sound like a task with the promise of low returns. As you work with your assessor in your placement locality, however, you will observe activities which aim to help patients to cope with their illness. This is a basic requirement of all community nurses, who should be able to recognise the need for this type of activity, and ensure that it is an integral part of their work with individuals and families. For example, helping patients to regain control of their lives could take a variety of forms. It may involve sharing relevant information about matters relating to the patient's illness which will contribute to the decision-making process. McDermott (1995) argues that optimising quality of life in chronic illness, along with meeting health promotion needs, have not always been adequately catered for. Policy should ensure that emotional and rehabilitation needs are being met through appropriate access to care. The patient with a venous leg ulcer would need to be informed about the value of particular types of treatment following appropriate assessment of the wound. Collier (1999) stated that optimising the healing potential of the patient is important. While he did not discuss the role of health promotion specifically, one could argue that any activity that is optimising the healing potential must, by its very nature, include an element of health promotion. In order to promote an understanding of why a treatment (which may not be too popular with the patient) is being recommended, the DN will have to engage in discussion with the patient. It is possible that this approach may help the patient become more compliant. Ensuring that patients are better informed about treatment regimes and the reasons for them is an important part of the process of promoting health.

If the majority of patients suffering from chronic illnesses are older people, the health promotion possibilities will be quite extensive. This will involve the DN in understanding how a sedentary lifestyle may have contributed to the patient's condition, and give suggestions of ways of alleviating the problem.

The opportunities for helping patients to achieve better health outcomes through health promotion activities have the potential of increasing the confidence of patients and carers, thus helping to reduce feelings of powerlessness, which may have accompanied their illness (Miller, 1992). The role of the DN is not just to provide physical care, but to be aware of the other factors which may have an impact on patients, and be able to mobilise support individually or with other members of the primary health care team to ensure that patients have the option of achieving the best outcomes possible in terms of their condition. The same is true for family carers and their needs. DNs may have to be the ones to identify potential problems or risks to the health of family carers, and this may need to be discussed, with appropriate action being planned. For example, advice on burnout, and providing information about respite care services to carers, could be seen as health promotion activities. With the needs of carers now forming a major part of the requirement, this role is essential, and needs to be identifiable in practice settings. (See Chapter 9 for further background into the need for health promotion activities in the community.)

Leveille and colleagues (1998) argue that in order to reduce disability risks and promote self-management of chronic illness, greater partnership with primary care teams (the equivalent of the PHCT in the UK) is essential for community nurses. Their study found that where an integrated programme of health promotion, functioning and health care utilisation was set up and delivered, this actually improved the function of those suffering with a chronic illness, and reduced the numbers becoming in-patients.

It is imperative that DNs recognise the important part they have to play in this process, and take steps to ensure that this is an integral part of their work with patients and their carers.

Conclusion

This chapter has considered the way that chronic illnesses impact on the lives of individuals and their carers in the community. The way care is being provided, and the support networks, which help people to cope within their own environments have been discussed. The legal frameworks, which identify new roles for community nurses, aim to ensure that the carers of chronically sick patients are given special priority in terms of their important role as caregivers. Because the bulk of the DN's work involves caring for the side effects of most chronic conditions, he or she is an important key worker who should participate in the development of policies, which will shape the way services develop to patients who are chronically sick. To do this effectively, an awareness of the legislative requirements, and application of the evidence from the literature should provide a sound basis from which to structure services, which will improve health outcomes for patients and their significant caregivers. The challenges of providing care to chronically sick patients have to be recognised by DNs, and the use of models, which tend to reflect intervention for acute care needs to be revised (Nolan and Nolan, 1995).

Further reading

Biegel, D., Sales, E. and Schulz, R. (1991) *Family Care-giving in Chronic Illness*. London, Sage.

References

Anionwu, E. and At, K, (2000) *The Politics of Sickle Cell and Thalassaemia*. Buckinghamshire, Open University Press.
Biegel, D., Sales, E. and Schultz, R. (1991) *Family Care-giving in Chronic Illness*. London, Sage.
Bull, M.J. and Jervis, L.L. (1997) Strategies used by chronically ill older women and their caregiving daughters in managing post hospital care. *Journal of Advanced Nursing*, **25**(3): 541–7.

Butler, B. (1997) *Ageing Beyond the Millennium*. London, Nuffield Trust, Age Concern, Cymru Wales.

Collier, M. (1999) Venous leg ulceration. In Miller, M. and Glover, D. (1999) *Wound Management: Theory and Practice*. London, NursingTimes books.

Corbin, J.M. and Strauss, A. (1991) A nursing model for chronic illness management based upon the trajectory framework. *Scholarly Inquiry for Nursing Practice*, 5(3): 155–74.

Cullum, N. and Roe, B. (1995) *Leg Ulcers: Nursing Management*. London, Scutari Press.

Department of Health (1990) *The NHS and Community Care Act*. London, HMSO.

Department of Health (1997) *The New NHS: Modern, Dependable*. London, DoH.

Department of Health (1999) *Making a Difference: Strengthening the Nursing, Midwifery and Health Visiting Contribution to Health and Health Care*. London, HMSO.

Department of Health and Social Security (1986) *Neighbourhood Nursing* (The Cumberlege Report). London, HMSO.

Dimond, M. and Jones, S.L. (1983) *Chronic Illness Across the Life Span*. USA, Appleton Century Crofts.

Donnellan, C. (1995) *Our Ageing Generation: Issues for the Nineties*. Cambridge, Independence Education Publishers.

Equal Opportunities Commission (1982) *Who Cares for the Carers?* Manchester, EOC.

King, E. (1985) *Long-term Care*. London, Churchill Livingstone.

Leveille, S.G., Wagner, E.H., Davis, C., Grothaus, L., Wallace, J., Logerfo, M. and Kent, D. (1998) Preventing disability and managing chronic illness in frail older adults: a randomized trial of a community based partnership with primary care. *Journal of American Geriatrics Society*, 46(10): 1191–8.

Loeb, S., Cahill, M., and McVan, B. (1992) *Teaching Patients with Chronic Conditions*. Boston, Springhouse Cooperation.

Lubkin, I.M. (1990) *Chronic Illness Impact and Interventions*, 2nd edn. Boston, Jones and Bartlett.

McDermott, S. (1995) The health promotion needs of older people. *Professional Nurse*, 10(8): 530–3.

Miller, J.F. (1992) *Coping with Chronic Illness: Overcoming Powerlessness*, 2nd edn. Philadelphia, F.A. Davis.

Murray, C.J. and Lopez, D. (1996) *Quantifying Global Health Risks: Estimates of the Burden of Disease Attributable to Selected Risk Factors*. Cambridge, Mass: Harvard University Press.

Nolan, M. and Nolan, J. (1995) Responding to the challenge of chronic illness. *British Journal of Nursing*, 4(3): 145–7.

Nolan, M., Grant, G. and Keady, J. (1996) *Understanding Family Care*. Buckinghamshire, Open University Press.

Smith, C.M. and Maurer, F.A. (2000) *Community Health Nursing, Theory and Practice*, 2nd edn. London, W.B. Saunders.

Strauss, A.L., Corbin, J., Fagerhaugh, S., Glaser, B., Maines, D., Suczek, B. and Weiner, C. (1984) *Chronic Illness and the Quality of Life*, 2nd edn. St Louis, Mosby.

Thorne, S. (1993) *Negotiating Health Care – The Social Context of Chronic Illness*. London, Sage.

Warner, M. , Langley, M., Gould, E. and Picek, A. (1998) *Health Care Futures 2001*. Cardiff, Welsh Institute for Health and Social Care.

11 Promoting mental health in primary care

CAROL WILKINSON
and SAM MAURIMOOTOO

Learning outcomes

By the end of this chapter you will have been introduced to:

- An awareness of mental health as an issue which may have an impact on the physical health of adult patients.
- The policy implications of more effective partnerships between health care professionals in the community.
- The available support for patients with mental health problems in the community, and the role of the community psychiatric nurse (CPN) within this framework.
- The meanings of some common terms used within the context of mental health.
- Mental health promotion and its likely benefits in improving and maintaining positive health outcomes for patients in the community.
- Issues and implications relating to the mental health care of older people, as raised in the Audit Commission's report (2000).

Introduction

This chapter is intended to provide a general introduction to some of the mental health issues you are likely to encounter during your placement in the community. Specific roles in mental health care will be highlighted, particularly that of the community psychiatric nurse (CPN) in maintaining health and well-being. The multidisciplinary relationships are considered within the context of the policy requirements, which expect all care providers to collaborate effectively to ensure the best health outcomes for all patients (DoH, 1993). As an adult nurse caring for sick adults, you are likely to encounter patients with a wide range of health care needs. It is imperative that, as a student, you are able to understand the likely impact of physical illness on mental health, and the appropriate support that may be needed by patients with mental health needs. Mental health promotion as a concept is also introduced in light of recent developments in community health care.

History and background

Mental illness has a long history of being shrouded in fear and revulsion, and throughout the centuries there has been a perception that those suffering from a mental illness were evil. This goes back to biblical and other ancient documents, which contain many references to madness or mental illness.

These are usually described in terms of possession by devils or evil spirits. The misapprehension that mental illness is governed by the moon (hence the term 'lunatic') became formally adopted during the 19th century and is still commonly held by some people.

This fear arising out of ignorance of the causes of mental illness, together with the use of excessive measures of treatment and types of custodial 'care' led to appalling treatment of the mentally ill. In the 18th century those considered to be afflicted were locked up in gaols, poor houses and lunatics' prisons in insanitary conditions. They were often chained up, starved and beaten. It was by no means uncommon for people to visit the so called 'madhouses' to taunt and provoke the unfortunate inmates as a form of entertainment. The private sector also ran mental institutions for profit and it became commonplace for people to be detained in them wrongfully. This might happen, for example, if a man wanted to get rid of his wife, or if a woman had fallen pregnant and was not in a legitimate relationship. They were hidden away to prevent social stigma. The laws of the day permitted the insane to be locked up in some secure place for as long as their madness was deemed to continue. Their property was often seized to pay for their main-tenance (Busfield, 1986).

By the 19th century, changes in legislation permitted the erection of county asylums. These were large prison-like constructions, located in remote rural areas. They were a safe distance away from centres of population. Many of these remain today, still used as psychiatric hospitals, improved and upgraded to allow for modern standards and methods of treatment.

Further legislation passed during the 1850s meant protection for people being wrongfully detained in asylums. The effect, however, was not apparent until well into the 20th century. The pattern of care of the mentally ill devel-oped as long-term custodial care. People committed to these institutions remained there for life. The prime entry into mental institutions was through admission by certification or compulsory detention. It was not until 1930 that it became possible for individuals to choose to enter hospital as voluntary patients, and to make their own decision to leave. Until 1948, voluntary patients had to give 72 hours notice of their intention to leave hospital. Certification remained a judicial rather than a medical phenom-enon (Fraser, 1975).

By the 1950s, progress in the treatment of the mentally ill took various approaches. Pharmacological research had produced a range of tranquillising drugs which replaced many of the physical restraints such as padded cells or straightjackets. Anti-depressant and neuroleptic drugs (for the treatment of schizophrenia) became available. Electro-convulsive therapy became the treatment of choice for depression. Mental illness came to be perceived as something that was episodic as opposed to life-long. It was now seen as a condition that could be treated (the medicalisation of mental health). Psychotherapy became a popular phenomenon during the 1970s and was regarded as a useful aid to recovery (Baly, 1980).

The Mental Health Act 1959 removed the concept of certification of insanity, replacing it with that of compulsory admission to hospital for observation and treatment. The grounds for compulsory admission were that a person had to be deemed mentally disordered, was unwilling to be admitted to or to stay in hospital and was a danger to him or herself, or to others. The procedure for admission was taken from the courts and placed in the hands of doctors and social workers. It also placed considerable restriction on the length of time for which anyone could be detained.

The 1983 Mental Health Act was similar in essence to the 1959 Act. It introduced further safeguards for the rights of the individual. However:

- It strengthened the previous legislation in that it shortened the length of time people could be detained without review.

- It strengthened patients' rights to appeal against detention.

- It instituted independent reviews of some patients detained for the longer periods permissible.

- It required independent medical second opinions with regard to some treatments such as electro-convulsive therapy (ECT).

- It also removed alcoholism as a sufficient medical reason for detention in hospital.

Mental health in primary care

Mental health problems may be experienced by one in seven people, and the precipitating factors often include loneliness, isolation, loss of social contacts, poor social networks and homelessness. Goldberg (1991) believes that these problems may occur as a result of stressful life events including bereavement, divorce, separation, new additions to the family, redundancy and unemploy-

---

Student Activity 11.1

- ◆ Find out from your DN assessor whether there are any awareness sessions for those who may have to care for the physical illness of a patient who also has a mental health problem.

- ◆ How are assessments planned?

- ◆ Who does the referral?

- ◆ Find out if there are any patients on your assessor/supervisor's caseload who have, or are likely to have, a mental health problem.

ment, and that at least one in four adults will experience mental health problems in any one year.

The most common health problems tend to be depression, eating disorders and anxiety disorders. Many of these can be treated effectively in primary care, although some may need quick referral to specialist services (DoH, 1998, 1999).

Clarifying meanings

Mental illness is that form of illness which presents mainly psychological symptoms and/or disturbances of behaviour, which may be incompatible with normal social functioning. But some forms of mental illness are not so clearly defined. *Mental health* is a positive sense of well-being that encompasses the spiritual and emotional resilience which enables individuals to enjoy their lives. It is about self-worth and surviving sadness, pain and disappointment with a sense of dignity. *Community mental health promotion* aims to build social networks, developing and enhancing life skills that will enable people to cope and be supportive to their families and friends in their locality. Within the community a variety of terms are commonly used within the context of mental health care. You will need to be familiar with them. These terms become relevant if you have to provide care for the physical illnesses of a patient who may have been identified as having mental health needs. Your assessor may have to work closely with one or more of these care workers.

- *Key worker*: the identified individual from a team (uni or multi-disciplinary) who will provide the focal point for service provision from that team and link with the potential service providers for the individual (Meteyard, 1990).
- *Case manager*: a similarly identified role to the key worker, with a more comprehensively addressed degree of responsibility for assessment, potential direct service provisions and co-ordination of other service providers across the full range of individual client needs and strengths (Ryan et al., 1991; Onyett, 1992).
- *Care manager*: has an identified duty to make a broad overview assessment of the community needs of an individual client, calling for specialist assessment in priority areas, develop the package of care and commission specific services, which may or may not involve direct service provision. Review may remain with the care manager or be shared with others such as case managers or key workers.
- *Community psychiatric nurse (CPN)*: a qualified psychiatric nurse working in the community.

The various health professionals will all be contributing towards a *care programme*. This is a process established for psychiatric patients in hospital to ensure discharge to adequately assessed and developed care. It requires close co-operation of health care and social care providers in hospital and in the community. The responsibility for developing the plan lies with the consultant psychiatrist. Some liaison work is taken forward with case managers or key workers (Ryan et al., 1991; Onyett, 1992).

As a student nurse, you will be involved in the process of maintaining well-being. With help from your assessor or supervisor, you will need to demonstrate knowledge of the client group in their care and empathy. Observation and communication will be a vital part of this role. Observing how members of the primary health care team (PHCT) collaborate to benefit patients will be vital. The same is true of the ability to observe the effects of physical illness on the mental state of patients, in order to be able to take appropriate action on the patient's behalf.

Mental health promotion

Mental health promotion involves a number of approaches to improving well-being:

1. It is strengthening the capacity of individuals to cope with emotional problems through building self-esteem, enhancing life skills and developing coping mechanisms.

2. It is enabling communities to develop strategies to assist well-being. For example, policies, strategies, training and skills to prevent and stop bullying at schools and in the workplace.

3. It is about removing barriers and promoting inclusion, which covers access to services and acknowledging the rights and capacities of the user.

4. It is about ensuring that physical illness does not contribute to a deterioration of the patient's mental health.

The importance of social networks

Those people most susceptible to mental health problems in the community are the ones who tend towards social isolation and a lack of support networks. Increasing social mobility in Britain over the last 30 years, family breakdown and an increase in lone parent communities has precipitated part of the picture in this growing isolation. The individual's nearest relative may be 40 miles away. The only daily contact may be with their next door neighbour. Some may live with just a pet for company, and would welcome the opportunity of a visit even for a cup of tea and a chat for half an hour. Making use of local amenities, for example leisure centres or shops, can be encouraged where possible (see Chapter 8 for community profiling).

Social support can encompass the interpersonal transactions that include love and respect (affect), acknowledgement of appropriateness of actions or statements (affirmation) and the provision of aid by way of information, money and so forth. Social networks enable people to maintain their individual social identity as well as to receive emotional support and contact with others.

Student Activity 11.2

- ◆ Read Mick Carpenter's Chapter 'Asylum Nursing Before 1914: A Chapter in the History of Labour' in *Rewriting Nursing History*, edited by Celia Davies (1980).

- ◆ Compare the distinct impressions created by Carpenter of psychiatric nursing during that period with today.

- ◆ How do you think this has changed?

- ◆ Discuss with one or more of your peers.

- ◆ Make notes in your portfolio.

Characteristics of long-term mental illness

People with long-term mental illness are living in the community, with or without stable accommodation. Some of them will have spent long periods of time in hospital. Others will have had regular contact with formal psychiatric services over long periods of time, including many short hospital admissions. In a few cases distress will have been experienced over a long time, but without the person having much, if any, previous contact with formal services.

In psychiatric terms, the majority of these clients have been described as suffering from psychotic illness, usually schizophrenia. They are often also characterised by a long history with multiple diagnoses, reflecting both the complexities of the clinical manifestation and the difficulties in achieving a consensus of opinion.

Patients with long-term mental illness are likely to have experienced difficulty in establishing and maintaining personal relationships, often resulting in poor networks of support and social isolation. Family relationships can vary from offering the very highest quality support to being severely critical,

Student Activity 11.3

- ◆ Talk to your assessor about a patient on the caseload who has a mental illness.

- ◆ Look at the profile of the patient, for example age, sex, support network and so on.

- ◆ Find out whether the patient's physical condition has had any impact on their emotional state.

- ◆ Keep a record of your findings.

rejecting and intensifying the wider felt social stigma associated with society's views of serious mental disturbance.

They have complex multiple needs, including a high incidence of ill health resulting from serious social and economic disadvantages in addition to the personal disadvantages implicit in the experience of severe distress. Inevitably, these patients will crop up on the DN's caseload, and the appropriate skills will be necessary to ensure that their needs are satisfactorily identified and met within the PHCT.

In the professional context, the value of specific training and the core skills of each profession must be recognised and remain vitally important. However, in a client-centred context they must be seen in a realistic light. The person with a long history of severe mental distress and fragmented relationships will find great difficulty separating out his or her own needs on professionally defined lines. Satisfactory models of care and treatment for the long-term mentally ill are still being developed (Bugge et al., 1999). There will be a need to establish close working relationships with each individual professional who deals with special areas of need. In the majority of cases, the client will respond to one professional as a focal point for discussing wants, needs and the wider range of services that may be available. Working closely with key workers is an absolute necessity for the DN, as this is the only way to ensure that care is as seamless as possible.

Establishing a rapport

It is necessary for you as a student nurse to build relationships with clients. First impressions are important on both sides so caution and an open approach are likely to yield a positive response in the first instance. You will obviously be working very closely with your assessor, and should be observant of the skills needed in these circumstances. Some are as follows:

- Avoid paperwork wherever possible, as this is about sharing basic information to establish a rapport.

- Create a positive atmosphere, attempting to focus on strengths, abilities and interests, not deficits and weaknesses.

- As far as possible, ensure equal power, through attempting to establish similar agendas.

- Create a comfortable atmosphere, by attention to the tone of your voice, your rate of speech and through active listening skills.

- Facilitate the breaking down of barriers, through appropriate worker self-disclosure that highlights similarities as well as differences in circumstances.

- Inject fun through discussion of lighter subjects or by using humour.

Case Study 11.1

Mrs Jay has recently returned home from hospital following the birth of her second daughter. Her husband was made redundant from his place of work four months ago and has been unable to find suitable employment. Over the last few weeks he has become increasingly agitated, has been drinking rather more alcohol than usual and arriving home at unpredictable hours. Their elder daughter has been responsible for her own needs and visits her next door neighbour after school for her evening meal.

Discuss the likely problems that may develop in this household. How might they be alleviated?

Mental illnesses

This section provides a brief summary of some types of mental illnesses that you may encounter in the community. This list is not exhaustive, and further reading will be necessary, depending on the type of symptoms which present themselves.

Neurosis

Neurosis is a mental disorder which does not affect the whole personality. It is characterised by exaggerated anxiety and tension. For example, in anxiety neurosis there is persistent anxiety and the accompanying symptoms of fear,

rapid pulse, sweating, trembling, loss of appetite and insomnia.
Obsessive/compulsive neurosis is characterised by compulsions and rumination (there is usually some pondering or meditation on the same idea continuously).

Psychosis

This is a severe mental illness affecting the whole personality. For example, manic depression where there are mild or severe attacks of elation or depression or both alternating.

Classifications

The field of mental disorders is a broad ranging one. However, for ease of explanation there are a series of disorders which come under the following classification.

Mental disorders are classified thus:

- Severe mental impairment, formerly known as mental handicap
- Psychopathy
- Neurotic illness
- Sexual disorders
- Functional psychoses.

Severe mental impairment

This is characterised by a failure to develop a normal degree of intelligence. As intelligence is a measure of a person's ability both to solve intellectual problems and acquire special skills, this failure means that the patient will experience more difficulties in dealing with life than those who are more fortunate.

Psychopathic personality

A person with a psychopathic personality will be unable to learn from his or her mistakes. Such an individual will also have difficulty in tolerating even mild degrees of frustration, find it hard to appreciate other people's emotional needs, and is likely to come into conflict with society. Treatment is usually requested by society rather than the individual. However, many people with these difficulties have insight into their behaviour and become depressed or anxious when they realise the mess they are making of their own and other people's lives. Such people may ask for treatment for their depression or anxiety.

Neurotic illness

Neurotic illnesses are divided into (i) anxiety states (ii) obsessional states and (iii) hysteria. The basic nature of the condition is a feeling of anxiety, which the individual attempts to reduce unconsciously by developing some form of symptom. The symptom may lead to the patient's escape from the stressful situation; it may represent the problems in a symbolic form, or it may be a somatic consequence of anxiety. The type of symptom developed will depend on the individual underlying personality and the nature of the stress he or she is experiencing.

Sexual disorders

These conditions do not really form a separate group. Sexual deviations may result from neurotic conditions or as a part of a general psychopathic problem. The sexual relationship is the most intense and thus, the most difficult of all human relationships. It is a potent source of stress. This is increased because of the moralistic aspects that equate sex and sin.

Functional psychoses

These are illnesses in which it is thought, but not proven, that there is an underlying malfunction of the brain, probably of a biochemical cause. This malfunction may be the cause of illness or it may lead to the persistence of symptoms when the situation that precipitated the illness no longer exists. These are subdivided as follows:

- *Affective disorders:* this includes endogenous depression, hypomania and mania. The primary feature of these is in the patient's mood. All the symptoms are understandable in terms of this changed mood.

- *Schizophrenias:* this is a diffuse and ill defined group of conditions that can be subdivided in a number of ways, the most common being *hebephrenic, catatonic, paranoid and simple.*

Organic psychoses

Organic psychoses are caused by a temporary or permanent interference with the function of brain cells. They are subdivided on the basis of the length of time for which the failure of function persists into acute and chronic. Both may be due to one or more of the following causes:

- Trauma
- Infection, for example syphilis, encephalitis

- Neoplasm
- Degradation of brain tissue in old age
- Vascular disorders, for example ischaemia, arteriosclerosis
- Toxins
- Metabolic disorders
- Endocrine disorders
- Heat or cold
- Autoimmunity.

Dementia

This is a condition of permanent mental deterioration as a result of organic cerebral disease.

- *Arteriosclerotic dementia* is due to insufficient blood supply to the brain caused by arteriosclerosis.
- *Dementia praecox* is an obsolete term for schizophrenia, implying the early onset of dementia.
- *Pre-senile dementia* is of unknown cause, often occurring before the age of 60. It is characterised by cerebral atrophy and histological changes of a distinct nature. (Now referred to as *Alzheimer's disease* – see below.)
- *Senile dementia* occurs in old age due to cerebral atrophy.

The common features associated with dementia include:

- Decreased reasoning ability. There is tendency to reflect on the past and there is an inability to come to terms with activities in the present. Short-term memory is lost whereas long-term memory is restored.
- Headaches and dizziness.
- Explosive emotional outbursts.
- Progressive personality deterioration. The person is no longer able to hold a coherent conversation, actions are abnormal and answers are inappropriate. The person doesn't make eye contact, and appears to be in a world of their own.

Care regime

- Those presenting with senile psychosis require reduction in environmental demands, which includes assisting in acceptance of the limitations imposed by this form of mental disorder (for example, assistance with washing, dressing, feeding, toileting). Provide a quiet non-stimulating environment and limit interaction with others. Stimulating environments can exaggerate the illness.

- The drug treatment is usually dependent on the extent of the condition. The use of histamines and nicotinic acid can help to relax the walls of the blood vessels, improving the blood supply to the cortical cells.

- The patient will need protected physical and social environments.

- Knowledge of previous personality patterns and responsibilities can assist in providing appropriate care. This will mean communicating with the client's family and long-term friends and associates wherever possible. Involving a partner is also helpful in this situation as partners will have the most knowledge in terms of day-to-day needs.

- Mobility is important. Taking the client out for walks and ensuring plenty of fresh air whenever possible will decrease confusion and physical deterioration. Places that are familiar will provide comfort to the client.

- Occupational therapy and group psychotherapy will be beneficial for some. This helps to relieve boredom, prevents dwelling on inner thoughts, assists in appreciation of their condition and facilitates the forming of friendships.

- The use of sedatives can aid insomnia and general restlessness.

- The provision of a good night light can help to alleviate fears and apprehension associated with the dark.

Depression

Endogenous depression

This condition arises from within the individual without any known obvious cause. Clients often say they have nothing to be depressed about. The manifestations of this condition are as follows:

- Sadness, feelings which differ from the normal response to unhappy events.

- Weeping without apparent cause.

- Lowness of spirit, lowering of interest in things and a loss of desire for former interests.

- Food intake becomes reduced as there are feelings of distaste and eating ceases to be a pleasure.

- Hobbies and pastimes are neglected, even reading the newspaper or watching television becomes a chore, too much effort.

- The person experiences an inability to concentrate and difficulty in making simple decisions.

- At work, tasks eventually become too arduous, leading to accumulation. This increases the feelings of guilt and hopelessness, exacerbating the depression.

- Dwelling on the same continuous thoughts leading to fixed ideas, often concerned with death and morbidity. The individual often wishes to be dead and dwells on the death of a friend or relative. This may progress on to the wish to commit suicide and the formulation of plans for carrying out this wish.

- Withdrawal is inevitable, sometimes to the extent that there is no speaking.

Reactive depression

This form of depression manifests in changes in mood, which arise from events happening to the person concerned. This largely involves the loss of someone or something for whom we have strong feelings of love or affection. The patient is able to explain their feelings and will give specific dates of the onset of the illness from a particular event. The clinical manifestations are:

- Feelings of sadness and tearfulness.
- Benefit is derived from crying.
- Preoccupation with thoughts concerning loss with often underlying thoughts of anger and resentment usually directed at other people rather than self. Others are blamed for the loss.
- Feelings are worse during the evening.
- Difficulty getting off to sleep at night, but once asleep tends to remain so for the entire duration.
- Can be cheered up for a while and is able to respond to company.
- Loss of appetite, constipation, weight loss, physiological changes (which are usually slight).

Assessment of needs of patients with a mental illness

- *Self-awareness:* note the significance of behaviour and body language.
- *Observation:* be aware of language, communication, interaction with others, general appearance, especially signs of neglect.
- *Interview:* patient and relatives. Note descriptions of behaviour patterns, preoccupation of thoughts and thought processes, social ties, religious convictions.

Care regime

- Encourage intake of fluids and a light, balanced diet with supplements where necessary.
- Encourage activity, for example hobbies, light exercise or sport and gradually build up to comfortable level of activity. The patient may benefit from occupational and/or art therapy.
- Observe fluid output.
- Observe sleeping pattern.
- Encourage hygiene and grooming. Maintaining self-image is important.
- There is likely to be low self-esteem. Listen to the required needs, encourage to participate in an activity enjoyed and give praise without being patronising.
- Medication should be taken as prescribed. Monitoring is to be undertaken noting effects on the individual. The medication regimen should be reviewed periodically.
- Partners and children should be actively encouraged in the care where appropriate.

Anxiety

Normal anxiety

This is a normal reaction of alertness that occurs under certain conditions. The reactions and responses can vary from person to person and whether it be preparation for marriage, awaiting examination results or being interviewed for a job. The usual experience involves nervousness, apprehension, sweaty palms, tension, and even nausea.

Abnormal anxiety

This is a prolonged and exaggerated state. This condition can make the individual physically ill, and interfere with normal activities of daily living. There is likely to be failure to meet the demands of self-care.

The anxiety state presents a number of physical, social and psychological manifestations.

Physical effects

This affects the central (CNS) and autonomic (ANS) nervous systems:

CNS: tension, aching limbs, fatigue, tremor, headache and emotional tension.

A NS: increased heart rate, pulse and blood pressure leading to palpitations. Pupils become over dilated leading to blurred vision. Decreased salivation, decreased gastro-intestinal motility leading to tension of stomach muscles. There is nausea and loss of appetite (anorexia). Drive is reduced, increased respiratory activity and increased sweat production.

Psychological effects

- Feelings of inferiority
- Difficulty in decision making
- Difficulty in concentration
- Feeling tired
- Irritability, feeling ill at ease
- Excessive wariness and suspicion.

Body language

- Restlessness
- Rate and tone of speech increases, pitch raises and stammering is possible
- Lack of eye contact
- Clasped hands or excessive fidgeting.

Care regime

- A calm, confident and sympathetic approach is required
- Accept the client as a sick person who needs help and tailor the care to suit specific need. Discuss problems when they are ready to do so
- Provide opportunity for rest and recuperation
- Establish what produces the anxiety and remove it if possible
- Provide support, guidance and reassurance
- Provide medication as prescribed, and monitor effectiveness
- Observe any alteration in mood or behaviour.

The role of the community psychiatric nurse (CPN)

It has taken many years for the role of the community psychiatric nurse to become established. Indeed, recent legislation has served to strengthen the autonomy and function. Legislation introduced in April 1996, and known as the Mental Health (Patients in the Community) Act 1995, gave designated CPNs the power to insist that certain people with mental health problems could attend a specified place for treatment or be required to live in a specified place. The emphasis of the legislation is for the CPN to work in partnership with others in the health care team and be involved in service provision for the mentally ill.

The role of the CPN began to gain prominence during the 1950s when the phenothiazine group of drugs were introduced to treat traditionally long-term hospitalised schizophrenic patients. It was the duty of the CPN to continue to administer medication to clients in their home following discharge from hospital. The role is sometimes perceived as a 'follow-up function'. The CPN also provides support, advice and guidance in the care and treatment of the mentally ill. The nurse is expected to work in the community, with some interface with the institution, taking referrals from the consultant psychiatrist. To date, there is no known chronicled evidence to suggest that CPNs have ever been attached to or involved with PHCTs (Gilmore et al., 1974; Lamb, 1976).

One reason relates to information quoted in a 1977 DHSS circular noting that specialist mental health nurses who give advice to the PHCT are best based in hospitals, and should maintain their expertise (Kratz, 1980).

The decision to run down large mental hospitals came during the early 1960s when the government initially suggested provision of care for the mentally ill in the community setting. It was at this stage that CPNs came to be situated in primary health care rather than in hospitals. It was considered appropriate for intervention in health care of the mentally ill to be made at various stages in care and treatment without the necessity for entry to secondary care (Wing and Olsen, 1979). Early preventive care would, it was thought, be likely to enhance the effectiveness of treatment. Although this policy decision was taken more than thirty years ago, the transition period has been slow.

Leopoldt (1979), Sharpe (1982) and Dyke (1984) all found that GPs thought it would be beneficial to have CPNs attached to their practices as members of the PHCT. Research undertaken in the 1970s and 1980s indicated that there was a desire to have CPNs based in primary care, but it had not yet happened in many places.

The models for developing the professional multidisciplinary practice in the community grew largely out of the co-operation of the different professions working together within the hospital settings. It has been extended in the community to implement more innovative practice through sharing tasks and skills across professional boundaries. This latter move has not been without criticism and has resulted in the professions looking more introspectively at their own skills base. Such a move also has an element of inevitability, both from the perspective of individual professionals wishing to extend the boundaries of their own skills and from the greater organisational demands imposed by the community setting as opposed to the more insular hospital setting.

The skills required by the CPN as with all mental health staff have been stipulated as follows (DoH, 1993, p. 119–20):

- Appropriate care and treatment of postnatal mental illness, eating disorders and pre-senile dementias.
- Counselling techniques.
- Behavioural, cognitive and family therapies.
- Equal opportunities – particularly for women and ethnic minority users of services.
- Communication and presentation skills.
- Restraint techniques.

The role of the CPN is extensive although there is still room for improvement (White, 1991). Generally speaking, however, it encompasses the following activities.

- *Counselling*: This role is extended to clients and their families, although the expertise is still developing. Some places have better provision than others. Additionally, Naughton (1993) reports that over 25 per cent of GP fundholders brought private counsellors into their surgeries and Monkley-Poole (1995) revealed that 55 per cent in his study employed counsellors. Naughton (1993) suggests that this should send alarm bells ringing in CPN quarters, because the counsellor role might also supplant that of community psychiatric nurses.

- *Neuroleptic medication*: The move to put people with mental health problems out into the community is their opportunity to sell their expertise to GPs. In fact, Monkley-Poole (1995) argues that the key role for CPNs may be the administration of neuroleptic depot injections, a role predominantly belonging to CPNs prior to working with PHCTs. This task-orientated, GP defined role may seriously reduce the effectiveness of the CPN professionally, particularly as it is focused on technological interventions rather than holistic care.

- *Taking care opportunities:* When attached to PHCTs, CPNs have the opportunity to be in contact with people before psychological problems become too disabling (Sharpe, 1975; Brooker and Jayne, 1984; Skidmore and Friend, 1984; Clist and Brandt, 1986). Scott and Robinson (1986) reported that when GPs referred patients to CPNs over half the problems were resolved within three months and only a limited number of patients needed to be sent for further psychiatric investigations.

- *Prevention and health promotion*: Dixon (1995) believes that the PHCT is an ideal base for the CPN, especially in terms of primary and preventive work. Whereas mental illness as opposed to mental health has been the traditional concern of the psychiatric nurses, community psychiatric nursing is adopting the concept of preventive care and health education. New forms of practice are expanding their interest into the social settings of everyday life, and are concerned with structural issues which have the potential to disrupt psychological health.

Role of the key worker

Meteyard (1990) defines the key worker simply as 'an identified person who is charged with a defined responsibility towards a specific service user'. The range of activities that a key worker may perform on behalf of an individual client may be many and varied:

- Providing access to the services of other team members
- Problem solving
- Explaining clients' needs and advocating for them
- Explaining the intricacies of the system to the client
- Preparing necessary referral arrangements
- Supporting service users through specialist core skills
- Advocating for new services.

Essentially, the individual worker will hold clinical and managerial responsibilities for the people to whom they are designated as key worker as well as providing core skills to the users of the service when another team member (key worker) requests the input. The finer details of the role would be determined by the operational policies agreed for the particular service.

Øvretveit (1991) notes involvement in organising multiprofessional teams:

- To ensure that clients receive a service which is better than the one which they would receive if each profession and agency were helping them independently.
- To promote a better understanding of the special skills of each profession and of the resources available, through working more closely with other professions in the team.
- To achieve better planning proposals from teams and improve their ability to identify gaps in services.
- To ensure easier workload management and to establish common priorities across professions.
- To offer specialist support from different professions with common interests.

Case Study 11.2

Jim, a 40-year-old schizophrenic, has been diagnosed as an insulin-dependent diabetic.

The DN has been asked to visit him at home to ensure stability and appropriate use of his medication.

How should she approach the care of this patient?

Case management functions

A case manager is in a position to build the strongest relationship with, and acquire the most knowledge about, a patient. In building a network of support to meet the client's needs, he or she may also provide the strongest links in the structure – facilitating communication between the client and medical services and between the different services themselves.

This liaison role often involves substantial amounts of groundwork to promote the delivery of services necessary to meet the client's specific needs, such as regular communication with the GP, psychiatrist, community psychiatric nurse and others. This groundwork may include:

- Identifying members of the target population
- Engaging new participants
- Conducting assessments
- Planning interventions
- Assuming ultimate responsibility for developing individualised packages of care
- Assertive outreach mode of working
- Providing assistance and training
- Arranging psychiatric and other medical services
- Providing inter-agency resource brokering and advocacy
- Developing community resources
- Facilitating readmissions to hospital, if necessary
- Working in partnership with families and other carers.

Mental health and older people

The Audit Commission (2000) identified that the number of older people with mental health problems is not only rising, but that there will be a greater increase of problems among those over 80 years, who will suffer from dementia, and the over 65s rising by 10 per cent over ten years, to 2.3 million. The major risk to their mental health will be the risk of depression, with suicidal tendencies. The problem of dementia is a great risk, and appropriate support for carers is essential. There is a particular need for rapid response from health care workers, when carers identify a problem that needs to be clarified. DNs who have older clients on their caseload will need to be responsive to these needs, and ensure that these are identified as part of the initial assessment process. A knowledge of support services will help to ensure that the appropriate information and/or referral can be readily made when this is needed. The fact that the Commission has recognised that appropriate services are not forthcoming, with specialist help being patchy and unco-ordinated, should alert nurses to the need for vigilance when working with patients on their caseload. Working closely with voluntary providers of services to those needing mental health support will help to strengthen service provision. This is a positive way of contributing to good care delivery practices.

The role of the PHCT is crucial in early identification of possible problems, and ensuring that help is available as soon as possible. Specialist mental health service providers have a responsibility to ensure that contact with family, carers and the GP is made. Access to specialist assessments and specialist services is best facilitated by the whole team, where this is appropriate, in order to provide education, training and support (Audit Commission, 2000).

Case Study 11.3

Mrs Jones is a 70-year-old lady who was admitted to hospital following a fall at home. Her husband said that she had been depressed, and had eventually become confused, wandering about at nights, hence her fall.

Her fall created a large sore on her leg, which the DN was asked to dress after her discharge.

Mr Jones reported that his wife was getting even more confused, and he didn't feel able to cope.

How do you think the DN may be able to support this family?

Late 20th-century care in the community

In the 1970s, the government committed to a radical shift in the treatment of mental illness, moving from institutionalised care to care in the community (DHSS, 1975). Individuals who were particularly acutely ill remained in hospitals, but were transferred to mental illness units or wards in local district general hospitals. This had the advantage of providing care in local centres of population and thus removing the stigma, which still attaches to the old mental institutions.

Residential care was also increasingly popular under private (and housing association) and statutory bodies for the long-term chronically mentally ill and the elderly mentally frail (mainly dementias). Senile dementia is one area of increase in the ageing population. These people require permanent care provided in small units close to where they live.

This is also applicable to inmates with schizophrenia. Many of these people have been in hospital since early adulthood and are expected to remain there forever. Various forms of accommodation to suit levels of dependency are required. This will vary from hostels with a fairly high level of staffing, through to group homes three or four people share or to individual flats.

These people will require easy access to services for food, medication, occupation and their families and friends. This also includes day hospitals, day centres, occupational and industrial therapy units and drop-in social centres. Access to forms of benefit is also necessary. Care in the community has thus lent itself to the necessity of partnership between health authorities and social services in particular, but also housing departments, housing associations and voluntary associations such as MIND.

Housing and mental health

There is a likelihood of encountering the mentally ill in a number of settings in the community. These can vary from their own homes where they enjoy their individual independence. Alternatively, there may be more collective/communal types of living. Attention has been drawn to specific housing needs for the mentally ill. This is underlined by the fact that conditions are felt to have some influence on precipitating illness and relapse, but again the research evidence tends to be inconclusive (Etherington, 1983):

- Where people are living on housing estates, particularly in high rise flats, it has been suggested that social isolation and the lack of garden space can contribute to stress.
- Overcrowding is believed to cause stress through the associated loss of privacy.
- Noise and disputes between tenants contribute to stress and some feelings of persecution.

- Cold and damp housing reduces habitable space resulting in overcrowding and reduced privacy.

Residential services

Since the late 1950s, psychiatric services in the UK for people experiencing long-term mental health problems have undergone a gradual but progressive process of deinstitutionalisation, characterised by an ever-growing range of residential services to replace the long stay ward.

The focus on grouping people together has naturally given rise to some loose guidelines for the provision of mental health aftercare. Garety (1988) has indicated that broadly, it appeared that group homes were largely serving an older deinstitutionalised clientele, while staffed hostels tended to serve younger clients with a wider range of problems, some of whom had not spent any long periods in hospital.

Hostel ward

Hostel wards were a development of the 1970s to accommodate the people perceived as being the most needy – the 'new long stay'. These units were designated to accommodate between 10 and 20 residents, providing 24 hour nursing care. They were closely linked with the hospital services and occasionally organised to share the nursing staff of the local hospital. The most widely known examples are the Maudsley on-site facility (Wykes, 1982) and Douglas House, an example of the off-site facility (Goldberg et al., 1985).

Mental aftercare hostels

Hostels accommodating in excess of 20 residents have been a common feature of community residential provision since the policy for closing the psychiatric hospitals came into being.

Group homes

Group homes began to be established in the 1950s and 60s in an attempt to tackle the stigma associated with institutional care. They have varied in size from three to eight places. Residents have their own single bedroom with shared communal rooms and an expectation of supporting the sharing of daily living skills. Closer proximity to family homes is more suited to older clients.

Sheltered accommodation

Sheltered units offer independent flats within a larger block, with shared day room facilities. They are characterised by a front line of supervision through wardens and alarm systems in each flat to call for assistance if needed. Such services are generally associated with a more elderly and physically frail client group and, to date, little use is made of such facilities for people with severe mental health difficulties. Their suitability could be improved by the provision of outside specialist support services.

Conclusion

This chapter has provided an insight into the issues which need to be considered when caring for patients in the community, who may be at risk of mental health problems. It may be argued that all patients are at risk, as physical illness of any sort may contribute not only to stress but to a range of other clinical problems affecting one's mental state.

As a student, your work with your supervisor should help you to identify good practice in working relationships across the PHCT, and the positive impact this can have on patient care and health outcomes. Mental health, for older people in particular, is now a government priority (DoH, 1997; NHSE, 1998; Welsh Office, 1998; Audit Commission, 2000). It is therefore imperative that all nurses, including DNs who are likely to have large numbers of older patients on their caseloads, are able to recognise the mental health needs of these patients, and work in partnership with families, carers, policy makers and other members of the PHCT, to ensure that awareness of needs can be translated into action to promote and develop good practice.

Further reading

Audit Commission (2000) *Forget Me Not – Mental Health Services for Older People*. London, Audit Commission.

Bruce, J., Watson, D., van Teijlingen, E.R., Lawton, K., Watson, M.S. and Palin, A.N. (1999) Dedicated psychiatric care within general practice: health outcome and service providers' views. *Journal of Advanced Nursing*, 29(5): 1060–7.

USEFUL WEB SITES

Depression Alliance www.depressionalliance.org

MIND – The Mental Health Charity www.mind.org.uk

National Schizophrenia Fellowship www.nsf.org.uk

References

Audit Commission (2000) *Forget Me Not – Mental Health Services for Older People.* London, Audit Commission.

Baly, M. E. (1980) *Nursing and Social Change.* London, Baillière Tindall.

Brooker, C. and Jayne, D. (1984) Time to rethink. *Nursing Times, Community Outlook,* April 11: 132–4.

Bugge, C., Smith, L.N. and Shanley, E. (1999) A descriptive survey to identify the perceived skills and community skill requirements of mental health staff. *Journal of Advanced Nursing,* 29(1): 218–28.

Busfield, J. (1986) *Managing Madness.* London, Hutchinson.

Carpenter, M. (1980) Asylum nursing before 1914: a chapter in the history of labour. In Davies, C. (ed.) *Rewriting Nursing History.* London, Croom Helm.

Clist, L. and Brandt, S. (1986) A new direction for CPNs in the PHCT? *Nursing Times, Community Outlook,* 82, September 19: 310–12.

Department of Health (1993) *Targeting Practice: The Contribution of Nurses Midwives and Health Visitors.* London, HMSO.

Department of Health (1997) *A Handbook on the Mental Health of Older People.* London, HMSO.

Department of Health (1998) *Our Healthier Nation.* London, HMSO.

Department of Health (1999) *National Service Framework for Mental Health.* London, HMSO.

Department of Health and Social Security (1975) *Better Services for the Mentally Ill.* London, HMSO.

Dixon, K. (1995) The future of a community psychiatric nurse: an identifiable philosophy, *Community Psychiatric Nursing Journal* (CPNJ), 5(2): 30–3.

Dyke, B. (1984) CPNs and the primary health care attachment, *Nursing Times,* 80(8): 55–7.

Etherington, S. (1983) *Housing and Mental Health,* London, MIND and Circle 33 Housing Trust.

Fraser, D. (1975) *The Evolution of the British Welfare State.* London and Basingstoke, Macmillan – now Palgrave.

Garety, P. (1988) Housing. In Lavender, A. and Holloway, F. (eds) *Community Care Practice: Services for Continuing Care Clients.* Chichester, John Wiley.

Gilmore, M., Bruce, N. and Hunt, M. (1974) *The Work of the Nursing Team in General Practice.* London, CETHV.

Goldberg, D.B. (1991) *Rethinking Rehabilitation. Life after Mental Illness.* London, MIND, pp. 8–10.

Goldberg, D.B., Bridges, K. and Cooper, W. (1985) Douglas House: a new type of hostel for chronic psychiatric patients, *British Journal of Psychiatry,* 147: 383–8.

Kratz, C. (1980) Other members of the PHCT. In Barber, J. and Kratz, C. (eds) *Towards Team Care.* Edinburgh, Churchill Livingstone.

Lacey, I. (1999) The role of the child primary mental health worker, *Journal of Advanced Nursing,* 30(1): 220–8.

Lamb, A. (1976) *Primary Health Care Nursing.* London, Baillière Tindall.

Leopoldt, H. (1979) Community psychiatric nursing, *Nursing Times,* 75(13): 53–6.

Meteyard, B. (1990) *The Community Care Worker Manual.* London, Longman.

Monkley-Poole, S. (1995) The attitudes of British fund-holding general practitioners to community psychiatric nursing services, *Journal of Advanced Nursing,* 21: 238–47.

NHS Executive (1998) *Partnership in Action.* London, HMSO.

Naughton, B. (1993) The marketing imperative, *Nursing Times*, **89**(19): 52–3.

Onyett, S. (1992) *Case Management in Mental Health*. London, Chapman & Hall.

Øvretveit, J. (1991) *Essentials of Multiprofessional Community Team Organisation*. London, Brunel Institute of Organisation and Social Studies.

Ryan, P., Ford, R. and Clifford, P. (1991) *Case Management and Community Care*. London, Research and Development for Psychiatry.

Scott, D. and Robinson, H. (1986) Community psychiatric nursing: a survey of patients and problems. *Journal of the College of General Practitioners*, March, pp. 130–2.

Sharpe, D. (1975) Views of the community psychiatric nurse, *Nursing Times, Community Outlook*, 11 April, pp. 132–4.

Sharpe, D. (1982) GPs' views of the CPN. *Nursing Times*, 6 October, pp. 1664–6.

Skidmore, D. and Friend, W. (1984) Should CPNs be in the PHCT? *Nursing Times, Community Outlook*, 19 September, pp. 310–12.

Sloan, G. (1999) Good characteristics of a clinical supervisor: a community mental health nurse perspective, *Journal of Advanced Nursing*, **30**(3): 713–22.

Welsh Office (1998) *Partnership for Improvement*. Cardiff, HMSO.

White, E. (1991) Practice nurses and CPNs: changing places? *Practice Nurse*, February, 4777–8.

Wing, J. and Oslen, R. (1979) *Community Care for the Mentally Disabled*. Oxford, Oxford University Press.

Wykes, T. (1982) A hostel-ward for new long stay patients in long-term community care. (J.K.Wing, ed.) *Psychological Medicine*, Monograph Supplement 2.

12

Patients with complex needs in primary care: people with learning disabilities

TOM TAIT and LESLEY STYRING

Learning outcomes

By the end of this chapter you will be able to:

■ Explore the philosophical ideologies that underpin caring for people with learning disability who have complex needs.

■ Appreciate the impact learning disability can have upon the individual, their family and those who provide services for them.

■ Explore the ambiguous position that informal carers hold within society.

■ Consider the role of the practitioner in providing individualised care to the person with a learning disability who has complex care needs.

■ Demonstrate good understanding of the roles and responsibilities of key professionals involved in supporting learning-disabled people with complex needs living in the community.

■ Value the interrelationships between the dimensions of learning disability and the importance of devising care strategies based upon holistic principles.

Introduction

The purpose of this chapter is to consider ways in which practitioners and service providers support people with learning disabilities who have complex care needs and their families living in the community. As a student of the adult branch, you will undoubtedly encounter a range of sick adults, including those who may have a learning disability. The need to work closely with the patient, family and key workers is as applicable here as it is to other patients. There are important factors to be considered if care is to be delivered appropriately, taking into consideration all relevant legislation. In particular, the patient and his or her carer should be at the centre of assessment and delivery of care.

Definition of terms

Learning disability: people with severe or profound adaptive behaviour problems associated with a moderate, severe or profound developmental impairment, and who are dependent upon specialist services, are said to have a 'learning disability'.

Service users: the people in this chapter who have a learning disability will be referred to as 'service users'.

Carer: the term 'carer' refers to informal carers who are usually the family of the person with a learning disability.

What are complex needs?

The term 'complex needs' can encompass a range of conditions associated with learning disability. What is important is that all concerned understand the language used by practitioners to describe complex needs. To date there has been no universal definition of complex need that appears common to all professional agencies involved in care delivery. The authors offer the following definition in the firm belief that it identifies general terminology and aids understanding in describing this particular group:

> People who by virtue of their learning disability and additional physical, emotional or behavioural problems require a co-ordinated approach to meeting their every-day needs.

For example, children who are born prematurely with cerebral palsy, visual impairment, severe epilepsy and feeding problems will require synchronised assistance at various levels and a range of support services at different times during their development, and throughout their lives (Figures 12.1 and 12.2).

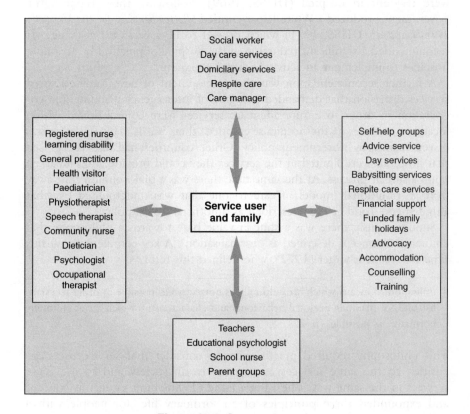

Figure 12.1 Support networks

Looking back

Historically, society demanded that people whose needs could not be met within local communities were housed away from them, normally in large institutions loosely described as hospitals. The medical model that prevailed was instrumental in ensuring that meeting physical needs was a prime objective of those working within the institution. (Read Chapter 1 of this text for a better overview of the historical context generally.)

Even today, there is still debate surrounding the advantages and disadvantages of caring for service users in hospital settings or supporting service users in their local communities, and the cost effectiveness of chosen settings.

While hospitals provided a safe and secure environment they did not meet all the needs of the service users. Specialised treatment was not available and very often service users with complex needs did not receive care and attention appropriate to their requirements.

During the late 1960s and early 1970s, hospital care came under scrutiny as official enquiries were instigated in response to a series of allegations surrounding the care and treatment of people with learning disabilities who were resident in hospital (DHSS, 1969). Following these reports, the government produced a White Paper entitled '*Better Services for the Mentally Handicapped*' (DHSS, 1971) which proved to be a catalyst for change. It recommended a significant reduction in the hospital population by actioning hospitals to implement an active discharge programme.

A further recommendation was the development of new, localised social services provision that demanded a degree of inter-agency planning and co-operation in order to ensure adequate services were commissioned within local communities as the hospitals 'emptied' their wards. This initiative was driven mainly by government policy. Other countries had also recognised that hospitals were limited in the services they could provide and embarked upon a similar process. At the same time there was a philosophical shift away from a 'traditional' model of care to one that was underpinned by what Brigden and Todd (1993) described as 'unofficial' social policy.

Simultaneously there was a shift in value base towards a philosophy that embraced a concept described as 'normalisation'. A key commentator at this time was Wolfensberger (1972), who defined this term as:

> utilisation of means which are culturally as normative as possible in order to establish and/or maintain personal behaviours and characteristics which are as culturally normative as possible. (p. 27)

This philosophy required practitioners to consider that service users are entitled to the same services as anyone else in society and to use these services in the same way. The King's Fund (1980) built upon this concept and expounded three principles of an 'ordinary life' for people with a learning disability:

1. People with learning disabilities have the same human value as anyone else and so the same human rights.

2. People with learning disabilities have a right and a need to live like others in the community.

3. Services must recognise the individuality of people with learning disabilities.

Although over two decades old now, these principles are still as valid today as they were then.

This philosophy required hospitals to actively restructure the residential services they provided by commissioning a range of smaller, community-based 'units' for service users ranging in size from one-bedroomed accommodation to 24-bed hostels. At the same time, nurse training was undergoing a radical change in response to the emerging new model of community care with a major shift away from focusing upon aetiology, anatomy and physiology towards greater emphasis upon the social sciences. As more service users moved into local communities and admissions to hospitals reduced, this put greater demand upon primary health care teams (PHCTs). In response, community learning disability teams developed with community learning disability nurses taking a lead role in providing practical support to service users and their families.

At the same time changes in the education system brought children who were previously considered to be uneducable into mainstream education. This was an acknowledgement that a child with a learning disability could acquire new skills with the appropriate levels of support, thus exposing them to a range of new life experiences.

Each of these initiatives was significant in its own right. Collectively they provided the foundations of a new community-based service for people with learning disabilities and their families. Unfortunately, the increased impetus that had arisen to use mainstream community services has frequently failed to acknowledge the uniqueness of the individual with complex care needs; resulting in a 'piecemeal' service for users and their families from this group. It is therefore essential that people with complex care needs have available to them a comprehensive network of support to ensure care in the community is successful.

In summary, this section has offered a brief historical overview of the development of services to people with learning disabilities in the United Kingdom. Recent government reports (NHS Executive, 1998, 1999) have made many exciting recommendations including greater collaboration between primary health care and social services. As services re-configure to meet the challenges these recommendations present, service providers must acknowledge that people with learning disabilities have the same rights and responsibilities as any other members of the community in which they live. For people with complex care needs, these rights can only be enjoyed if the correct level of specialist health and social services within the community are available to them.

The impact of learning disability upon the family

'A handicapped child means a handicapped family'

Although arguably a sweeping generalisation, this statement encapsulates the potential impact of disability upon the family as a whole. Twigg and Atkin (1994) suggest that informal carers occupy an ambiguous position within the care system as services are normally structured around the service user rather than the carer, yet Pike (1999) argues that some services provided are for the benefit of the carer, not the service user. What is clear is the absence of any single co-ordinated approach that acknowledges the potential tensions between the needs of the family and the needs of the service user, and the way agencies should react to them.

Student Activity 12.1

Think of your life and any bad times you have faced. Some you will have overcome without any help from anyone while others may have required you to seek guidance and support from a variety of sources.

- Identify the significant people in your life and the role they have played in helping you.

- Imagine your neighbour has just given birth to a baby boy who has a range of complex needs. Using Figure 12.1 to guide you, identify the help and support the child and family members may require and who might provide that assistance.

The issue of practitioners' interaction with informal carers was highlighted by Summerton (2000) who argues that relationships between formal and informal carers need to be more constructive. The King's Fund (1998) recommends eight components of good practice, when working in partnership with carers:

- Information
- Recognition
- Quality services
- Time off

- Emotional support
- Training to care
- Financial security
- A voice.

In 1998, the UKCC suggested that the majority of care provided within a community setting is given by informal carers. These carers will require guidance, encouragement and resources to ensure continuity of care between the formal and informal support networks. To achieve this continuity, the relationship that develops between the practitioner and informal carer must be built upon a foundation of mutual respect, trust and understanding. These components will build a partnership that can help empower both partners to deliver care that acknowledges the tensions that can exist and devise strategies to overcome them.

Discovery of complex needs

Most families experience some emotional distress when a diagnosis of learning disability is made. Kubler-Ross (1970) identified five stages of grief experienced by a person who is dying. Similar stages can also be experienced by parents following their child's diagnosis of learning disability. Often their reactions mirror those of the bereaved (see Chapter 14 for further discussion of this concept).

The first stage is *denial and isolation*. A parent's hopes and aspirations for their child's potential are dashed and the immediate future may be too bleak to contemplate. Initially, the parents may even deny that there is anything wrong with the child and refuse any contact with the appropriate practitioner. It is important to be aware that denial is normally a temporary defence and will be replaced by partial acceptance. It is essential, therefore, that practitioners allow parents and siblings the opportunity to explore and express their feelings in their own ways.

The potential problem of isolation should not be ignored. Despite changing attitudes towards disability, there is still a possibility that the reactions of extended family members and friends will reinforce the feelings of inadequacy. For example, parents receive fewer congratulations cards, as friends are unsure whether these are appropriate. Sensitivity is required and there are now a small number of dedicated groups that offer advice and support during this difficult time.

The second stage is *anger*. Parents find it difficult to cope with the situation and become angry and resentful. This is a difficult time for the practitioner, as the anger may be displaced in many different directions. Parents, relatives and siblings may find fault with everything the practitioner does and may alienate themselves from the very people who are trying to help. It is very important that the practitioner does not take this anger personally, however it may feel at the time. It is a crucial stage in coming to terms with disability. If parents are made to suppress their anger, there can be negative repercussions in the future.

The next stage is described by Kubler-Ross as *bargaining*. 'Please God, I will never do it again, please make my baby all right'. These thoughts are not untypical as parents strive to come to terms with their child's disability. The practitioner should realise that this type of promise is usually associated with guilt and any such comments from the parents should be treated seriously. A skilled counsellor may be able to explore any unresolved issues that are causing the anxiety and distress.

Depression is the fourth stage that occurs when the parents realise the full implications of having a child with learning disabilities. Parental expectations will not be realised and feelings of disappointment, failure and hopelessness will ensue. These feelings can interfere with the normal bonding processes that take place and if left unresolved can ultimately lead to rejection. The practitioner can make a valuable contribution by affirming the parent's negative feelings, as it is OK to feel bad. Facilitating access to appropriate services, as well as contact with others who can relate their positive experiences of learning disability, is an appropriate strategy to use. The emphasis must shift away from the negative towards hope in the knowledge that there are the appropriate services available to support the family.

Finally, the last stage is *acceptance* but it could be argued that only a very few parents ever truly accept their child's disability. Unresolved problems can go back many years. At this time parents require assistance in 'mapping out' their child's future, finding out about the types of services available, where these are located and when they are accessible. For the child with complex disability, a 'life plan' will help professionals to focus the appropriate care and support at the appropriate time in an appropriate manner.

A life plan is a systematic approach to planning a learning disabled child's future. It ensures continuity of care and acknowledges significant life events, thereby ensuring that the child has the best possible opportunity to reach his or her full potential. The approach is multidisciplinary and requires co-ordination of care. A registered nurse for people with learning disabilities normally undertakes this role. Figure 12.2 identifies key agency involvement and the timescale of participation.

This section has explored the potential impact that the birth of a learning disabled child can have upon the nuclear and extended family. What is vital for practitioners is the acknowledgement that family members will require support that is dissimilar from the support required by their learning disabled child. However, although the needs of the child and the family may be different, they are equally important and support should not be provided to one to the detriment of the other.

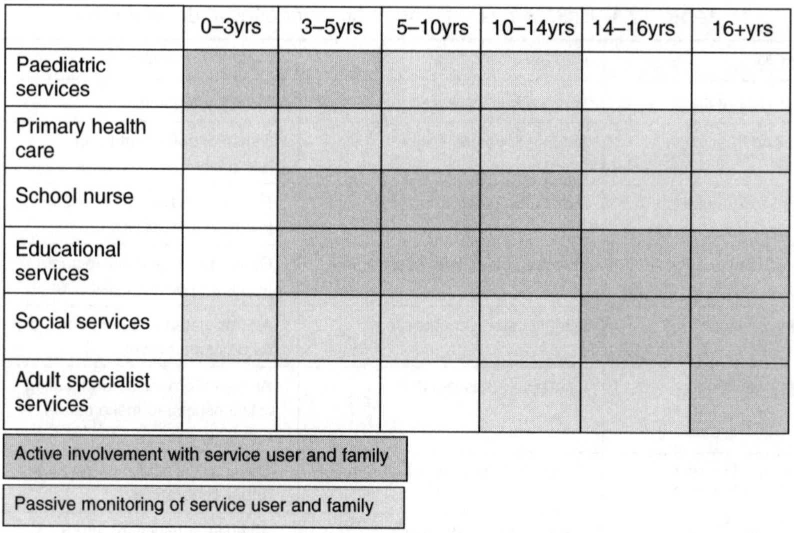

	0–3yrs	3–5yrs	5–10yrs	10–14yrs	14–16yrs	16+yrs
Paediatric services						
Primary health care						
School nurse						
Educational services						
Social services						
Adult specialist services						

Active involvement with service user and family
Passive monitoring of service user and family

Figure 12.2 Inter-agency involvement
Source: Hutchinson and Styring (1998).

'Growing pains'

The period of transition from childhood to adulthood is not without its problems. Atkinson and colleagues (1996) state that during this period the young person develops to sexual maturity and establishes an identity as an individual apart from the family. Table 12.1 identifies Erikson's (1963) eight stages of psychosocial development.

Adolescence is a turbulent time for any young person. However, for a service user the problems surrounding 'normal' psychosocial development are often masked by their complex needs. This is often compounded by the cause of the learning disability. For example the abnormal sexual characteristics of children with Turner's syndrome, Kleinfelter's syndrome and fragile-X syndrome become more apparent at puberty, a time when positive personal image is crucial. The danger exists that service users will become more aware of their sexual differences, and this will be detrimental to the development of a positive self-concept.

The emotional turmoil often associated with adolescence applies equally to those with learning disabilities. This is particularly evident in those people with mild learning disabilities who may yearn for a 'normal' lifestyle. While their aspirations are often to gain meaningful employment, get married and have children, they become increasingly aware of their disability and how this will impact upon them in the future.

Their struggle for independence often brings them into conflict with carers as the service user tries to maintain control. For example, the person may

Table 12.1 Erikson's eight stages of psychosocial development

Stages	Psychosocial crises	Favourable outcome
First year of life	Trust versus mistrust	Trust and optimism
Second Year	Autonomy versus doubt	Sense of self-control and adequacy
Third to fifth years	Initiative versus guilt	Purpose and direction; ability to initiate one's activities.
Sixth year to puberty	Industry versus inferiority	Competence and intellectual, social and physical skills
Adolescence	Identity versus confusion	An integrated image of one's self as a unique person
Early adulthood	Intimacy versus isolation	Ability to form close and lasting relationships; to make career commitments
Middle adulthood	Generativity versus self-absorption	Concern for family, society and future generations
The ageing years	Integrity versus despair	A sense of fulfilment and a satisfaction of one's life

want to engage in a sexual relationship while this is against the wishes of their carers. Health care professionals must be aware that this is a crucial time in terms of mental health and recognise that there are a growing number of people with learning disabilities and mental health problems who are at risk of self-harm during this stage.

As well as the psychosocial aspects of adolescence, health care professionals need to acknowledge the physiological problems which can occur at this time. For example a child with epilepsy who has been well controlled on medication can suddenly experience an increase in seizures due to the hormonal changes that occur in puberty. Similarly, someone with diabetes can experience instability and become insulin dependent when they have only required oral medication before. When such changes apply to people with learning disabilities, they will need support and readily accessible information.

It is important to be aware that some conditions are 'ignored' because they are an 'accepted' part of disability. One example of this is incontinence. A 15-year-old boy with enuresis and no learning disability will almost certainly be

Student Activity 12.2

♦ Spend a moment considering the conflicts and resolutions in your own adolescence and reflect upon those that caused you the most distress.

♦ Make notes on your thoughts in your portfolio.

referred to a specialist for further investigations. But if the 15-year-old boy has Down's syndrome, his 'problem' will be associated with his learning disability, therefore it will not assume such significance and he may not be given access to specialist treatment.

This section has explored the complex and often painful issues surrounding adolescence. It is important for the practitioner to be aware that development is a life-long process, no matter how disabled the person may appear. People with complex needs will change both physically and psychologically. Their social support networks will also change as they come into contact with new life experiences and formal and informal support systems. They will also have to adjust to cope with this potentially difficult period in their lives that may place added strain upon their family and the professionals involved in their care.

Case Study 12.1

John is 17 years old and suffers from Down's syndrome. He has diabetes mellitus, which is normally well controlled by insulin injection that his mother administers. He attends a local special school and stays in a local authority respite unit on a regular basis. John's mother lives on her own, looking after John and his younger sister.

The staff at the respite unit have reported that John's behaviour is deteriorating, with him becoming unco-operative and verbally aggressive.

Under these headings identify possible reasons for John's behaviour:

PHYSICAL   PSYCHOLOGICAL   ENVIRONMENTAL

Adulthood: delivering holistic care

While the National Health Service was founded upon the principle that good quality health care should be available to all, some groups of individuals (including those with learning disabilities) are not getting a fair deal (NHS Executive, 1999). It is essential therefore that practitioners working with people with complex needs understand the special needs of this client group.

If a practitioner is to provide care that is both effective and dignified to people with learning disabilities, it is important to acknowledge that people are different. Just because two people with a learning disability have the same condition, this does not mean that their care should be the same. (Chapter 6 explores further the issues involved when working with differences and diversity in primary care settings.)

People are individuals in their own right. The care provided will need to address the many different areas that, put together, make us who we are. These areas can be grouped into five dimensions:

- Psychological
- Physical
- Sociological
- Educational
- Spiritual.

A major principle in the provision of holistic care is to maintain a service user's dignity at all times.

- Look for the human worth of the person with a learning disability. See the person, not their disability.
- Respect the racial and cultural origin of the people in your care at all times.
- Respect the gender and sexual orientation of the person in your care.
- Accept the person's values and attitudes in an non-judgemental way.
- Regardless of circumstances, respect a person's uniqueness and recognise their personal care needs.

A holistic approach to care affirms that people are different. Health professionals must recognise these differences and provide care that focuses upon personal needs. There are different dimensions to being human. Holistic care for people with complex needs, therefore, must be based around the identification of personal requirements in each of these dimensions.

Trans-professional working

In today's modern health services a person's needs may not be met by just one single agency. The structure of the health, education and social services as illustrated in Figure 12.2 suggests that meeting complex needs will require an input from many different professionals, at different times. It has been known for a nurse, doctor, social worker and voluntary visitor to be involved with one service user, all trying to meet the same need. This duplication is costly to the service provider not to mention very frustrating to the service user. Thomas (1992) suggests that too often the many different facets of community care are a maze through which service users have to plot a path. Much of the policy from the last 15 years or so emphasises the need for improved collaboration among all primary care workers, so that care delivery can be as seamless as possible for the benefit of patients (NHS and Community Care Act 1990; DoH, 1999, 2000).

As community care progressed, a framework developed in response to a need to co-ordinate professional input as well as to ensure the care delivered was flexible and responsive to individual need. This was to ensure that 'packages' of care could be constructed, embracing the concept of sharing responsibility across professional boundaries.

Care management can be organised in different ways but essentially the care manager is responsible for developing action plans following recommendations of the different practitioners, and organising resources and finance to implement the action plan.

Walker and colleagues (1994) suggest that need is defined primarily by people who provide services, rather than by service users and their families. Care management can place professionals in positions of 'gate keeping' services. This can give care managers more power than service users, which places the service user at a disadvantage. The voices of service users and/or their informal carers are not as powerful as those of professional carers. So it is important that a series of checks is in place that redresses this imbalance and provides opportunities for professionals, service users and their families to work in equal partnerships where contributions are equally valued.

As previously stated, meeting the needs of people who have a learning disability will require a co-ordinated approach. Care management will provide a vehicle to deliver such an objective and, if done properly, will ensure that the service user receives appropriate and effective care.

In summary, as the health service re-organises in response to a rapidly developing community-based sector, practitioners will be required to undertake a variety of different roles including one that co-ordinates the input from a range of health and social care agencies. Care management can help to deliver individualised, harmonised packages of care.

Student Activity 12.3

◆ Consider the role of a care manager and identify the key skills required to fulfil this important role.

◆ Discuss your thoughts and queries with your assessor/supervisor.

◆ Make notes in your portfolio.

An equal partnership

The challenge for practitioners and service providers in meeting the needs of people with learning disabilities is to engage in a meaningful relationship with the service users and their carers. In order to achieve this, professionals will have to use inventive and novel approaches to present information in ways that service users understand. Holmes (1995) suggests professionals need to guard against assumptions of intellectual impairment as these could lead to us automatically denying information and choice (see Chapter 11, Case Study 11.3, for example).

The principles of leading 'an ordinary life' in the community should acknowledge that people with learning disabilities have the right to make decisions about their own life. Historically, Spackman and colleagues (1995) suggest that decision making has been denied to service users because they were seen as being incapable of developing the relevant skills. It is not surprising, given their paid carers' low expectations, that adults with learning disabilities today still have low expectations of themselves.

Spackman et al. (1995) believe the advocacy movement has done much to improve the situation and it is fair to assume that service users can make decisions given the opportunity to do so. Although this can take considerable time and effort on the part of the professional, it is worth remembering that recent government initiatives have focused upon service user involvement (DoH, 1997), and people with learning disabilities are no exception. This initiative will require practitioners to acquire and develop their skills in advocacy and self-advocacy. However, the assumption that professional carers can be true advocates has been challenged as the advocate role requires an objective stance with no professional interests that may dilute arguments and compromise outcomes.

Case Study 12.2

Mrs Higginson has just given birth to Anna who has been diagnosed as having Down's syndrome. Mr Higginson has refused to accompany his wife to any outpatient appointments with the consultant paediatrician and will not talk about his feelings towards Anna.

With this scenario in mind you may wish to consider why Mr Higginson is behaving this way, and explore possible strategies the community practitioner can adopt to overcome the present problems. It is important to remember that each family will have an individual set of problems that will require a co-ordinated approach to meeting their needs.

This chapter had been able to cover only some of the aspects of caring for a person who has a learning disability and complex needs, and who is living in the community. In many ways, this chapter perhaps raises more questions and issues than it answers. Speak to any experienced practitioner in this field and they will probably suggest that this is the very nature of caring for a person with a learning disability. There are no easy answers or magic wands to wave.

It is only with planned, systematic care interventions that complex problems can be analysed, and strategies implemented to provide nursing support that focuses upon real need.

The requirements for clear comprehensive lines of communication between the family, the service user and different professionals are crucial to a successful community care package. The care management role can assist in ensuring the service user remains as the central focus of any care provision. It should be remembered that the learning disability practitioner might be one of many professionals supporting a service user and their family. In the case of intervention because of the physical illness of a disabled person, close collaboration is essential. A district nurse (DN) who may be delivering care will need to be aware of the contribution of the primary health care team, and the requirement that members of that team who are involved in the care are consulted.

People are different, and this is equally true for people with a learning disability. Just because two people have the same diagnosis it does not mean their needs will be the same. Patterns of support will differ from region to region too. How the service user and their family relate to the local community will also be dependent upon a variety of factors that will shape the type of relationship and role the community practitioner develops with the family.

The challenge for the practitioner is to be aware of the different factors that contribute to a person requiring a co-ordinated approach to meet their everyday needs and to work with others in devising strategies that enhance a service user's quality of life. Turton and Orr (1993) suggest that delivering nursing care in a community setting is evidently not high technology care but it is essential care and preventive care 'par excellence'. If your assessor has learning disabled service users with a physical illness on his or her caseload, you will be intimately involved in their lives, and the lives of their families. Sharing their disappointments and successes is what makes caring in the community such a challenging, exciting and rewarding experience.

USEFUL WEB SITES

British Institute of Learning Disabilities http://www.bild.org.uk

Headway National Head Injuries Association http://www.headway.org.uk

Mencap http://www.mencap.org.uk

References

Atkinson, R., Atkinson, R., Smith, E., Dern, D. and Nolen-Hoeksema, S. (1996) *Hilgard's Introduction to Psychology*, 8th edn. London, Harcourt Brace.

Brigden, P. and Todd, M. (1993) *Concepts in Community Care for People with a Learning Difficulty*. London, Macmillan – now Palgrave.

Department of Health (1997) *The New NHS: Modern, Dependable*. London, HMSO.

Department of Health (1999) *The Health Act*. London, HMSO.

Department of Health (2000) *The NHS Plan*. London, HMSO.

Department of Health and Social Security (1969) Report of the Committee of Inquiry into Allegations of Patients and Other Irregularities at Ely Hospital, Cardiff. London, HMSO.

Department of Health and Social Security (1971) *Better Services for the Mentally Handicapped*. London, HMSO.

Erikson, E.H. (1963) *Childhood and Society*, 2nd edn. New York, Norton.

Holmes, A. (1995) Self-advocacy in learning disabilities, *British Journal of Nursing*, 4(8): 448–50.

Hutchinson, R. and Styring, L. (1998) The net has holes in: finding children with multiple disabilities and complex needs who will challenge services in the future. Paper given at the ENB Learning Disability Conference: Partnership, Priorities and Progress, Lancaster University 13–14 July 1998.

King's Fund (1980) *An Ordinary Life*. London, King's Fund.

King's Fund (1998) *The Carers Compass – Directions for Improving Support to Carers*. London, King's Fund.

Kubler-Ross, E. (1970) *On Death and Dying*. London, Tavistock.

NHS Executive (1998) *Signposts for Success*. London, HMSO.

NHS Executive (1999) *Once a Day*. London, HMSO.

Pike, N. (1999) All we are really here for is storage dear. Psychodynamic approaches to the short-term care of children with learning disabilities, *Journal of Learning Disabilities for Nursing Health and Social Care*, 3(1): 3–11.

Spackman, T., Goddard, A., Ingham R. (1995) Developing decision making skills for people with learning disabilities, *Nursing Standard*, 9(19) : 28–31.

Summerton, H. (2000) Who cares? *Nursing Times*. 96(1): 24–5.

Thomas, J. (1992) Package deals, *Nursing Times*, 88(29): 48–9.

Turton, P. and Orr, J. (1993) *Learning to Care in the Community*, 2nd edn. London, Arnold.

Twigg, J. and Atkin, K. (1994) *Carers Perceived: Policy and Practice in Informal Care*. Milton Keynes, Open University Press, pp. 30–1.

United Kingdom Central Council for Nursing, Midwifery and Health Visiting (1998) *Standards for Specialist Education and Practice*. London, UKCC.

Walker, C., Walker, A. and Ryan, T. (1994) Services for People with Learning Difficulties – Balancing the Interests of Users, their Families and Service Providers. Social Services Research 1994 – 1. The University of Birmingham.

Wolfensberger, W. (1972) *Normalisation. The Principle of Normalisation in Human Services*, National Institute of Mental Retardation, Toronto, p. 27.

13

Older people in society: sociopolitical implications and the impact on health care delivery

EILEEN BUCHANAN

Learning outcomes

By the end of this chapter you will be able to:

- Identify ways in which individuals have been defined as 'elderly' in society.

- Appreciate the problem of stereotyping older people and how this may impact on care delivery.

- Discuss characteristics of older people that influence their perception and acceptance of care.

- Identify and discuss developments in social policy specifically aimed at the care of older people in the community.

- Identify and explain the variety of agencies responsible for the provision of care in the community.

- Discuss the advantages of collaborative care, and recognise possible barriers to effective collaboration, which need to be addressed.

Introduction

Community care according to the White Paper *Caring for People* (DoH, 1989) emphasised the need to provide the right level of intervention and support to enable everyone to achieve maximum independence and control over their own lives. This is a particularly appropriate definition in relation to older people, whose health care needs have become an important subject for debate. Increasing longevity and a desire to ensure that those extra years should be characterised by an acceptable level of social physical and mental health has both social and political implications in society.

The definition reflects, in part, current political philosophy that emphasises the value of providing a choice of care services for older people as and when their health needs change. It also reflects a change in the way society has come to view the care of frail older people. The 1990s have witnessed a consistent move away from long-term institutional care, to health and social care provision within the community. Current policy, it is argued, aims to enable older people to remain for as long as possible in their own homes. The central focus of policy is on the value of self-reliance and on families as the bulwark of community care provision (Davey, 1999). Whether or not this is an appropriate focus has been a subject of debate and, some would argue, is open to question.

In terms of demographic change, population forecasts identify a considerable increase in the number of the very old as the 21st century continues, and this has inevitable consequences in terms of health care provision. The potential economic consequences of providing long-term care have to be considered as part of the cost of the overall health care system, and health care policy is influenced by both political and social concerns. While it may be argued that old age does not automatically result in failing health, the possibility of having to rely on health care services does increase with age. In an ageing society the cost of long-term care will fall largely on a decreasing number of younger working adults, and many of those who carry much of the care burden of elderly relatives in the community today will themselves be approaching old age.

From a nursing perspective, such factors lead us to consider aspects of the process of care in which nurses may play a leading role. The promotion and maintenance of good physical and mental health, for example, is essential if older people are to remain independent for as long as possible. Community nurses, already identified as key providers of care to older people, will have a crucial role to play in health needs assessment, in the provision of evidence of health need, and in the implementation of strategies to promote health and improve the quality of life.

Ageing and society: defining old age

One of the problems faced by policy makers is how to gain an accurate definition of the specific group for which the policy is to be formulated. This is particularly true of older people. They clearly represent 'the whole of a generation who have survived to a certain age', but they are also no more than a cross-section of ordinary people in society, with different life experiences and expectations, who in any other circumstances would not be linked as a group (Tinker, 1992).

Attaching labels such as 'the elderly' has enabled policy makers and professionals to define older people as a group for whom resources may be identified. As the number of older people in society steadily increases, however, an all-embracing term becomes less viable. This is especially true in terms of the nurse–patient relationship where it becomes important for nurses interacting with individual patients or clients to be aware of the way in which the use of stereotypes of 'the elderly' persist, despite evidence that this group can never be seen as homogeneous.

> Everyone faces at all times two fateful possibilities: one is to grow older, the other not. Anonymous. (BBC Online – Health and Fitness – Ageing)

Ageing is a natural biological process that begins in early adulthood, but only becomes obvious several decades later. In modern society being old is generally associated with the official age of retirement from paid work,

Student Activity 13.1

◆ How old is 'old'? Give reasons for your answer.

◆ List some characteristics that you associate with being old and group them into:

   – Positive characteristics

   – Negative characteristics.

◆ Discuss with your peers.

◆ Make notes in your portfolio.

currently 65 years for men and 60 years for women, when the State pension becomes payable. Many people, however, continue to work beyond 65 years and would not consider themselves to be old. Equally, many women who have never worked outside the home continue in the role they have developed for themselves within the family and community. One way of looking at ageing is covered in the old French proverb which tells us that 'Forty is the old age of youth; fifty is the youth of old age'. It is this idea, which underlies current attempts to resolve the problem of a clear definition by defining old age in terms of categories, for example:

● The young elderly (60–74)

● The elderly (75–84)

● The old elderly (85+).

The social and biological characteristics associated with the three groups highlighted above are sufficiently distinct for them to be acceptable as a guide when considering the needs of older people. It is as well to remember, however, that some people appear to be old long before they are 60, and some retain younger characteristics well into 'old' old age.

Defining old age in positive terms is most often linked with social characteristics, for example:

● Being regarded as wise and experienced in life (in traditional societies).

● The ability to teach skills to young people (for example apprenticeship).

● Not being dependent on paid work.

● Having more time available for leisure or educational activities.

● Having time to travel with friends or family.

● Developing family relationships – getting to know grandchildren.

In recent years some commercial companies, especially in the retail sector, have developed positive policies towards the employment of older people, recognising skills and characteristics which benefit both the organisation and the individual. Research by Forster (1993) supports this positive attitude showing that older employees have less absenteeism, more job stability and greater output than younger workers.

Negative perspectives tend to focus on biological changes which affect appearance, or manner, such as:

- Grey hair, or wrinkled skin
- Poor mobility
- Poor posture.

Some loss of faculties – both mental and physical – may also be associated with getting older, for example:

- Poor memory, or loss of hearing
- Being slow to respond to questions or requests
- Misunderstanding questions or requests
- Slowness in completing tasks such as personal hygiene, or dressing
- Increased risk of accidents.

The problem of ageism

When we make associations between old age and particular characteristics this may then lead us to make generalised negative assumptions about how 'old people' look, how they are likely to behave, and the extent of their physical and intellectual capabilities. Despite the diversity of older people, there remains a tendency, among nurses as among others, to lump them together as if they were a homogeneous group, and to act in a way which means that the older person is not treated as an individual with individual rights and needs. This is referred to as 'ageism', and may be defined as, 'Attitudes and beliefs that present negative stereotypes of older people, and actions, which result in discrimination'.

During the latter part of the 20th century, researchers in social gerontology (the study of ageing in society) produced a variety of explanations of how negative stereotypes have developed and why they persist in Western societies.

We have already identified retirement from paid work as one of the ways in which we define being old but social gerontologists have considered the concept of retirement from two perspectives. These are structured dependence and the political economy of old age.

Student Activity 13.2

♦ Why do stereotypes of old age persist?

♦ Identify as many sources of stereotypes as you can.

♦ Make notes in your portfolio.

1. Structured dependence

In the agricultural and developing industrial society of the 19th century, older workers were generally accepted as valuable teachers passing on traditional skills to young people in the workplace (apprenticeship). Late industrial society, however, is characterised by:

• A highly specialised division of labour

• Mandatory retirement, encouraged or enforced by state pension schemes

• Marginalisation of older people, and dependence on the state for survival.

Walker (1981) further suggests that retirement has increased in importance and is a deliberate process of 'social engineering' to remove older workers from the labour force with the result that older people in British society have become increasingly dependent. Townsend (1981) highlights the close link between structured dependence and inequalities in social class. He argues that the quality of life in retirement reflects the structured inequalities of income and resources in the occupational system.

2. A political economy of old age

Smith (1984) represents a school of thought, which argues that there has always been some form of 'retirement', dependent on the ratio of old to young people in society.

The nature of society's response is determined by how much money is available in the public purse:

• *1908 and 1948:* periods in which we can identify a positive response to old age and an emphasis on the need for collective provision to support older people.

• *1980s–1990s:* a view of older people as a 'burden' on society and a return to policies which focus on the need for greater reliance on family support and private provision in their care.

Johnson (1991), however, is somewhat critical of such explanations. He suggests that they have helped to perpetuate negative stereotypes, because they focus on a very small group, mostly of older people living in institutions. Welfare payments and pensions, Johnson argues, could be looked at in a more positive light, and may be more accurately regarded as simply providing a source of security for older people.

When seeking to provide adequate and relevant support, the needs of economically and socially independent older people must also be considered. Concentration on the concept of the 'structured dependency' of older people, it may be argued, has tended to deflect attention away from more progressive and optimistic views of the economic and social status of the elderly in Britain today. We need to redress this balance.

Clearly, the tendency to stereotype anyone over a certain age – to characterise or categorise a person too readily or simplistically according to a conventional image, reflects the kind of society we live in. What we see and hear around us – most frequently from the media in modern society, but also in everyday conversations – influences the images we have of old people. For example:

- Television sit-coms such as *One Foot in the Grave*
- News items of elderly patients not receiving adequate care
- Documentaries of old people sitting staring into space in residential care
- News stories of elder abuse.

It does seem that healthy, happy and productive old people are less newsworthy than those falling ill and left waiting on trolleys in hospital corridors. Eccentric old people may make us laugh, but old people who are forgetful or slow in their responses can make us impatient, and lack of patience can lead to a lack of adequate or appropriate care. Dimond (2000) points out that current research on elder abuse highlights the danger that older people being abused may be neglected by existing service provision.

Negative stereotyping is frequently reinforced through everyday conversation, and nurses need to be aware of the ease with which happens. Most will have heard older people referred to in negative, patronising and derogatory terms such as:

- 'Poor old thing'
- 'Sweet'
- 'Past it'
- 'Has been'
- 'Over the hill'.

Such phrases may seem innocent in themselves, but they are symptomatic of an attitude to older people that denies their dignity as individuals. In addition, it may be argued that ageism among nurses can reinforce the structured dependence imposed upon older people by society (Jones, 1993).

Too often, ageist attitudes result in the assumption that older people may readily be described as:

- Of little value
- Unable to look after themselves
- Slow to accept change
- Intolerant and lacking understanding of the young.

Another aspect of growing older is a certain ambivalence towards visible changes, which tends to be gender related. Women, for example, prompted by the cosmetic and 'beauty' industries, are encouraged to conceal signs of ageing, such as grey hair or wrinkles. On the other hand, the phrase 'mutton dressed as lamb' is used often enough to be readily understood as a negative comment on the appearance of some older women. Older men attract less negative stereotyping but may, nevertheless, find themselves patronised as often as older women.

Given the significant number of older people represented in the caseloads of community nurses, it is essential that nurses are able to identify and remain aware of the extent of stereotyping. It is important on the one hand because such negative images make it easy to underestimate the ability of older people to enjoy a normal happy and healthy lifestyle. In addition, it can add to the difficulty of assessing the ability of older people to deal adequately, in their own terms, with adverse situations. Nurses need to think carefully about the most appropriate care to offer, especially when an older person has become vulnerable through a temporary illness, or perhaps is grieving the loss of a partner (see Chapter 14 for more information on grief reactions and bereavement). It is very easy to take over when the best response might be to allow time for the individual to adjust to a new situation and to give only the appropriate level of support and encouragement to help maintain independence.

Somerville (1987) highlights three examples of quite normal behaviour patterns in older people which, if they are misinterpreted can cause 'irreparable damage' to well-being:

- A tendency to be slow at performing tasks may be interpreted as evidence of impairment and intellectual decline, whereas when given sufficient time there is no reason why an older person cannot perform and complete the task as well as a younger person.

- Forgetfulness in the old is often interpreted as a negative age-related impairment – yet forgetfulness is a normal behaviour pattern at any age.

- Poor motivation and lack of concentration can be symptomatic of depression (which may occur at any age) rather than of dementia. Mental changes are more often a manifestation of illness than of normal ageing.

By developing an awareness of the assumptions underlying ageism, nurses reduce the risk of older people being treated in a way that can limit and disempower them. Good nursing care in the form of relevant interventions can contribute considerably to the achievement of a better quality lifestyle. It is equally important, however, that such understanding is accompanied by an ability to distinguish quite clearly between the assumptions of ageism, and the physiological changes due to the ageing process. Such changes can be detrimental to an individual's ability to maintain independence unless they are identified and adequately treated.

Medical aspects of ageing

As noted earlier, ageing is a normal biological process and in a healthy individual may present few major health problems. However, gradual degeneration in physiological function may be exacerbated by genetic inheritance and/or adverse environmental factors and lead to increased vulnerability to the diseases of old age. Slowing down of cell division in old age, for example, can reduce the response of the immune system. Reduced immunity means that infections more readily take hold, and dormant infections may be reactivated. Bones and joints are the two parts of the musculoskeletal system most affected by ageing, and the older person with these problems may often

Student Activity 13.3

- ◆ Identify possible medical problems associated with an ageing body.

- ◆ Identify age-associated factors that may exacerbate medical conditions.

- ◆ Do these correlate with older patients on your assessor's caseload?

- ◆ Discuss with one or two of your peers.

- ◆ Make notes in your portfolio.

be in pain and have poor mobility. This in turn may result in poor nutrition, or lack of exercise, which further diminishes the ability of the ageing body to cope adequately with normal lifestyle needs.

You may have identified a variety of medical problems including respiratory and/or circulatory impairment, osteoporosis, osteoarthritis, all of which are disabling conditions, leading to poor or lack of mobility and attendant problems. Johnson (2000) notes, for example, that increasing age is a contributory risk factor in the development of osteoarthritis. The onset is usually insidious, and some 10 per cent of women over the age of 80 present with osteoarthritis of the hip. The condition is associated with reduced quality of life, disability, chronic pain and social isolation. These factors can lead to depression, especially when they happen to someone who has led an active and interesting life largely involved with other people.

You may also have noted the possibility of dementia, vertigo, a tendency to fall, and have considered urinary tract infections, constipation, or diabetes. Assessing the health of older people, you will have discovered, is a complex activity and you may have identified some important factors as outlined below.

- *Multiple diseases:* failure in one system may lead to failure in another – no one disease dominates the clinical picture.

- *Symptoms* which are common to a number of diseases include:
  - Confusion
  - Falls
  - Incontinence
  - Immobility.

- *Complications* can be caused by multiple drug use.

- *Failure to seek medical help* may be because individuals:
  - Are afraid of the consequences
  - Fear possible treatment or hospitalisation
  - Have low expectations of health
  - Experience insensitivity on the part of health professionals to their cultural needs.

- *Inability to communicate due to intellectual failure* may cause problems with:
  - History-taking

– Diagnosis

– Management.

Multiple health problems in older people can be the result of the failure of health professionals to identify the initial problem, partly because of a tendency to define some conditions as an inevitable result of the ageing process. A further contributory factor, however, is the failure of health professionals to listen to what individuals themselves see as important issues. Gunaratnam (1997) provides examples of the experiences of Asian clients and carers who found that service providers consistently failed to recognise and respond to the central concerns in their lives. This raises further issues in relation to myths and stereotypes of ethnic minority groups, that there is inevitably an extended family network offering support, for example. But lack of accessible information about services and inappropriate provision can render 'care in the community' meaningless to any individual or group, and can lead to a rejection of much needed help and support.

Research by the Royal Commission for Long-term Care (DoH, 1999) showed that demand for ethnic minority elders was not for 'different or special' services, but for more responsive and culturally sensitive mainstream services which will benefit all older people who need care. The potential increase in the number of frail older patients, and the intended outcome of policy that 'the quality of care must increase so that older people will continue to share in the improvements, choice and greater flexibility' as experienced by the rest of society (paragraphs 8.4 and 8.35) present a challenge to nurses to make the most effective use of their skills and knowledge.

Case study

The following case study presents a scenario that will give you the opportunity to explore your understanding and awareness of the problem of 'ageism' discussed above, and it allows you to use your knowledge and understanding of possible medical conditions associated with the ageing process. You should refer to the principles of needs assessment discussed in Chapter 8 as you identify specific health care needs of the client in this case study.

Your assessment will undoubtedly highlight a number of factors to be considered in relation to this client, including her previous lifestyle and the need for exploration of the cause of the fractured femur. You would, no doubt, consider her lack of interest in her books, and note the causes and consequences of a poor appetite. You will also have identified the difficulties faced by a son giving advice regarding personal care to his mother; the fact that he works shifts, and has a hobby that takes him away from home. You would also have noted that although her daughter lives in the same town, she has a career and a home of her own.

Case Study 13.1

Mrs Ellen Ford, a 78-year-old widow, lives in an inner city terraced house, which she shares with her 36-year-old son, Richard. They have lived in the house for 20 years and Mrs Ford is a well-known member of the local community. Richard is a laboratory assistant with a large firm and works shifts. He is also a keen amateur archaeologist, and travels whenever possible to interesting archaeological sites both here and abroad. His 39-year-old sister, a financial advisor, lives in the same town with her partner. They lead a busy life but telephone regularly and visit each month.

Mrs Ford retired from teaching at the local grammar school at 65, has never suffered any major illness, and until recently led a busy life as a voluntary worker for a local charity and held reading sessions for children at the local public library.

Richard contacted the GP following the discharge of his mother from hospital due to a fractured neck of femur. He expressed some concern that his mother was not recovering well. She appeared to have lost interest in reading – formerly her favourite hobby. She lacked interest in her personal hygiene and appearance, was not eating properly, and yet became irritated if questioned, insisting that she did not require help.

The district nurse has very little information from the hospital, except to say that Mrs Ford was anxious to get home and had been interviewed by a social worker.

Your conclusions would be based on your awareness of the kind of lifestyle led by Mrs Ford until her accident; the extent to which she was able and willing to listen to, and to consider an assessment of her current state of health; discussion with her son and daughter and most likely with her GP and DN. One particular aspect of the situation, which needs further exploration, relates to her discharge from hospital. What information was she given? Were her condition and treatment explained? Was she offered a care package? The new guidance on hospital discharge emphasises that patients, their families and their carers should be given adequate information to enable them to understand the discharge process and to take sensible decisions about continuing care (Richards, 1996). However, Smith's (1997) report on the dissatisfaction of patients discharged from hospital following a stroke or fractured neck of femur concluded that hospital staff need reminding to be particularly vigilant in ensuring that frail older people have clear and concise information and instructions on discharge.

You may have considered several possible medical problems which might be diagnosed by Mrs Ford's GP, including osteoporosis, dementia, visual impairment or clinical depression. You would also be aware that she was an independent, intelligent woman, used to being treated with respect, and accustomed to making decisions for herself and others. Is her current apathetic state the result of depression? She has certainly experienced a drastic change of lifestyle. Was it changing before the accident? Is she presenting with symptoms of a more serious underlying disease?

Clearly, this situation requires careful thought about the most appropriate approach to take if problems are to be resolved and Mrs Ford is to regain or improve on her original health status and lifestyle. Whatever the conclusions drawn about the causes of the current situation, and the possible consequences of her changed lifestyle, the plan of care devised would reflect the intention to provide services and care designed to enable Mrs Ford to achieve a better quality of life.

It may be that you see a clear role for the community nursing services, but you will also have identified the possibility of involving other professionals and agencies in the care of this client. It would seem to be important to offer Mrs Ford only that care which she sees as relevant in helping her to maintain independence at the moment. The situation may change if the cause of Mrs Ford's current health status is related to a major health problem such as dementia. The knowledge that she is well known within the neighbourhood, would be another factor to consider. It may be important to establish whether Mrs Ford, whose friends and neighbours are likely to be interested in her well-being, would be prepared to accept their help and support where appropriate, together with the support of her son and daughter, rather than or in addition to statutory or voluntary services.

The identification of a variety of sources of care, and the kind of decision making required to ensure that appropriate care is offered, brings into focus the whole concept of community care and what it means for older people. It also highlights the need for adequate education and preparation of community nurses as significant participants in the process of assessing health needs and implementing care in the community. In an environment of seemingly continuous change, as policy makers seek to adjust social and political theories to meet the expectations and practical care needs of the growing number of older people in the community, it is important for nurses to become more politically and socially aware. As a student, you have the opportunity of developing skills in practice to which the application of the theory you receive on your programme, when applied, will help to better equip you for this awareness. The development of skills necessary for the newly envisaged commissioning/purchaser role will be easier if nurses have a clear understanding of developments in social policy specifically aimed at the care of older people in the community.

Student Activity 13.4

♦ Identify reasons why community care for older people has become a significant element of social policy.

♦ Discuss this with your assessor.

♦ Make notes in your portfolio.

Social policy and community care

Community care is a phrase that is frequently used but rarely clearly defined (see Chapter 1). In the definition noted at the beginning of this chapter emphasis is placed on the view of community care as a support system intended to promote independence and empower people to take control of their own lives.

The concept of community care has a long history, but in relation to older people in society it became a significant element of social policy only in the latter part of the 20th century.

Despite the lack of a precise meaning, Victor (1997) suggests that it is possible to identify several key features, which define community care. The first key element, and perhaps original meaning, of the term is the desire to provide care outside institutions such as hospitals and long-stay facilities. A second key element is the provision of services in the client or patient's own home. The third element is the desire to provide care in a setting that is as 'normal' as is possible given the client's needs. Fourth is an emphasis on the involvement of lay and voluntary carers within the community giving support to individuals who are unable to adequately care for themselves either temporarily or permanently because of illness or lack of personal resources. Doyal (1997) emphasises the value of good quality care and points out that:

> good community care necessitates access to those goods and services that are necessary for the satisfaction of the basic human need for health and autonomy. Unless these needs are optimally met, individuals will be unable to do their best to flourish as persons and as good citizens. (p. 192)

The way in which these needs are met, however, is closely related to current political and economic theory and this in turn determines the choice of a particular type of social policy. It has been argued that, while policy is what happens in theory, practice is what happens in reality and there may be very little relationship between the two. Such a view is supported by the changes in community care policy highlighted in the White Paper *Caring for*

People (DoH, 1989). Changes reflect the criticisms of previous policy decisions which, it is argued, left gaps in care and inadequate provision of services for older people.

Nevertheless, as Walker (1997) points out, the importance of policy is that it does reflect the values of current society, it represents how people think, and how governments 'endeavour to engineer change'. The case study above provided an opportunity to explore the best possible response to the needs of an individual for effective care within a range of options made available through current community care policy. It may also, however, have high-lighted the difficulties which can arise in identifying who will provide the services, especially where needs are not clearly defined, as is often the case with older people.

There is a widely held view that in the past, older people were largely cared for by their families, and that current provision of care for older people is now, or should be, the responsibility of the state. A review of historical research, however, suggests a much more complex picture of community care and it seems that policy makers have consistently failed to articulate clear and precise strategies on how the needs of older people in society may be adequately met.

The growth of community care for older people in Britain has been sporadic and may be seen as a series of responses to demographic, social and economic changes. These three factors have influenced the way in which older people have been perceived, how we might best care for them, and how resources should be distributed. It is possible to distinguish three main elements to the growth of community care (Malin et al., 1999):

- Deinstitutionalisation.

- The development of planning and provision for priority groups (of professional and voluntary services in the community to support older people and their carers).
- Care provided by, rather than 'in', the community: the continuum of formal and informal care.

Historically, long-term care provision for older people by the National Health Service (NHS), and by local authorities meant institutionalisation (Audit Commission, 1997). The principle of care 'from the cradle to the grave', which underpinned the NHS, was taken very seriously. Hospitals developed specialist wards or units devoted to 'geriatric' care, and local authority 'homes' provided residential care to those older people without visible means of support. Little attention was paid, however, to the needs of older people who were living in their own homes. In addition, the significant contribution to the care of older people by informal carers went largely unrecognised.

By the late 1950s, the establishment of some professional and voluntary services underpinned the second element in the development of community care – the provision of social care in the community. The intention was to seek alternative ways of caring for older people, and to promote care *in* the community rather than care in institutional settings. A new principle – that it was in the best interests of older people to remain in their own homes for as long as possible – gave added impetus, and services to help maintain people at home became increasingly available. The 1962 Hospital Plan, for example, was designed to prevent expensive hospital admissions by increasing community health services (DHSS, 1962).

During the 1960s and 1970s, however, successive reports and policy statements highlighted the fact that despite the policy intentions, in reality, the input of professional services, supported only by fragmented voluntary services, had been inadequate in meeting the needs of older people in the community (Seebohm Committee, 1968). Questions were raised as to why the policy had been largely ineffective, and some commentators identified a failure to develop a clear central strategy in planning care, or to provide effective financial support for community care services. Part of the problem, they argued, was the simplistic perception of the care needs of older people. In addition, the contribution of families to care had been simply taken for granted in policy debates, without sufficient consideration of the fact that this was not always readily available (Walker, 1982; Parker, 1990).

The White Paper *A Happier Old Age* (DHSS, 1978) acknowledged the wish of 'most elderly people' to remain in their own homes, and stated that the intention of current policy was to 'promote an active approach to treatment and rehabilitation'. The paper also pronounced that families could not be expected to shoulder the entire care burden for the growing number of frail older people, and they should be able to look to the wider community for support. Thus the beginning of the 1980s heralded the third element in the development of community care – that of care *by* the community, where informal carers and the voluntary sector are viewed as integral to the provision of social care.

Student Activity 13.5

- ◆ Write down as many agencies on your placement patch you can think of that provide care or resources for older people in the community.

- ◆ Identify the providers as either statutory or voluntary services.

- ◆ Compare your list with one or two of your peers in another patch.

- ◆ Make notes in your portfolio.

You will, no doubt be able to identify a number of agencies that provide care, from the statutory health services including nursing, medical and other therapeutic services, to voluntary agencies and pressure groups concerned specifically with older people. Services may be accessed from four sources:

1. Local authorities
2. NHS community health services } **Statutory Sector***
3. The independent sector: voluntary agencies and commercial enterprises
4. Informal carers.

- Local authority social services* arrange for provision of:
  - Housing department and welfare rights
  - Advice and social work support
  - Domiciliary care and personal care
  - Day care and residential care
  - Meals/lunch clubs/recreation
  - Warden services/financial advice/telephone.

- Community health services* include:
  - District nursing and health visiting
  - General practitioner and practice nursing services
  - Specialist services: continence advisers/clinical nurse specialists/community psychiatric nurse
  - Pharmaceutical services
  - Chiropody/dental/optical services
  - Occupational therapy/physiotherapy/speech therapy
  - Screening and preventive services
  - Respite care.

- The independent sector/voluntary agencies include:
  - Private nursing homes and residential homes
  - Age Concern
  - Help the Aged
  - Carers National Association
  - Red Cross

- Alzheimer's Disease Society
- Royal National Institute for the Blind
- Care and Repair England/Scotland/Wales.

Legislative changes in the 1990s established a role for social services as purchasers rather than providers of services, with an emphasis on the need to use the independent sector as providers. A distinction was also made between health care (free at the point of delivery) and social care (means tested). This division resulted in some conflict in decisions as to which agency (health or social services) was responsible for 'personal care' because of difficulties of definition. In their *Report on Long-term Care* (DoH, 1999) the Royal Commission noted that such care fell within the internationally recognised definition of nursing:

> because it directly involves touching a person's body, incorporates issues of intimacy, personal dignity and confidentiality. Because of risks associated with poor personal care (e.g. risks of infection or skin breakdown) it is important that careful assessment is made of how best it can be provided and by whom. (paras 6.43/6.44)

The Commission nevertheless thought that personal care (which they recommended should be exempt from means testing) could be:

> delivered by many people who are not nurses, in particular care assistants employed by social services departments or agencies. (para 6.43)

Such decisions highlight the trend in current policy, to place emphasis on the need to be flexible in the provision of care. Nurses might reflect on the fact that in such situations, the decision-making process requires close collaboration between health services and social services, to ensure that the 'careful assessments' are made by people with appropriate skills and experience. Kendrick (1999) argues that to see the maintenance of a patient's personal hygiene as basic 'and belonging to the emerging skills of inexperienced or unqualified staff', is to deny the importance of the host of assessment and interpersonal skills inherent in such care. The very fact that an individual has to accept assistance with personal needs, he points out, tends to threaten or compromise their sense of dignity, individuality and autonomy.

Current policy sees an effective joint consultation process as the cornerstone of community care planning, and new initiatives such as the establishment of primary care groups and trusts (PCGs/PCTs) are designed to encourage collaborative care. In their White Paper *The New NHS: Modern, Dependable* (DoH, 1997) the government placed great emphasis on the need for a truly 'national' health service, in which local provision matches the goals set at national level. The PCG is a group comprising representatives of a variety of agencies within a defined community, including community nurses.

A central function of the group is to consider the overall or 'holistic' health needs of a population. In theory, regional variations in provision should disappear as each 'community' should be funded according to the needs identified by the PCG, which are then incorporated by the relevant health authority in its Health Improvement Programme. As PCTs (and later care trusts) replace PCGs, you should be able to observe a more participative approach to the provision of care for people in the community. Better inter-agency collaboration between the professionals and increased participation by community nurses should be a positive feature within the new structure.

Your review of service provision for older people will have included the important part played by lay carers, such as family members, friends and neighbours, in the provision of care. The results of a survey of carers of dependent older people commissioned by the European Commission in 1993 showed that the family is 'overwhelmingly the main source of care for older people'. Adult children were most frequently mentioned (40 per cent) followed by spouses (32 per cent). Further research has consistently found that most informal carers are women – the proportion varying between 60 per cent and 80 per cent among the member states (McGlone and Cronin, 1995).

The role and contribution of lay carers was finally recognised by government in the Carers (Recognition and Services) Act 1995. Under the Act local authorities are obliged on request to recognise and assess the needs of carers. As a direct consequence of the Act health and social service professionals have a collective responsibility to ensure that families receive the services to which they are entitled (Adcock, 2000). It may also be argued that greater public awareness encouraged by the media, and documents such as The Patient's Charter (DoH, 1993) which emphasise individual rights and the benefits of health services, has increased the pressure on community nurses to provide flexible and individually responsive care to patients in the community.

A recent study by the Policy Studies Institute, of the care of older people following discharge from hospital, however, suggests that some nurses are not responding adequately to the needs of older patients. One problem appeared to be the reluctance of nurses in hospital elderly care units to refer people to other professions (O'Dowd, 2000). Clearly it is of great help to community nurses if patients are discharged with adequate and appropriate care packages, and it would seem as important to improve communication between hospital and community as it is to improve and enhance communication and collaboration between different agencies within the community.

Collaborative care

It is a characteristic of community care that it is provided by a number of agencies, both statutory and voluntary, and additionally by lay carers. It has also been characteristic of each development of social policy that good, effective community care is seen to be dependent on the ability of the various organisations and agencies to work together in the assessment, planning and delivery of community care services. Close liaison and effective collaboration are regarded as essential to ensure smooth and comprehensive care delivery. In addition, current social policy emphasises the importance of patient/client/carer participation in the decision-making process if patient-centred individualised care is to be achieved.

You will no doubt identify the importance of regular, effective communication between agencies as a good foundation for liaison and collaboration. This is not always easy to achieve with heavy caseloads, professional responsibilities, and the need to make an active contribution to meetings within your own sphere.

Student Activity 13.6

♦ What factors would you consider to be important in achieving close liaison and effective collaboration?

♦ What factors might cause difficulty in the achievement of effective collaborative care?

The achievement of good communication depends on a number of factors:

- Commitment to the process
- A sound knowledge of the factors involved
- Good time management
- Valuing your own contribution to the process
- A willingness to listen to and value the contribution of colleagues
- Prompt distribution of accurate minutes of meetings to those involved.

Important factors in ensuring effective collaboration would include:

- Knowledge and understanding of the role and function of other agencies
- Being aware of and accepting different perspectives of a problem
- Efficient and effective documentation
- Willingness to share knowledge
- Clear understanding of boundaries and responsibilities
- A common philosophy based on the empowerment of patients and clients.

Effective collaborative care requires a good working knowledge of the roles and functions of all agencies involved. This is particularly important where there are budgetary constraints, but there are factors relating to professional agendas and boundaries that can affect care delivery both positively and negatively, and these must be carefully considered when planning future service provision. Malin and colleagues (1999) note the different character-istics and values of professional groups, but suggest that they could be put to good use.

The collectivist and rights-based values of social work, for example, are different from the more individualist values based on care and obligation that are central to nursing, and both differ from the medical model approach of GPs whose core knowledge-base is rooted in the physical sciences. However, Malin and colleagues (1999) argue that although consensus decisions may be difficult to achieve, professional expertise of various sorts is an essential element in assessing a diversity of need. Differences, even conflicts, they suggest, can be utilised as 'sources of energy and advantage, rather than of disruption', if participants can establish an agreed sense of obligation to providing care that is of most benefit to the patient or client.

A practical example of a successful initiative in improved inter-agency collaboration is provided by Redworth and colleagues (1999) in their discus-sion of a programme of education initiated by a district nursing team for social service home carers. The rationale for the project was that 'successful planning of education leads to a coherent delivery of services for patients in practice'.

Their experience of implementing the project supports the view of Malin et al. (1999) that an important factor in improving collaboration is the devel-opment of a fundamental philosophy of care common to both groups, and that it should incorporate the concept of patient empowerment. In this instance, the issue of empowerment had caused a problem for the home care workers. They felt it was a philosophy that should underpin their work, but it became apparent that traditional influences meant that, in practice, their role was one of acting for their clients rather than encouraging them to develop their potential for self-care. This perception of care tended to increase patient dependence, and the education programme was developed to bring about change. Teachers with diverse roles, from social workers, clinical nurse specialists, community nurses and the community pharmacist, were recruited, and the process was supported through regular meetings and sharing of ideas and activities.

Effective collaboration also involves equal participation in the decision-making process, and this is a relatively new area for nurses. The new methods of commissioning care provision in the community, discussed above, are still being tried and tested. But community nurses have the opportunity to make a very positive contribution, especially with regard to arguing for adequate resources for preventive health care and the promotion of health in older

people. If the problems of 'ageism' are to be finally conquered, nurses must
lead the way in developing positive attitudes to ageing. As recognised
promoters of health, they are in a key position to challenge negative attitudes
to old age through positive programmes of rehabilitative and health
enhancing activities. The continuing development of skills in appropriate
needs assessment, and more clearly defined opportunities for discussion with
other agencies will be of crucial importance in enabling them to provide the
'right level of intervention and support' in this important aspect of the care
of older people.

Health promotion and older people

Our beliefs and values about health develop from our experiences of life, and
many older people today will have been influenced by their parents and
grandparents whose lifestyle and life expectancy were very different from
those of today. Beliefs about the ageing process and the 'place' of older
people in society that have been gained in the early years of life can be very
significant in influencing the views of older people regarding their ability to
maintain and improve their health status. Roberts (1990) identifies certain
beliefs which may have an influence on how older people perceive their
health. These include such issues as immediacy, where health strategies
promising future benefits are not likely to be considered useful. Others
include believing they are too old for it to matter, and overvaluing 'rest'.

Although nurses need to be aware that older people may have entrenched
beliefs about health, they must be equally aware of the dangers of ageism
when assessing health need. Once again it is important not to treat older
people as a homogeneous group. Ginn and colleagues (1997) remind us that
there is a reciprocal relationship between behaviour and health in that a
person's state of health may influence their capacity to engage in health
promoting behaviours. They review research into health promotion issues
and old age, and stress that the health of older people, as with people in any
other age group, reflects structural influences such as social class, material
circumstances, gender, ethnicity and area of residence. Thus any approach to
health promotion among older people must recognise this diversity.

Clearly, an important factor in searching for appropriate health promoting
activities is to use observational skills and to listen to the individual
concerned. Some older people, for example, have a very active life because
they are involved with their extended family. Others have good social
networks and are able to maintain outside contacts with a variety of friends
and associates. Many continue to work either in paid employment or in a
voluntary capacity for many years after 'retirement' age.

The health of older people can be most effectively promoted through a
partnership approach combining individual health education with social poli-

cies to improve standards of living and access to appropriate health and social care (Ginn et al., 1997). As noted above, this approach should be facilitated by new commissioning structures in which nurses can be active participants. In addition, nurses are already well placed to reduce the risk of illness in old age by encouraging preventive health care activities such as health checks, immunisation and screening.

Factors related to lifestyle habits that are important to restoring, maintaining and promoting health in old age are unlikely to differ substantially from the needs of other groups, and your approach would undoubtedly be based on a model identified in Chapter 9. It is, however, important to recognise that the concept of health should include a sense of well-being, and

---

Student Activity 13.7

♦ What factors are important to the maintenance and improvement of health in later life?

♦ How would you encourage health awareness in older people?

---

among older people this is closely related to satisfaction with social aspects of life and the supportive quality of their environment (Ginn et al., 1997). Bearing in mind what has been said regarding influences on health outside the control of individuals, some factors you might have considered are:

● Adequate nutritional intake:

- An adequate well-balanced diet – especially fruit/vegetables (or juice)
- Adequate fluid intake – regular hot drinks in cold weather
- Immunisation – influenza vaccine
- Regular checks (including screening).

● Regular exercise:

- A daily walk
- Swimming
- Dancing
- Housework/gardening.

Regular (even if gentle) exercise has many benefits for older people. It helps maintain bone density and mobility – diminishes the risk of osteoporosis; reduces the risk of falls/fractures, of obesity, high blood pressure; diminishes the risk of cardiovascular disease and stroke.

- Caution in relation to:
  - Smoking
  - Alcohol
  - High fat/high sugar content foods.

Additional factors:

- The importance of social activities in preventing isolation/raising self-esteem.
- Educational/recreational courses and activities:
  - Help to maintain intellectual interest
  - Provide another source of participative or social activity
  - Can often be very satisfying to those people who did not have the opportunity to pursue such interests when they were younger.

The *Report on Long-term Care* makes particular reference to opportunities for education and access to leisure opportunities for older people stating that they should 'continue to be a high priority in all aspects of public provision' (DoH, 1999, para. 10.9).

There should be little difficulty in raising awareness of health issues among older people, despite ageist assumptions that this group are cautious and inflexible. Wiles (1999) found older people to be 'significantly more open-minded, cheerful and accepting' of new ideas and change. On the other hand, good observational and communication skills, as discussed in Chapter 7, are essential in situations where health has been compromised by illness or accident, for example where assistance is clearly needed but is not acceptable to the older person.

This can be particularly important where finance is concerned, since many older people find it difficult to accept what they regard as 'charity', and may need to be persuaded to accept state benefits. An attempt to raise awareness and to encourage a more positive outlook often involves seeking ways to prompt discussion in which the older person retains control. Many older people may find it easier to look at their current lifestyle in terms of how they managed life when they were younger. Remembering and talking about the past – 'reminiscing' – can be a therapeutic activity in itself when used appropriately. Buchanan (1997, p. 5) suggests that effective reminiscence may be used to 'promote social inclusion ... being counted as a member of a social group, and counting oneself as a member'. When used appropriately, reminiscence is a process which could help reduce social isolation and encourage older people to begin to value their contribution to their local community and to society, providing a positive means of health promotion.

Conclusion

Increases in the average life span mean that a large proportion of life is now spent in old age. From a positive perspective, new technology, developments in health knowledge and a keen interest in health and fitness in a large part of the population, should mean that an increasing number of these years will be spent in relatively good health. However, in increasingly ageing societies – it is a worldwide phenomenon – the health of older people has become a social and political issue. The persistence of 'ageism', at least in British society, is apparent in government approaches to policy, which continue to take a pessimistic view of the potential 'burden' of health care needs in later life. Although community care provides essential service provision for a variety of groups, it has become inextricably linked with the health and social care needs of older people. More importantly, it is seen largely in terms of the acceptance of disability and dependence in old age.

There is no doubt that an increase in the frail elderly population (85 and over) could mean greater demand for health and social services to enable people to remain in their own homes. And it may also be argued that for the (minority) of older people who do require clinical care, the community nursing services are often essential in improving quality of life, and that they also provide an important link with the wider community. The role of the nurse as a health promoter to older people in general, however, has enormous potential. In an ageing society, the prevention of preventable diseases of old age becomes increasingly important. Community nurses are in a prime position to assess needs, to plan appropriately and with sufficient support from health authorities to implement care which encourages older people to maintain their independence for as long as possible. As put so neatly by Oscar Wilde: 'One can survive everything nowadays, except death.' But for older people it is the quality of survival which is important, and skilled, self-aware and knowledgeable community nurses present the best way of achieving this.

Further reading

Audit Commission Briefing (1997) *The Coming of Age*. Abingdon, ACP.
Bright, R. (1997) *Wholeness in Later Life*. London, Jessica Kingsley: Chapters 1 and 2.
Tinker, A. (1992) *Elderly People in Modern Society*, 4th edn. London, Longman: Chapters 2, 6 and 8.

USEFUL WEB SITES

Age Concern www.ace.org.uk

BBC's Page on Positive Ageing www.bbc.co.uk/health/ageing

British Geriatric Society www.bgs.org.uk

Health and Age The Novartis Foundation for Gerontology www.healthandage.com/
edu/primer

References

Adcock, L. (2000) Assessing the needs of carers. *Journal of Community Nursing*,
14(3): 4–6.
Appleby, J. and Harrison, A. (1999) *Health Care UK 1999/2000: The King's Fund
Review of Health Policy*. London, King's Fund.
Arber, S. and Ginn, J. (1990) The meaning of informal care: gender and the contrib-
ution of elderly people. *Ageing and Society*, 10: 429–54.
Audit Commission Briefing (1997) *The Coming of Age*. Abingdon, ACP.
Bornat, J., Johnson, J., Pereira, C., Pilgrim, D. and Williams, F. (1997) *Community
Care – A Reader*, 2nd edn. Basingstoke, Macmillan – now Palgrave, in association
with The Open University.
Buchanan, K. (1997) Reminiscence and social exclusion, *Reminiscence*, 15 (August),
3–5.
Bytheway, B. (1995) *Ageism*. Buckingham, OUP.
Davey, B. (1999) Solving economic, social and environmental problems together: an
empowerment strategy for losers. In Barnes, M. and Warren, L. (eds) *Paths to
Empowerment*. Bristol, Policy Press.
Denham, M.J. (1997) *Continuing Care for Older People*. Cheltenham, Stanley
Thornes.
Department of Health (1989) *Caring For People: Community Care in the Next
Decade and Beyond*. London, HMSO.
Department of Health (1990) The NHS and Community Care Act (1990). London,
HMSO.
Department of Health (1993) *The Patient's Charter*. London, DoH.
Department of Health (1997) *The New NHS: Modern, Dependable*. London, HMSO.
Department of Health (1999) Royal Commission on Long-term Care *With Respect to
Old Age*. London, HMSO.
Department of Health (2001) *National Service Framework for Older People*. London,
DoH.
Department of Health and Social Security (1962) Hospital Plan for England and
Wales. CMND 1604. London, HMSO.
Department of Health and Social Security (1978) *A Happier Old Age*. London,
HMSO.
Dimond, B. (2000) Legal issues arising in community nursing 5: elder abuse. *British
Journal of Community Nursing*, 5(3): 118–21.
Doyal, L. (1997) Human need and the moral right to optimal community care. In
Bornat, J., Johnson, J., Pereira, C., Pilgrim, D. and Williams, F. (eds) (1997)
Community Care – A Reader, 2nd edn. Basingstoke, Macmillan – now Palgrave, in
association with The Open University.
Forster, P. (1993) The forty something barrier: medicine and age discrimination.
British Medical Journal, 306(3): 637–9, February.
Ginn, J, Arber, S. and Cooper, H. (1997) *Researching Older People's Health Needs
and Health Promotion Issues*. London, Health Education Authority.

Gunaratnam, Y. (1997) Breaking the silence. Black and ethnic minority carers and service provsion. In Bornat, J., Johnson, J., Pereira, C., Pilgrim, D. and Williams, F. (eds) (1997) *Community Care – A Reader,* 2nd edn. Basingstoke, Macmillan – now Palgrave, in association with The Open University.

Jeffreys, M. (1991) *Growing Old in the Twentieth Century.* London, Routledge.

Johnson, W. (1991) The structured dependency of the elderly: a critical note. In Jeffreys, M. (ed.) *Growing Old in the Twentieth Century.* London, Routledge.

Johnson, W. (2000) How osteoarthritis can affect quality of life. *Practice Nurse,* 19(5).

Jones, H. (1993) Altered images. *Nursing Times,* 89(5): 58–60.

Kendrick, K. (1999) Patient washing: a skill, not a task. *Professional Nurse,* 14(5): 304.

Linton, T., Woods, B. and Phair, L. (2000) Training is not enough to change care practice. *Journal of Dementia Care,* March/April, 15–17.

Malin, N., Manthorpe, J., Race, D. and Wilmot, S. (1999) *Community Care for Nurses and the Caring Professions.* Buckingham, Open University Press.

McGlone, F. and Cronin, N. (1995) *A Crisis in Care? The Future of Family and State Care for Older People in the European Union.* London, Family Policy Studies Centre.

Meads, G. (1997) *Health and Social Services in Primary Care: An Effective Combination?* London, FT Health Care.

Means, R. and Smith, R. (1998) *Community Care: Policy and Practice,* 2nd edn. Basingstoke, Macmillan – now Palgrave.

NHS Executive (1996) *Evidence-based Purchasing: Rehabilitation for Older People.* London, NHSE.

NHS Health and Advisory Service (1997) *Services for People who are Elderly.* London, HMSO.

Nolan, J. (1999) Working with older people: opportunities for community nursing. *British Journal of Community Nursing,* 4(2): 86–9.

O'Dowd, A. (2000) Nurses slow to meet older patients' needs. *Nursing Times,* 6(13): 5.

Parker, G. (1990) *With Due Care and Attention: A Review of Research on Informal Care.* London, Family Policy Studies Centre.

Redworth, F., Jones-Tatum, L. and Atkin, J. (1999) District nurses and home carers 2: collaborative education. *British Journal of Community Nursing,* 4(10): 538–42.

Richards, M. (1996) *Community Care for Older People.* Bristol, Jordan.

Roberts, A. (1990) Systems of life: Number 186. *Nursing Times,* 86(32): 59–62.

Seebohm Committee (1968) *Report of the Committee on Local Authority and Allied Personal Social Services.* CMND.3703. London, HMSO.

Smith, M. (1997) Are older people satisfied with discharge information? *Nursing Times,* 93(43): 52–3.

Smith, R. (1984) The structured dependence of the elderly as a recent development: Some sceptical historical thoughts. *Ageing and Society,* 4(4): 409–28.

Somerville, F. (1987) Towards a better understanding of the elderly. *Senior Nurse,* 7(3): 44–6.

Tinker, A. (1992) *Elderly People in Modern Society,* 4th edn. London, Longman.

Townsend, P. (1981) The structured dependency of the elderly: a creation of social policy in the twentieth century. *Ageing and Society,* 1(1): 5–28.

Victor, C.R. (1997) Community care. In Denham, M.J. (1997) (ed.) *Continuing Care for Older People.* Cheltenham, Stanley Thornes.

Walker, A. (1981) Towards a political economy of old age. *Ageing and Society,* 1(1): 73–94.

Walker, A. (1982) *Community Care: The Family, the State and Social Policy.* Oxford, Blackwell Science.

Walker, A. (1997) Community care policy. From consensus to conflict. In Bornat, J., Johnson, J., Pereira, C., Pilgrim, D. and Williams, F. (eds) (1997) *Community Care – A Reader,* 2nd edn. Basingstoke, Macmillan – now Palgrave, in association with The Open University.

Wiles, J. (1999) 'Age cannot wither her ...'. *Elderly Care,* 11(5): 11–14.

14

Death, dying and bereavement

CLAIRE HENRY

Learning outcomes

By the end of this chapter you will be able to:

- Understand the emotional processes likely to be encountered by patients and family members when death is unavoidable.
- Explain the coping mechanisms used to help the patients and family cope with death.
- Discuss the role of the nurse in caring for a patient who is dying using a holistic approach.
- Discuss the role of the nurse in bereavement support for the family.
- Be aware of the effect that caring for a dying patient and family may have on the nurse and how to access appropriate support.

Introduction

Death, dying and bereavement are situations we all experience on either a personal or professional level. These experiences can happen in a variety of situations at home, in hospital, at work, during play or even on holiday. Death may occur as a result of a chronic debilitating illness, where it is expected, or it may be sudden and unexpected. Wherever or however it occurs, its effects on the bereaved are immediate and in some cases long-term.

This chapter will examine the effects of death, dying and bereavement on patients and their family, friends and others they come into contact with, including health care professionals. For the purpose of this chapter the focus will be on the role of the nurse. This will relate to various care settings primarily focusing on the community.

While you are reading this chapter it is important that you reflect on any experiences you have had during your training, or in your everyday life,

Student Activity 14.1

Think of an experience you have had either personally, or as a student nurse, where you have had to deal with death, dying or impending bereavement.

- ◆ What was the situation?
- ◆ How were you supported?
- ◆ How did you feel?
- ◆ Make notes about your experience in your portfolio.

relating to death, dying and bereavement. This will help you to understand what the patient and their family may be experiencing. It is also important to recognise the fact that you are an individual and will have feelings and needs. Often this type of care can be difficult to deal with, as there is a large amount of fear associated with these issues. It also highlights to us our own mortality.

Death in the United Kingdom

In the UK there are on average 640,000 deaths per year. People die from many different causes, and deaths may be expected or unexpected.

Expected death

Expected death may be caused by one of the following:

- Cancer
- HIV and AIDS
- Neurological diseases such as motor neurone disease and multiple sclerosis
- Chronic heart failure
- Respiratory conditions such as bronchiectasis
- End stage renal failure.

All the diseases mentioned above present problems in predicting life expectancy. Many of these diseases have long illness trajectories and it is difficult for any member of the health care team to assess accurately when a patient is in the palliative phase of their disease. Even when it is evident, many doctors are reluctant to tell patients that the focus of their treatment has changed from curative to palliative.

Unexpected death

Unexpected deaths can result in a variety of problems. They can be caused by, for example:

- Road traffic accidents
- Accidents in the home
- Natural disasters such as earthquakes or hurricanes
- Disasters such as aeroplane crashes or terrorist activity
- Myocardial infarctions

- Cerebral vascular accidents
- Gastrointestinal bleeds
- Meningitis
- Drug or solvent abuse
- Miscarriages
- Murder
- Suicide.

These are just some examples, there are obviously many more. Both expected and unexpected deaths give rise to similar reactions.

Palliative care

Palliative care has developed in response to the needs of cancer patients and covers certain other diseases. This type of care aims to provide for, and manage patients and their families, faced with a terminal disease. This can only be provided when it is known that the patient is going to die from their disease. Patients who are expected to die can access these services, which provide support for them and their family prior to death. Where death is unexpected, however, palliative care services can be accessed for bereavement care.

A simplistic approach is to define palliative care as the desire to alleviate for patients the most distressing symptoms of the dying process. A more complete view, as defined by the World Health Organization (1990) refers to the patient as a whole, and identifies palliative care as the active total care of patients where the disease is not responsive to curative treatment. Pain control, and responding to physical symptoms along with psychological, social and spiritual problems are paramount. The WHO identifies the goal of palliative care as the achievement of the best quality of life for patients and their families.

Palliative interventions aim to control distressing symptoms and improve a patient's quality of life, for example through the use of palliative radiotherapy, chemotherapy, surgical procedures and anaesthetic techniques for pain relief.

Student Activity 14.2

♦ With your peers, see if you can come up with any other definitions of palliative care. This can be based on experiences you
  have had, or on patients you have cared for.

♦ Make notes for your portfolio.

Terminal care is an important part of palliative care. It usually refers to the management of patients during the last few days, weeks or even months of life, from a point where it has become clear that the patient is in a progressive state of decline.

Specialist palliative care services can be provided in a number of ways:

- Direct contact either in a specialist unit or by a member of the team visiting at home or in the outpatient setting
- Indirectly through advice to a patient's present professional advisers or carers.

As with other health care services, the focus emphasises the team approach. Services provide physical, psychological, social and spiritual support. The team includes practitioners with a broad mix of skills, including medical and nursing skills, social work, pastoral and spiritual care, physiotherapy, occupational therapy, and pharmacy and related specialities.

The key principles underpinning palliative care, which should be practised by all nurses in all care settings, include:

- Focusing on quality of life which includes good symptom control.
- A whole person approach, taking into account the person's past life experiences and current situation.
- Care that encompasses both the person with life-threatening disease and those that matter to that person.
- Respect for patients' autonomy and choice over place of care, treatment options and access to specialist palliative care.
- Emphasis on open and sensitive communication, which extends to patients, informal carers and professional colleagues (see Chapter 7 for more information about communication).

These principles are key when providing palliative care to patients and their families. However, even though the principles are still applicable, traditionalists in palliative care feel the focus of care has changed. Previously synonymous with terminal cancer care, palliative care has broadened its scope in some areas to encompass cancer patients at an earlier stage of their illness. A recent model of palliative care has suggested that many patients need palliative care early in the course of their disease and sometimes from diagnosis (Ahmedzai, 1996). Some palliative care providers have challenged this, stating that the needs of the dying may once again be overlooked (Biswas, 1993). What can be seen from this debate is that the timing of the involvement of the palliative care service in a patient's disease trajectory is under scrutiny.

With palliative care now beginning at diagnosis, more individuals have been exposed to the services. It is no surprise, therefore, that others outside the cancer care field are becoming increasingly interested in the service. There have been examples such as in AIDS and motor neurone disease where palliative care has already been widely offered. However, the pace of interest from other areas is now increasing notably for cases of chronic circulatory and respiratory disease. There are areas into which palliative care has not had a significant impact yet, for example, where older people are dying in residential or nursing homes (Katz et al., 1999). It could be that pockets of excellence become available in certain localities whereas nothing is available elsewhere. This highlights that all is by no means perfect or equitable in contemporary palliative care developments.

There is a growing body of evidence to show that many patients who die from non-malignant diseases have unmet needs for symptom control,

---

Student Activity 14.3

♦ Find out at what point palliative care services are accessed in your area.

♦ Compare this to another area locally, and make notes in your portfolio.

---

psychological support, open communication, control over their final days and choice about what sort of care they receive (Addington-Hall, 1998). There have been numerous studies examining specific diseases and dying. These include motor neurone disease, dementia, chronic obstructive disease, stroke and heart disease (Wilkes, 1984; Barby and Leigh, 1995; Beattie et al., 1995; Lloyd-Williams, 1996; Skilbeck et al., 1997.)

It has now been recognised that inequality in service exists. However, what has to be addressed is the question of the transferability of current services for cancer patients to non-malignant patients and their carers.

Understanding the emotional processes likely to be encountered by patients and family members when death is unavoidable

Communication

Communication with the patient and all team members is a vital. The focus on communication must be open so that most terminally ill patients are at least told they are dying and have the options discussed openly with them (Glaser and Strauss, 1968; Kubler-Ross, 1970). This is important when the diagnosis is given, and when other issues arise along the patient's journey. For example, patients will need to consider where they want to die. At such

Student Activity 14.4

◆ Discuss with your supervisor what level of choice is available for patients wishing to have palliative care in your area.

◆ Compare this with your peers in another area.

◆ Make notes in your portfolio.

points it is important for the nurse to know what services are available, as it is no good offering patients services and support that cannot be provided within your area.

The use of open and honest communication with patients and families may be difficult. This gets no easier once the patient has been diagnosed. Many health care professionals have concerns about telling patients they are going to die of their disease. They often feel that by informing the patient that the focus of their care is palliative, they will take away hope and cause an enormous amount of distress. The patient and family will of course be distressed, but they need to be informed about what is happening if they are to be able to plan the time they have and take more control. Honesty with patients and their families is an important part of care. If health care professionals are honest about treatment the patient can make decisions, whereas if they are not told that the treatment is palliative, they may suffer terrible side effects believing that they may be cured.

This type of communication causes great stress to most health care professionals. Some may feel that not being honest with patients and families will protect them from having to cope with the emotions that are unleashed. This is an unacceptable strategy, however.

Student Activity 14.5

◆ Read Chapter 36 in Dickinson and Johnson (1993) *Death, Dying and Bereavement*.

◆ Discuss the implications with your assessor and one or two of your peers.

◆ Make notes in your portfolio.

Breaking bad news

No one likes having to break bad news, particularly bad news that will change the way patients and their families will view their future. There are many reasons why this may be so.

It may be because the newsgiver is fearful of the reactions they will unleash in the patient and/or relative. There may be concerns that answers, or a plan of care, are not readily available. There may be discomfort in saying 'I do not know'. There could also be a feeling of failure and fear of being blamed by patients and their relatives. Other reasons may include wanting to protect the patient and feeling embarrassed about giving the patient the bad news. There may not be enough time to spend with patients and their families, so the event is postponed or left for someone else.

All these factors are important and, in order to give some guidance, many models have been developed to aid this process and provide clarification on the best way to give the news.

Student Activity 14.6

◆ Read Chapter 35 in Dickenson and Johnson (1993) *Death, Dying and Bereavement*.

◆ Discuss with one or two of your peers.

◆ Make notes in your portfolio.

Grief and loss

Grief starts when the diagnosis is made. However, grief may also be considered to start before the diagnosis. Often the patient and a member of the family have noticed a change in behaviour, a loss of weight, or had a sense that something is wrong. When the diagnosis is given, even with the most optimistic outlook, the patient and relatives often fear the worst. All involved may talk about it and be optimistic for each other. The professional may only find out about this when the patient has died and relatives are discussing their feelings and experiences.

Grief has been defined by Rando (1984) as an individual's physical, psychological and social response to loss. But there are many ways that grief and loss can be interpreted. Grief is an individual experience through which many people move using their own unique resources and support network. It is a dynamic process, which is unlikely to proceed tidily along a line, or through the various stages of a model.

However, models can be useful in helping us as nurses to understand the reactions and stages an individual may go through in relation to grief, loss and bereavement.

'Bereavement' is the term used to pigeonhole the sense of loss that occurs when you sustain an important loss. The term is a neutral, bureaucratic one that covers any situation in which a relative or friend has lost a person they are attached to. Bereavement can be difficult for an individual as the emphasis has shifted from the patient to the relative and the bereaved becomes the focus of care (Gamlin, 1994).

Individual bereavement reactions are expressed through thoughts and feelings. The cultural and social background influences this (Cooley, 1992). As a student nurse, particularly one working with adults in community settings, it is important that you try to familiarise yourself with different cultural beliefs and rituals in relation to death and dying. A few examples of different cultures are given below. This does not, however, remove the requirement to ensure that individual family needs are recognised and catered for during their bereavement (Kinghorn and Gamlin, 2001).

Buddhism

Buddhists believe that dying is very much part of life; therefore they will appreciate very full and honest information to help them prepare. Their death should be talked about openly. The individual will want to retain as clear a state of consciousness as possible. This may affect what medication is given. It is important that a Buddhist monk or lay devotee should be informed of the impending death, and the family will usually undertake responsibility for this. Following the death it is vital that the family and the monk are left to ease the transition of the patient in silence or with quiet chanting.

Christianity

Roman Catholics and other Christians believe in life after death. Some Christians believe not in life immediately after death, but in a life to come. When a Roman Catholic or practising Church of England person is ill they can receive the sacrament of the sick. The sacrament is to symbolise forgiveness, healing and reconciliation. A small bottle of holy water may be placed near the bed; this should not be removed. It is important that the priest is either present at the moment of death or that he is called soon after to administer the 'last rites'.

Christians of any denomination may wish to receive holy communiun regularly, for as long as they are able, from a priest of their own tradition, and some Christian families may wish to perform their own last offices as a mark of respect for their loved one, and to have their priest or pastor present at the time of death. Sensitivity to the specific needs of people of different Christian denominations is as applicable as it is for people of other faiths. The wishes of families must be paramount and sensitivity is essential.

Hinduism

Hindus prefer to die at home. Before death a Hindu desires to offer food and other articles to the needy, religious persons or to the temple. A female calf may be offered and this can be represented symbolically by Kusha grass. A small peace of this sacred grass may be placed under the bed of the dying patient by their relatives.

Relatives may wish to read from the holy book and the patient may wish to lie on the floor to symbolise closeness with Mother Earth or to indicate the giving of the bed to someone in greater need.

A tulsi leaf may be placed in the patient's mouth along with water from the Ganges, which may be sprinkled over the patient. The relative or the Hindu priest may do this. A thread may be placed around the patient's neck or wrist, and these must not be removed. If a non-Hindu is to be involved in last offices, they must wear gloves so that they do not touch the body.

Islam

Muslims believe in life after death and believe that death is the will of Allah and should be accepted as such. You should not say to Muslim patients that they are going to die, but rather that they are very poorly as it is considered that only God knows when you are going to die. Death is seen as a change from this world to another and the patient's family will help with the transition. Religious leaders may be called by the family and, as for members of other faiths, this may need to be facilitated. The family will read from the holy Qur'an. The patient may wish to sit or lie facing Mecca. In the event of death the patient should be turned onto their right side, facing south-east. It is vital that non-Muslims do not touch the body, as it is considered sacred.

Judaism

The main emphasis of Judaism is on this life. They do believe in an afterlife although this takes different forms for different groups. Orthodox Jews believe in a bodily resurrection at the time of the coming of the Messiah, whereas for Reform Jews the emphasis is more on a spiritual afterlife. In accordance with Jewish faith, a dying person should not be left on their own. This gives the patient the chance to say a special prayer or confession and receive affirmation of faith. Involvement of the rabbi is as requested by the family.

Sikhism

Sikhs believe in reincarnation and death is seen as a step in life and therefore not necessarily a sad occasion. It is imperative that the family's wishes are adhered to, especially with regard to Sikh custom. Neither the hair nor the beard should be trimmed. Carers should ensure that consultation with the family takes place before any attempt is made to perform last offices.

Models of grief reaction

There are many models that have been developed in relation to grief reaction. These models are equally applicable to the person who is dying, the family and others who are associated with them. This can also be applied to individuals who have experienced an unexpected death.

While these models may be useful in helping you to understand what is happening to someone who is grieving, you should be aware that in practice grief does not fit into neat boxes. It may be very chaotic.

The models to be explored are:

Kubler-Ross (1970): The five stages of grief.

Parkes (1972): as revealed in *Bereavement Studies of Grief in Adult Life*.

Worden (1984): Grief counselling and grief therapy.

Cruse (1995) A generalised pattern of bereavement.

Kubler-Ross (1970) lists five stages:

1. Anger

2. Denial

3. Depression/guilt

4. Bargaining

5. Acceptance.

Parkes (1972) in *Bereavement Studies of Grief in Adult Life*. Parkes believes that bereavement is a process that has four distinct stages:

1. Experiencing the pain of grief

2. Fear, guilt, anger and resentment

3. Apathy, aimlessness and sadness

4. Gradual hope and movement in a new direction.

Worden (1984) *Grief Counselling and Grief Therapy*. Worden sees bereavement as a series of tasks, and believes that the person can influence their progress through it.
   The tasks are as follows:

1. To accept the reality of the loss

2. To experience pain and grief

3. To adjust to a new environment

4. To withdraw emotional energy and reinvest it in other relationships.

All the above models talk about reactions, some more simply than others. The individual experiencing grief loss and bereavement may have other reactions.

A generalised pattern of bereavement

Time	State
1–14 Days	Shock, numbness Disbelief Relief
Onset after 14 days	Fear Alarm Anger (repressed/misplaced) Guilt Denial (of death; of grief)
2–3 months	Yearning Searching
3–6 months	Emptiness Depression Loneliness Also guilt and anger persisting
1 year	Every day has been an anniversary
1–5 years	Acceptance Healing

Common reactions to grief

These manifest themselves in several ways: physically, emotionally, socially and spiritually.

Physical reactions:

- Weakness and fatigue
- Tachycardia
- Increased blood pressure
- Dry mouth
- Muscular tension
- Stomach ache
- Dizziness
- Changes in weight and appetite
- Susceptibility to illness
- Self-neglect
- Disturbed sleep patterns
- Headaches
- Hot and cold flushes

The physical reactions can be difficult to cope with and often the individual who is grieving does not always seek help with the symptoms. If the individual has underlying problems, the grief reaction can only exacerbate these. It is important that nurses look for these problems and suggest ways of coping. Most of the problems are interlinked so it is important that the individual feels someone is taking them seriously. Many individuals, when going through the grief reaction feel that the whole situation is not real and often cannot believe the way they are reacting to the loss of someone when they are faced with the fact that they are going to die.

Emotional reactions:

- Numbness
- Anger
- Despair
- Yearning
- Confusion
- Vindictiveness
- Denial

- Feeling of being lost
- Anxiety
- Crying
- Helplessness
- Bitterness
- Hopelessness
- Hysteria

- Rage
- Sadness
- Euphoria
- Peacefulness
- Guilt
- Relief
- Mood swings

Emotional reactions can be varied and difficult to deal with as many individual who are going through the grief reaction fluctuate between various emotions.

Anger

It is understandable to feel angry when you have lost someone. But this may be difficult for you, as a student or a nurse, to deal with – especially if the anger is directed at you. The most effective way to deal with anger is not to retaliate but just to let them shout. It is important to be aware that individuals may have a right to be angry, particularly if the cause of death of a loved one was a car accident or natural disaster.

Denial

While denial is often seen as a negative reaction, it does serve a function. When individuals cannot cope with what is happening they may, without realising it, use denial and continue in denial until they feel able to cope. Occasionally, this may be much stronger than expected. A relative may behave as though the patient does not have a life-threatening illness, or a bereaved person may appear to believe that their loved one is still alive. Continuous rejection of what is happening can be destructive. It is important for nurses to understand the difficulties, as trying to make an individual face up to a difficult situation before he or she feels ready to do so may have a detrimental effect.

Social reactions:

- Searching
- Disorientation
- Poor concentration
- Blaming others
- Preoccupation
- Increased activity

- Decreased physical activity
- Withdrawal from their own surroundings
- Withdrawal from friends and activities
- Forgetfulness
- Seeking isolation

Social reactions can be difficult. An individual may withdraw both from friends and from their surroundings as these remind them of the person who has been lost. This may be especially true if it is a child who has died, or where a couple have led closely intertwined lives and the bereaved partner does not feel able to carry on alone. Preoccupation with events or details becomes common, as does the tendency to become focused on one aspect of life.

Spiritual reactions:

- Searching for meaning
- Self-discovery
- Rituals/customs
- Unanswerable questions

Why?
Questioning one's own faith
Cultural concerns

* * *

The loss of a loved one can and does change individuals, sometimes in unexpected ways. For example, one teenager may appear to have grown up overnight after losing a parent, while another may turn to alcohol or other methods to help blot out the pain of loss.

The death of a loved one is not always seen as negative. Some may feel relieved from a terrible burden which they may have had, caring for this person for a considerable length of time, or they may be glad that their loved one is no longer suffering.

Dealing with all these reactions and questions can be a daunting prospect for any nurse. The grief process may also be compounded by some of the following factors:

1. Fear of the unknown – what will happen, unanswered questions, conspiracy

2. Depression

3. Loneliness

4. Reduced independence – loss of responsibilities

5. Pain – its control, acceptance of methods used

6. Altered body image

7. The timing and manner of death, loss of control.

Cancer presents its own degree of problems in relation to grief. With the ongoing developments in treatment, some patients may go into long periods of remission. This may increase the hope of a cure, when they have been told by a surgeon that most of the cancer has been taken away, only to be informed at a later date that the cancer has returned and no further treatment can be offered.

The reaction of family, friends and others to a death is very individual and varied. This may be directly related to the cause of death, or to the relationship shared with the person they have lost. You may be involved, with your DN assessor/supervisor, in supporting the parents and relatives of a child who is dying or has died. It is important that you have an understanding of the possible reactions and why they may be occurring. Make sure you find some time to discuss this with your assessor and one or two of your peers.

The loss of a child is in today's society often seen as unacceptable to the parents, as it appears to 'go against the natural order'. When a child dies, parents do not only mourn the present loss, but their future as well. Often when a family is faced with the death of a child, the parents' natural instincts are to protect that child. Even if this is due only to the level of grief the parents are experiencing, the child may perceive this as exclusion. The protection can also work in reverse and the child may try to protect the parents by appearing to be coping with the situation. It is important that children are allowed to go through the stages of grief and are able to say their goodbyes.

Case Study 14.1

Mr Smith is a 54-year-old married man who has been fit and active until recently when he has become increasingly lethargic and has been having difficulty with eating due to pain. He has also lost a large amount of weight. He is convinced that he has a stomach ulcer. However, not having any idea that he is being investigated for cancer he attends his outpatients' appointment alone following his endoscopy. He is seen by a different doctor from his last visit who tells him without any warning that he has cancer of the oesophagus and that it is inoperable and he should go home and sort out his affairs.

What reactions may he experienced?

How should he tell his wife?

What problems do you perceive in this scenario?

Suggest ways in which this situation could have been handled differently.

When a child dies it is important that the children remaining have the opportunity to talk and understand that death is final.

Children are naturally curious about all aspects of life and death and their imaginations can be highly developed. Where children have experienced loss or death and have been made to feel involved and treated honestly by their parents, they cope better with future bereavements. If children's feelings are ignored, however, this can lead to fear and anxieties, and may have profound implications on the surviving children.

The silent griever

The silent griever is difficult for professionals to cope with. For reasons known perhaps only to themselves, a patient who knows about his or her illness may not have informed relatives of the actual diagnosis or even the prognosis.

Student Activity 14.7

◆ Read Chapter 59 in Dickenson and Johnson (1993) *Death, Dying and Bereavement.*

◆ Make notes after discussion with your peers.

The hidden griever

This group of individuals can be very difficult to identify especially by professionals. Many people may have secret lives and these individuals, whether estranged or with a secret partner may not be able to grieve openly. This may manifest itself in other ways, such as health problems or changes in their behaviour.

Explaining the mechanisms used to help patients and family cope with death and dying

Team approach

There is plenty of evidence supporting the effectiveness of a multidisciplinary approach towards caring for patients and their families in all care settings (Caddow and Grayson, 1992; Harrow et al., 1994). Many of the national documents such as the Calman–Hine Report (1995) and a report

Student Activity 14.8

When you are providing palliative care for a terminally ill patient; think about who is in the team and what their roles are.

♦ Do the roles of the professionals and others involved in the patient's care change?

♦ Check who appears to be the leader of care and discuss with your peers and assessor why you feel this person is the right or wrong person to be leading the patient's care.

♦ Make notes in your portfolio.

from the National Council for Hospice and Specialist Palliative Care Services (1996) highlight the importance of a multidisciplinary approach to palliative care. When caring for patients who are facing a life-threatening illness, it is vital that this approach is used. This may include doctors, nurses, social workers, religious leaders, physiotherapists, occupational therapists, pharmacists and others in related specialties. Different disciplines can view patient care from a variety of perspectives, enabling the patient and family to receive the most appropriate range of response. It also means that, having an established and dedicated team, skills in palliative care can be improved and expertise developed.

A team is a group of individuals with a common purpose of working together with a common goal. In caring for dying patients and their family, the goal must be to improve quality of life for whatever time is left.

Each team member brings a particular skill and has a responsibility for making individual decisions within his or her area of expertise. Team members have the opportunity to share knowledge and information through discussion about the future care plans for the patient and family.

There could be considerable variation in what is defined as a team. It is not just a group put together in a room. An effective team may comprise just two or three, or a whole cross-section of health care professionals who meet on a regular basis.

When making arrangements for, and undertaking the needs assessment, it is vital that the patient and relevant family members are seen as an integral part of the care team, and take part in the decision-making process.

What are the roles of each member of the team?

The role of each team member will depend on the skills of others. It is important to remember that team members can change, but teamwork depends on each member's experience.

Doctors

- General practitioners (GPs) provide medical support in the primary care setting for symptom control and other underlying conditions. They prescribe the majority of the medication unless nurse prescribing (from a limited formulary only) has been implemented in their area.

- Specialist doctors may also be involved, to deal with specific symptoms. These include an anaesthetist, oncologists and surgeons. They provide medical supervision to other members of the team and along with other members provide education and undertake research to improve patient care.

District nurses (DNs)

The DN provides much of the day-to-day support. Most of the time spent with patients is used to perform several different functions. The DN undertakes the assessment to determine the level of need and may draw in clinical nurse specialists who have particular knowledge in this area to address identified needs.

Specialist nurses

These may include staff that are supported by charities, such as Macmillan nurses or Marie Curie nurses. Others may be funded directly via the health services. These posts may be specific (such as breast care nurses) or have a specialist role such as chemotherapy or palliative care.

Pharmacists

The pharmacist provides information on drugs, their function, interactions and cost. They also dispense the drugs themselves, as prescribed by the doctor.

Physiotherapists

Physiotherapists provide support for patient mobility and breathing problems. They can also provide relaxation therapy and various techniques to help with symptom control.

Occupational therapists

The role of the occupational therapist is to assess patients' ability to perform activities of daily living, ensure they are safe and provide aid and advice to enable the patient and family to regain independence.

Dietitian

The dietitian provides information on dietary needs. Nutritional requirements of patients are calculated. This is often difficult to achieve in some situations. The dietitian provides alternative ways of dealing with symptoms other than drugs for example constipation, dry sore mouth and nausea. Carers especially value their input as the dietitian provides practical advice on how to overcome difficulties associated with diet.

Social workers

The social worker provides practical support to patients and their families at home. The assessment of the physiotherapist and occupational therapist is vital as this provides the social worker with information on what activities of daily living the patient can manage. Support such as help with washing and dressing, meal preparation or the provision of mobile meals, help with shopping and collecting pensions are just a few of the tasks which will be provided by social services through their support networks, which include home help services, and the involvement of the voluntary sector where appropriate. Information on benefits is also available, allowing patients and their families to buy in more care.

Religious leaders

The chaplain or other religious leader provides spiritual support. The focus is not purely on patients' and families' religious beliefs, but on their whole spiritual being. Many patients and families when faced with a terminal disease seek out individuals, often a religious leader to help them find spiritual peace.

Psychologists

The psychologist provides support for patients and their families when they are having psychological problems that cannot be addressed by other team members. They may have behavioural problems or be withdrawn.

Access to members of the team can be initiated by the patient, the patient's relatives, or by key workers such as the GP and/or the DN.

Collaboration between the multidisciplinary team and other agencies is vital in the delivery of palliative care.

Community support

Various organisations provide a vast array of services. These services do vary across the country, but a few examples will be given here. Many are integrated into the NHS, are self-funded initially, but later on are taken over by the NHS. Some are, however, funded in partnership at the start, if they are able to offer a certain level of service with which the NHS is happy. Examples include:

● *Marie Curie Nursing Service*

Marie Curie nurses provide nursing care to patients and support carers in their own homes.

- *Hospital/hospice at home*

This type of scheme provides up to 24-hour support within the patient's own home for an agreed period of time, often 7–10 days.

- *Day care*

This provides social support and provides the carers with a break. Day care is provided by statutory service providers, for example social services, and voluntary services, for example Age Concern.

- *Voluntary organisations*

These types of organisation are often developed according to local need. There are many useful ways in which to obtain this type of information. These include national directories, and the local telephone directory or health centre noticeboard.

- *Information/helplines*

  This type of help is available nationally, provided by organisations such as CancerBACUP, Cancerlink and Macmillan Cancer Relief. Other helplines have been developed locally. These are often run by organisations that provide other services. NHS Direct is now available locally in most parts of the UK and provides up to date information and advice from qualified, experienced NHS nurses.

- *Patient advocacy services*

  These are provided by health or social services and are designed for people whose first language is not English or who have problems with communication. An interpreting service is provided, as well as a worker who can act on the patient's behalf to ensure their views are heard.

- *Complementary therapies*

  There are many avenues through which complementary therapies can be obtained. The NHS may provide some of the treatments, and these are also often provided in hospices where therapists provide the treatments free of charge. The important factor to consider here is that the treatment should be *complementary* and not alternative. These treatments can cost so this may exclude some patients. There are organisations that have been set up to provide combined programmes, for example the Bristol Centre.

- *Hospices*

  Hospices have been set up to care for the dying. They provide inpatient care for symptom control, respite care and terminal care. They may also have day care, outpatients, befriending services, sitting services, counselling and bereavement support. The services provided will vary across the country.

- *Nursing homes*
  These provide support for many palliative care patients. With the increase in the elderly population there is an increasing demand for this type of care. The hospices and the specialist and community nurses provide specialist support.

- *Financial organisations*
  These may be statutory, such as the Benefits Agency. Or national charities, such as Macmillan Cancer Relief, may provide grants for patients. Other local organisations may provide information and support in connection with all types of financial matters.

- *Support groups*
  These are often site specific and may be either part of a national organisation (for example Roy Castle support groups) or groups set up locally.

- *Befriending service*
  These services are often provided by voluntary organisations. Volunteers will spend time with inpatients and are matched with the patient in relation to interests. This service varies according to geographical area. The majority of these schemes provide training for all their volunteers.

- *Transport*
  Transport will be provided by the health service but often volunteers will take patients to the hospital in order to minimise the time they have to wait once there.

- *Bereavement services*
  These are provided by both statutory and voluntary organisations. *Cruse* is a national organisation that provides both one to one and group support. There are many other organisations that offer bereavement support depending on the nature of the death. Examples are the Child Bereavement Trust, the National Association of Victim Support Schemes and the Compassionate Friends.

Student Activity 14.9

- Find out what services are available in your area for patients with cancer and non-malignant diseases.

- Explore one of the local voluntary organisations in more detail finding out how it fits in with other services.

Case Study 14.2

Mr Smith, who has been diagnosed with cancer of the oesophagus, has informed his wife of his diagnosis. The GP has also received information about his diagnosis. Mr and Mrs Smith are concerned about their financial state and they still have two teenaged children at school. Mr Smith has seen an oncologist who has given him some radiotherapy to improve his symptoms. He is still having problems with eating and is very angry about his situation. His wife is becoming increasingly withdrawn. She is worried about getting out as she does not drive and the bus service is not very reliable.

How can this family be helped to deal with their situation?

What services and support could you suggest to help Mr and Mrs Smith?

The role of the nurse in caring for a patient who is dying

When caring for patients who are dying you may be faced with a number of dilemmas. These are important to consider before exploring the practical issues of care. Talk to your peers and your assessor to help you deal with the issues. Some of these are as follows:

Ethical issues relating to death and dying

Confidentiality

As with any other areas of nursing, information should not be divulged to a third party without the consent of the patient. This may prove problematic when the patient is unconscious or affected by cerebral metastases or chemical imbalances resulting in an inability to give consent. As a student, you will be working closely with your DN assessor, who will give careful consideration to the individual's particular circumstances. The patient's next of kin should then act in the capacity of executor so that information and consent can be given.

There may be practical difficulties here too, as some relatives may put pressure on health care professionals to give them the information and then proceed to request that the medical staff do not tell the patient. Often, relatives are doing this for very compassionate reasons, wanting to protect their loved one, and enabling them to plan for the future. This approach allows the relatives to do this but not the patient themselves. However, even though relatives go to great lengths to hide the fact that the patient is dying, Doyle and colleagues (1993) highlight the fact that many patients are aware of their diagnosis and prognosis, but the relatives refuse to acknowledge this. The situation can intensify as both parties convince themselves that the other has no knowledge.

The patient may not inform others about how much they know and while relatives appear to be happy with the fact that the patient is not given all the information, they expect to be told everything.

In order to address what can be a very difficult situation, the heath care professional must inform the relatives that the patient has the right to all information. This may be easier for doctors, but often the nurse in all care settings is perceived as being more approachable and understanding of the relatives' situation. This may be particularly true in the home when the nurse has given care to the patient and the relatives talk freely to him or her. There are possibilities for a breakdown in communication, or for relatives to misuse the information. The situation needs to be handled sensitively and professionally.

Another important aspect is regular communication between the health professionals involved in the patient's care, so that information given is consistent and all are respecting confidentiality.

Euthanasia

When patients or their relatives ask for euthanasia they are often asking for better care as their pain may not be being relieved or they are finding that they have no control over their lives. In most cases more can be done to improve symptom control.

Many patients will express what they want for treatment and when they wish to have treatment withdrawn.

Assessment

The clinical component of palliative care has widened beyond providing effective control of physical symptoms, to developing an individualised, patient centred approach. This means that in planning an individual patient's care, palliative care professionals try to appreciate the complex interactions between the physical, psychological, social and spiritual factors of the patient's circumstances, resulting in holistic care.

As nurses we cannot predict how individuals will react. It is part of the nurse's role to be aware of the possible reactions and to have an understanding of why they are happening. It is important that nurses consider all the factors that will have an effect on patients and their families when they are faced with the death of a loved one. Nurses need to have an insight into cultural and religious issues in order to assess individual family needs.

The DN plays a key role in undertaking an assessment and providing care, which will often involve other services in order to address patient needs appropriately. This is vital in order to plan for, and be able to deliver, care which is structured to the needs of the patient.

There should be an ongoing process of reassessment as needs are always changing. The situation may change on a daily basis making it difficult for patients and their families to cope.

Many of the patients with non-malignant conditions will gradually deteriorate and often their individual needs are not reassessed as the family tends to carry on regardless, often unaware themselves until the situation has become appallingly difficult. In such a case, the community nurse plays a key role in providing support, and has the opportunity to reassess the family situation continually, responding to changes and preventing a crisis situation.

Helping people to cope with a family member who is faced with a life-threatening disease can be very daunting. Individuals will all cope with it in a different way.

Symptom control

The control of symptoms plays an important role in palliative care and forms part of the holistic approach.

Advances in symptom control have become more sophisticated. The understanding of these is increasingly reliant on specialist knowledge. The palliative care multidisciplinary team provides access to specialists such as anaesthetists, oncologists and surgeons.

These specialists recognise the benefits of using their skills on patients who would not normally be referred to them. For example, anaesthetic pain control clinics offer invasive techniques such as epidurals and nerve blocks. Without collaborative working, these techniques are much less likely to be offered to help control the symptoms of a patient with cancer. Other examples include the use of palliative chemotherapy, radiotherapy, bronchial and oesophageal stents (Penson and Fisher, 1995; McPhail, 1999).

There are many symptoms experienced by patients. The following lists the most common in cancer and the terminal phase (Kaye, 1997):

- Weakness
- Pain
- Anorexia
- Constipation
- Dyspnoea
- Insomnia

- Sweats
- Oedema
- Dry/sore mouth
- Nausea/vomiting
- Anxiety
- Cough

Terminal symptoms in advanced cancer:

- Moist breathing

- Retention of urine

- Pain
- Agitation
- Incontinence of urine
- Dyspnoea

- Nausea and vomiting
- Sweating
- Jerking, twitching
- Confusion

When assessing these symptoms the following principles may be applied:

1. Listen to detail when the patient is explaining the problems.

2. Ask about all symptoms. Don't focus on just the ones the patient tells you about.

3. A detailed drug history is vital especially when asking for advice. It is pointless letting the patient start on drugs that have already been tried.

4. Ask yourself why the symptoms are occurring and look for possible reversible factors; for example, constipation may be caused by drugs.

5. Intersperse questions about physical symptoms with questions about feelings.

6. Treat symptoms quickly if they have no further benefit in the diagnostic processes in advanced disease.

7. Make one change at a time.

8. Explain the changes that have been made to the patient and their family.

9. Include the patient and family members in the decision making.

10. Make a plan.

11. Monitor regularly.

12. Remember emotional factors.

13. Reduce or stop drugs whenever possible.

Student Activity 14.10

◆ Read Chapter 4 in Twycross, R. (1997) Symptom Management II.

◆ Discuss with your peers.

◆ Make notes in your portfolio.

Pain

Pain is one of the many symptoms that may be experienced by patients during the palliative phase of their disease. The fear of pain can affect the patient and their family in all aspects of care – physical, psychological, social and spiritual. Pain management and control forms a very important part of the patient's care plan, and this should always be reflected in the approaches being used to assess, plan and deliver the care that is needed.

When patients with cancer and other life-threatening diseases experience pain, this is a constant reminder that they are not being cured of their disease. There are many factors that affect patients' experience of pain (Carr and Mann, 2000).

Often patients with chronic pain do not appear to be in pain when assessed, so it is important to undertake a holistic assessment.

Coping with physical pain is important but it is also important to remember the effects of psychological and social pain, and make allowances for these.

Student Activity 14.11

♦ Undertake a holistic assessment on a palliative care patient during your placement and discuss with your assessor what factors you think are compounding the patient's pain.

♦ When undertaking this assessment observe the family and find out how the patient's pain may be affecting them.

Case Study 14.3

Mr Smith's condition is deteriorating and, although the treatment was effective at first, now he is deteriorating rapidly. All members of the family, including Mr Smith, want him to die at home if possible. His main problems are pain and lack of mobility.

What would your role be as the community nurse visiting Mr Smith?

What services would you consider to help support Mr and Mrs Smith at home?

What are the other alternatives to dying at home?

Evaluation of services and care

The evaluation of health care services is vital and ensuring effectiveness is a key aspect of this. The main way to evaluate care for dying patients is to ask the family and patient themselves whether you have been able to address their needs. It is important that, if gaps are identified, they are highlighted and steps taken to address the issues.

What can you do to help?

There are many ways in which you can provide support and help.

- Provide information on all services, be they statutory or voluntary.
- Take time to listen both to the patient and to the family.
- Ensure a safe environment in which patients can express emotions, enabling them to cry, feel sad, and/or be angry.
- Provide the opportunity to have someone to talk to and ensure the information remains confidential between the nurse and either the patient or the family.
- If the person you are visiting has been bereaved, allow them to talk about the person they have lost by name.
- Provide the opportunity to talk about the current situation, and the events that may have led up to the death and bereavement.
- Help people to develop new interests if they have been bereaved.
- Provide private time for a family by not visiting too often and respecting the family's privacy.
- Help the family to share memories of their loved one and acknowledge that they each have a different way of coping. They may wish to grieve privately and alone and may often want their own space. Be sensitive to this.

Being aware of the effect that caring for a dying patient and family may have on the nurse and how to access appropriate support

In order to care for a patient and family who are facing impending death or have had a sudden bereavement it is vital that you look after yourself.

How to look after ourselves

You are no good to your patient and their family if you are not coping yourself. It is vital that you remember what you cannot do, and what support is there for you.

What you cannot do

You cannot change the outcome that the patient is going to die. You do not have magical powers or the ability to perform miracles and put everything right.

Do not set unrealistic goals. If you do this you could cause distress to the patient, the family and yourself.

Do not forget that you are only one part of the family's life.

You cannot solve all the patient's and family's problems.

You cannot be all things to all people.

What support is there for you

Support is available in a variety of ways, formal and informal, at home and at work. Examples include:

- Networks within the team
- Networks outside the team
- Staff support
- Peer supervision
- Recognising strengths and weakness
- Knowing how you react to people
- Debriefing discussion before and after difficult situations
- Keep your role clear
- Being able to finish the meetings/ 'closure'

- Team partnership
- Informal support
- Supervision
- Supervision from another person
- How does your own life situation impact?
- Do you tend to take on the role of 'rescuer'? Of 'victim'?
- Have days when you do not take work home
- Friendship versus professional relationship
- How long to carry on

Student Activity 14.12

♦ Identify and discuss with your peers the support, available in your placement, for your assessor, and you, when dealing with death and dying.

♦ How is the team able to take care of itself in these circumstances?

♦ Make notes in your portfolio.

Conclusion

Caring for dying patients and their families has been discussed in this chapter and has addressed some of the issues relating to assessing, planning and delivering care which is sensitive to the needs of dying patients and families who may be bereaved. However, it is important that as nurses, services and support for these patients and their families are constantly developed and the focus continues to be on the specific needs of patients and their families.

Further reading

Dickenson, D. and Johnson, M. (1993) *Death, Dying and Bereavement*. Buckingham, The Open University Press.

Doyle, D. (1996) *Domiciliary Palliative Care, A Guide for the Primary Care Team*. Oxford, Oxford University Press.

Green, J. (1989) Death with dignity. *Nursing Times*, **85**: 5–9.

Green, J. (1992) Death with dignity. *Nursing Times*, **88**: 9.

Prout, C. (1992) Death with dignity, paganism. *Nursing Times*, **88**: 33.

Twycross, R. (1997) *Introducing Palliative Care*, 2nd edn. Oxford, Radcliffe Medical Press.

Twycross, R., Wilcock, A. and Thorp, S. (1998) *Palliative Care Formulary. A to Z of Symptom Control*. Oxford, Radcliffe Medical Press.

Wright, B. (1996) *Sudden Death*. Edinburgh, Churchill Livingstone.

USEFUL WEB SITES

CancerBACUP www.cancerbacup.org.uk

Child Bereavement Trust www.childbereavement.org.uk

Growth House Inc (Care of the dying) www.growthhouse.org

Macmillan Cancer Relief www.macmillan.org.uk

Motor Neurone Disease Association www.businessconnections.com/MND/mnd.htm

National Kidney Federation www.kidney.org.uk

References

Addington-Hall, J.M. (1998) *Reaching Out: Specialist Palliative Care for Adults with Non-malignant Diseases*. London, Council for Hospice and Specialist Palliative Care Services.

Ahmedzai, S. (1996) Making a success out of life's failures. *Progress in Palliative Care*, **4**: 1–3.

Barby, T. and Leigh, P.N. (1995) Palliative care in motor neurone disease. *International Journal of Palliative Nursing*. **1**: 183–8.

Barnard, D., Towers, A., Boston, P. and Lambrinidou, Y. (2000) *Crossing Over. Narratives of Palliative Care*. London, Oxford University Press.

Beattie, J.M., Murray, R.G., Brittle, J. and Catamheira, T. (1995) Palliative care in terminal cardiac failure. Small numbers of patients with terminal cardiac failure may make considerable demands on services. *British Medical Journal*, 310: 1411.

Biswas, B. (1993) The medicalisation of dying: a nurse's view. In Clark, D. (ed.) *The Future for Palliative Care: Issues of Policy and Practice*. Buckinghamshire, Open University Press.

Caddow, P. and Grayson, G. (1992) A team to ensure sensitive continuing care: setting up a symptom control/support team. *Professional Nurse*, 7(11): 719–24.

Calman, K. and Hine, D. (1995) *A Policy Framework for Commissioning Cancer Services*. London, DoH/Welsh Office.

Carr, E. and Mann, E. (2000) *Pain: Creative Approaches to Effective Management*. Basingstoke, Macmillan – now Palgrave.

Cooley, M. (1992) Bereavement care. *Cancer Nursing*, 15(2): 125–9.

Cruse, J.M. (1995) *Illustrated Dictionary of Immunology*. London, CRC Press.

Dickenson, D. and Johnson, M. (1993) *Death, Dying and Bereavement*. Buckingham, Open University Press.

Doyle, D., Hanks, G.W. and MacDonald, N. (1993) *The Oxford Textbook of Palliative Medicine*. Oxford, Oxford Medical Publishers.

Gamlin, R. (1994) *Caring for the Bereaved*. Open learning guide. London, Formworld.

Glaser, B.G. and Strauss, A.L. (1968) *A Time for Dying*. Chicago, Aldine.

Harrow, T., Lempp, H. and McDermott, S. (1994) Managing change to improve outpatient care. *British Journal of Nursing*, 3(19): 1005–11.

Katz, J., Komaromy, C. and Sidell, M. (1999) Understanding palliative care in residential and nursing homes. *International Journal of Palliative Nursing*, 5(2): 58–64.

Kaye, P. (1997) *A to Z of Symptom Control*. Northampton, EPL Publications.

Kinghorn, S. and Gamlin, R. (2001) *Palliative Nursing: Bringing Comfort and Hope*. London, Baillière Tindall.

Kubler-Ross, E. (1970) *On Death and Dying*. London, Tavistock.

Lloyd-Williams, M. (1996) An audit of palliative care in dementia. *European Journal of Cancer Care*, 5: 53–5.

McPhail, G. (1999) Chemotherapy in palliative cancer care: changing perspectives. *International Journal of Palliative Nursing*, 5(2): 81–5.

National Council for Hospice and Specialist Palliative Care Services (1996) *Palliative Care in the Hospital Setting*. Occasional paper 10. London.

Parkes, C. (1972) *Bereavement Studies of Grief in Adult Life*. Harmondsworth, Penguin.

Penson, J. and Fisher, R.A. (1995) *Palliative Care for People with Cancer*, 2nd edn. London, Arnold.

Rando, T.A. (1984) *Grief, Dying and Death: Clinical Interventions for Caregivers*. Champaign Illinois, Research Press.

Skilbeck, J., Mott, L., Smith, D., Page, H. and Clark, D. (1997) Nursing care for people dying from chronic obstructive airways disease. *International Journal of Palliative Nursing*, 3: 100–6.

Twycross, R. (1997) *Introducing Palliative Care*, 2nd edn. Oxford, Radcliffe Medical Press.

Wilkes, E (1984) Dying now. *Lancet*, 1: 950–2.

Worden, W. (1984) *Grief Counselling and Grief Therapy*. London, Tavistock.

World Health Organization (1990) *Cancer Pain Relief and Palliative Care*. Technical Report series 804, Geneva, WHO.

Wright, S. (1985) Change in nursing: the application of change theory to practice. *Nursing Practice*, 2: 85–91.

15

The future of nursing in primary care

NAOMI A. WATSON

Learning outcomes

By the end of this chapter you will be able to:

■ Recognise the reasons for a continuous change in policy and practices, and the implications for community nursing, and its management in primary care.

■ Identify specific measures needed to ensure the continuation of an improvement in access to health and health care.

■ Examine the methods being considered to provide a more flexible, user-friendly service for the community.

■ Consider the role of primary care groups (PCGs) and primary care trusts, (PCTs) in the development of community nursing, and its implications for nurses of adult patients.

Introduction

This chapter aims to help you consolidate your learning by considering the contribution of a very high level of change to the way care has evolved in the community. Continuous change, especially if it is rapid, tends to result in anxiety and uncertainty. The reality of events, however, and the challenges they present, have to be understood within their contextual frameworks in order to help us all cope better with these events. Community nursing is set to change even further, and the information provided in the chapters of this text will help to give you a clear and concise understanding of the way forward, and of your contribution as practitioners of the future to the process. This concluding chapter should provide you with an overview of the trends according to policy, and the way they are set to develop, so that you can anticipate planned and possible changes. This should enable you to approach them with less anxiety and more confidence (Warner et al., 1998).

Recognising the reasons for a continuous change in policy and practices

When the NHS was set up in 1948, the overall aims of providing a comprehensive service for all from the cradle to the grave, free at the point of delivery, were noble and worthwhile concepts. The rapid developments which heralded the introduction of the service have been major contributors to the way it has evolved. For example, the industrial revolution, with the development of large cities bringing larger numbers of people together in smaller amounts of space and isolating people from traditional support networks, contributed to the creation of new types of illnesses. This may have resulted in the eventual excessive demand for health care which still characterises the NHS today. One could argue that this trend in terms of demand is set to continue for the future. If we stop to think of the advances in science and technology that dominated the 20th century, the need to find new ways of delivering a service, which is of the highest quality, relevant to the needs of the community, is a pressing priority.

Student Activity 15.1

Think about the types of health care services for adult patients that you have encountered since you started your community placement.

♦ Do you think a continuous change in policy and practice is needed? Why, or why not?

♦ Discuss this with one or more of your peers.

♦ Make notes in your portfolio.

Searching for new ways of working, and making decisions on the way forward, therefore, is an important part of planning for the present and the future. Working alongside your assessors on your community placement should already have exposed you to the initial stages of many of the changes taking place, or being planned. You are encouraged to make time to discuss your assessor's involvement in the changes, to ensure that you understand the contribution that the DN is expected to make, and possible ways of doing so. Considering the way community nursing is set to develop should help to ensure that future changes are recognised before they occur, that opportunities and/or threats to good service delivery practices can be anticipated and that community nurses have a major say in the way these services develop. All available options for delivering care to large numbers of patients in community settings will need to be explored, and community nurses will have the opportunity to lead the way in ensuring high standards of practice, based on innovative and creative concepts. These will be firmly set within the evidence from their practice, and supported by the literature.

There is another important point to remember about the early evolution of the NHS. The major focus of care delivery was actually on acute services, with most of the available funding going to hospitals, while services in the community became, in effect, 'Cinderella services'. This early emphasis on 'cure', as opposed to 'care' or prevention, may have been another contributory factor to the problems of the service today. Shifting the trends from acute sector focus to primary care has been a continuing feature of major policy since 1990 (DoH, 1990, 1997, 1999).

Warner and colleagues (1998) summarise the issues influencing change as follows:

- Economic and political
- Demographic
- Epidemiological.

Economic and political factors influencing change

Perhaps the most important factor that needs to be considered is the effect of globalisation on changes in health and health care practices. The UK, as a major Western country, continues to be involved in and affected by global events. The challenges these present for the future are driven by a technological age, which is breaking down some barriers in terms of culture, economy and lifestyles. At the same time, other barriers are being erected, for example in developing countries where the effects of the rising costs of debts are seen to have an impact on their ability to contain economic deprivation. Recent lobbying of Western governments by pressure groups such as Jubilee 2000 in the UK, and other groups internationally, has been in connection with demands for debts to be cancelled in order to give developing countries a better chance of establishing economic practices, which will contribute to sustainable developments in the reduction of poverty and its resultant effects on health outcomes, in particular, for children. Whatever the situation regarding their economic status and levels of debt, more nations are set to become independent, and an increasing number of people in nations across the world will live in towns and cities, as urbanisation escalates (OECD, 1997). It is easy to recognise the impact this will have on international health outcomes, and the need to understand, from a global analytical perspective, the connections between health and national and international development of nations (WHO, 1996).

On a national level, the increase in migration and the refugee problem present new challenges to planners, and force a consideration of innovative ways of dealing with what could be seen as a continuing persistent problem. Recent events in parts of Europe such as Bosnia, Kosovo and Albania, which led to large numbers of refugees arriving in the UK from these areas, have highlighted many problems, and raised sensitive issues relating to the way the refugee problem is managed nationally.

As a student, you will invariably be involved in the delivery of care to diverse groups in the community, many of whom will be refugees. The impact on local health policy and planning may vary depending on the methods used by individual localities to deal with the problem. As you work alongside your assessor, you should be able to recognise possible ways that the DN is able to influence policy and practice. For example, working sensitively with diverse groups who may be unpopular in local communities, and developing services specific to their needs based on sound evidence from practice, could provide the opportunity to generate new research in these areas from a nursing perspective (see Chapter 6 on differences and diversity).

Perhaps the major impact on the future of community nursing is the European perspective. The European Union now has a major impact on events in the UK, and this appears set to continue. The issues relating to a common market economy and free trade have also had implications for health care. For example, privatisation has had as much of an effect on health care as it has on other public sector services in the UK. Warner (1997) concludes that this trend will be a major focus in health care for the future, with markets being planned and managed in a regulatory manner.

To summarise, the effects on health and health care need to be considered on a global level. The technological age is contributing to a narrowing of some cultural and social gaps, while others are widening. The increase in numbers of refugees nationally and internationally forces a new look at how the problem is managed and new ways of working effectively. The impact of the European perspective and the increasing emphasis on privatisation is a feature across the public sector, including health and health care delivery. Community nurses can choose to participate actively in planning for these changes, given the fact that they are involved in care delivery and support to patients in a major way.

Demographic factors

Specific issues identified here include the increase in life expectancy and the fall in fertility rates, with a lowering of birth rates across Western Europe. There is an increasing population of older people, many of whom are living till they are 80 years old or over. Numbers are projected to increase by the year 2010, with over half the population of the UK predicted to be aged 45 and over. This is now a reality, with implications for care planning and service delivery. Donnellan (1995) argues that, given these statistics, it is imperative that we look again at our approach to ageing, and perhaps begin to focus not on the possible burden that older people may become (Butler, 1997), but on the many positive factors, and particularly on the way that society's perceptions may contribute more to creating a problem rather than a solution (see Chapter 13 for more information about caring for older people). There are other issues, however, which need to be considered here, for example, the increasing rates of divorce and single parent families, with an impact on traditional family values. The fall in fertility rates and lower birth rates indicate possible problems with future labour shortages, and a reduction in the numbers of informal carer networks, which have traditionally provided the bulk of caring in families and communities (Warner et al., 1998).

Epidemiological factors

These are identified as an increase in chronic non-communicable diseases (see Chapter 10), a growth in mental ill-health (see Chapter 11), overeating and obesity, and a new uprising of infectious diseases.

Warner and colleagues (1998) argue that changes in epidemiological perspectives are an inevitable consequence of changes to the demography. The increase in chronic illnesses is a further feature of future trends, being offset by lifestyle factors, which may tend to exaggerate the situation. For example, the increasing use of alcohol, tobacco, and drug use and abuse, and increasing sedentary lifestyles, will impact on the numbers of individuals with chronic illnesses (see chapter on chronic illnesses). DNs play a major role in providing health care to those suffering from chronic illnesses in the community, including supporting their families and carers. This indicates an increasing demand on the DN's time and resources, and an increasing need to be able to work innovatively and creatively.

Mental well-being has been identified by policy makers as a key requirement affecting present and future trends in health outcomes of individuals. The range of contributory issues affecting this include continuing unemployment, especially among men, the increasing narrowing of role demarcation between the sexes, and other pressures such as workplace stress. DNs will need to improve on present practices in terms of working collaboratively with other service providers to ensure that support for people in the community who are vulnerable to mental health problems is as seamless as possible. The awareness of the way factors combine to exacerbate or precipitate physical illnesses should help to ensure that services are structured to take this into consideration. For example, it is now recognised that mental ill-health among older people is increasing, but service response has not been forthcoming (Audit Commission, 2000). Given that the DN's caseload contains large numbers of older patients, this should indicate the possibility of contributing to a recognition of a problem and facilitating rapid responses for families and carers. To do this effectively, DNs will have to improve their own knowledge base about mental health, so that early signs can be identified and action taken quickly. (Chapter 11 in this text gives a good introduction on mental health issues for you as a student.)

The impact of lifestyle factors on the health outcomes of individuals is perhaps best observed in the increasing rates of dietary and nutritional problems. The problem of obesity has been identified as having major significance, along with the increasing numbers of people suffering from eating disorders at both ends of the continuum. Changes in the stages of the food chain which may result in further problems have also been identified (Calman, 1995). The role of the DN in the promotion of healthy lifestyles should be clear. Even when working with patients who are chronically sick, there is a requirement to ensure that they are encouraged to adopt a healthier approach to their illness, as this may contribute to a more positive health outcome.

For example, dietary advice for patients with problems such as coronary artery disease, circulatory problems, Asthma, among others, may help to alleviate some of the effects. Again, working closely with other members of the primary health care team (PHCT), in this instance the community dietitian, should ensure that patients receive as much support as possible to help them make better choices for more positive health outcomes. The recognition that it is now no longer possible for any community nurse just to deliver health care is a key aspect of understanding the changing roles of all the members of the PHCT, and specifically the DN (Trent Health, 1993). While the concept of the holistic approach is talked about widely in health service practice, it is imperative that it is seen in action, and that the methods used are both identifiable and quantifiable. This is the evidence which DNs will be able to use to influence policy and future planning of services.

Student Activity 15.2

◆ Make a list of alternative therapies that you are aware of, with types of known chronic illness that they may be used for.

◆ Using your list as a guide, talk to your assessor to find out whether there are any a) private practitioners, b) general practitioners, who are happy to prescribe for patients.

◆ Discuss your findings with one or two of your peers, to see how practice compares in different localities.

◆ Keep records of your findings in your portfolio.

The medical advances which have taken place throughout the last century, and which continue today, include an increasing reliance on (and possible overuse of) prescribed drugs. The case of antibiotics has been widely featured in the discussions (Warner et al., 1998). It has been suggested that new strains of infections that are resistant to antibiotics are set to affect individuals, while old strains return to become a major problem. This will be compounded by a reduction of investment in the development of, and research into new antibiotics. On the other hand, the increasing use of alternative and complementary therapies has now begun to have an effect on patient choice (Hunt and Zurek, 1997). Community nursing response will have to take into consideration the availability of and use of alternative forms of therapies. In many localities some GPs will now consider prescribing non-medical therapies. DNs should be able to help patients identify both medical and non-medical practitioners, so that patient choice can be maintained. They should also understand what these are, and their possible effects on different illnesses, so that they will be able to advise patients accordingly.

Improving access to health and health care

One of the key features of policy has been the recognition of the factors which affect the way services are accessed by different people in the community (DoH, 1990, 1998). It was acknowledged that community nurses have a major role to play in ensuring that everyone is able to access health care at the point of need. The Black Report (DHSS, 1980) and *The Health Divide* (Whitehead, 1987) provided evidence, which identified a range of barriers to access for specific groups. More recently, the Acheson Report (1998) shows that very little has changed in terms of real improvements in access at all levels. The new shift in emphasis is concerned with widening access, by providing a range of flexible services. This theme is further developed by the proposals in the NHS Plan, which are meant to strengthen the response of the NHS to patients and ensure that they are at the centre of planning for effective care delivery (DoH, 2000). In order to do this effectively, the following issues have to be acknowledged:

● Patient choice is now an integral part of all processes when access is being considered.

● Members of the public are now much better informed and hence, have become more demanding as consumers of services.

● The increasing awareness of the growing numbers of older people in society, and the potential for their empowerment, supported by powerful pressure groups such as Age Concern, among others.

● The ability of individuals to mount successful challenges to the autonomy of professionals.

Patient choice has been embedded in health care provision through policies such as The Patient's Charter, which give patients the right to appropriate information in order to make the right choices. Social class, among other factors, has been shown to have a major impact on how much infor-

Student Activity 15.3

◆ Read Chapter 13 of this text, and consider the extent to which older people are now being considered in a more positive light.

◆ What are the implications for the future?

◆ Talk to your assessor and find out what views are held about this, from the DN perspective.

◆ Discuss your findings with one or more of your peers.

◆ Make notes in your portfolio.

mation may be passed on. Community nurses may be able to ensure better access by acting on patients' behalf in this regard. However, the increasing use of the computer and Internet, along with other forms of electronic communication, means that patients are becoming better informed. In consequence, they also tend to be more demanding. This increase in capacity to access information from a variety of sources, usually independent of professionals, now means that there is a gradual shift from the professional dominance of the industrial age, to patient dominance with emphasis on self-care, the involvement of families, carers and other self-help networks and partnerships. As a result, professional roles would appear to be most effective when they are facilitative rather than dictating the way services are accessed (Jennings et al., 1997).

The economics of ageing have implications for the future (Donnellan, 1995). It has yet to be recognised that many older people in society lead active, busy lives contributing economically and remaining well rather than conforming to stereotype and being dependent on service provision. With the help of strong pressure groups, older people are gradually becoming more empowered, and are hence able to make their own demands in terms of their entitlements to services to which they would have contributed financially over their busy working years. They are also demanding their right to be considered and consulted individually, and as a group, in the planning and delivery of services appropriate to them.

Flexibility in health care access: issues to consider in primary care

Modernising access to health care has a number of components in terms of practical application. It involves considering a wider range of flexibility in work patterns, and the need for appropriate skill mixing to deliver care effectively (DoH, 1997; Warner et al., 1998) This includes a mixture of permanent and temporary staff working together to ensure that workforce planning reflects the actual needs of the population for which particular services have been designed. Embedded within this is the re-evaluation of professional roles as boundaries become unclear, and the increasing need for more collaborative working becomes imperative, and new roles being undertaken by all nurses. Within the community, nurse prescribing is now a regular feature of the work of the DN. The benefits for patients can be identified as part of the whole package of needs assessment and care delivery, although taking on roles that were previously the doctors' domain has brought its own controversies. *The Scope of Professional Practice* for nurses (UKCC, 1992) has already made a significant contribution to this debate. All nurses, including those in community settings, are being made more aware of their responsibilities to recognise their own strengths and possible areas for development. This is their full responsibility, with professional awareness requiring them to decline from undertaking activities for which they have not been appropriately prepared and ensuring that they make appropriate arrangements for professional and clinical development. The evidence for this is now a requirement for continuing registration and, as a student, you will notice that you have been encouraged to maintain a portfolio to show evidence of your learning, as a part of this process (UKCC, 1992).

Aspects of the nature of nursing which appear to have possible significance for future developments have been discussed as part of the Heathrow Debate (DoH, 1994). In terms of a significant contribution for the future, the report identifies the following issues:

- The need for nursing to have special responsibility for the frail and vulnerable in society.
- Concern not only for those who are sick, but also for those who are well.
- A teaching role that includes carers, patients and other professionals.
- The development and co-ordination of care programmes.
- A properly co-ordinated function.
- Technical expertise, exercised personally or through others.

Notice that all of the above will have significance for the role of the DN. With more people on their caseloads being older, their concern will have to be inclusive of the fact that as individuals become older, they may become more vulnerable, for example to hypothermia in the winter, or to other illnesses for which they may be able to get protection in the form of appropriate screening and vaccination. The needs of families and carers are already a requirement for consideration, with the Carers (Recognition and Services) Act 1995 identifying specific support that should be available for them. Teaching patients and their significant others about their illness and about ways of keeping well is also a function of the DN's role. Multiprofessional partnerships in learning, however, are emerging only slowly. DNs in some parts of the UK are becoming involved in the preparation of medical students, who undertake clinical placements in the community, and some pre-registration students share multi-agency learning with social workers and medical students at specific points in their learning menus. This aspect of role development for community nurses is still in its infancy, and may well become a key feature of future requirements.

The range of possibilities for improving access now forms part of all discussions on the subject, and includes not just the role of nurses, but also that of the GP and others who provide health care to the community. It is imperative, however, to be able to identify the possible impact of flexible access on community nurses. This will be invaluable evidence, which it may be possible to use in planning future services. One of the major issues for recognition may be the need for services to be available when the public need them;

hence continuous availability appears to be a particular focus. The setting up of services such as NHS Direct, which gives the community 24-hour access to health information, benefits them by giving advice quickly about the best course of action if they have a worrying health problem. This service is provided by nurses who have been appropriately prepared for the role. As an innovation, it forms part of the policy agenda to explore new concepts in flexible access. Evaluation of NHS Direct aims to ensure that performance and standard are informed, and targets can be set for national service (NHS Executive, 1998).

Student Activity 15.4

Visit your local library and find out about the new types of access to health services which are available in the locality of your placement.

♦ Is there a walk-in centre in the locality? If not, where is the nearest centre?

♦ Find out what types and levels of services are available.

♦ If possible, visit a walk-in centre, to see if you can get a feel of how services are organised and delivered in this setting.

♦ Discuss your findings with your assessor and one or two of your peers.

♦ Keep a record in your portfolio.

Other initiatives include walk-in centres based in the community, in places such as shops and supermarkets, and staffed by nurses. At these, members of the public can have consultations, receive health information, self-help advice and simple treatments, with advice for any further referrals that may be needed. Primary care walk-in centres were designed to help members of the community make better use of the NHS, and professionals to make better use of their skills. This is in response to modern lifestyles, with opening times reflecting flexibility of access, and including early mornings, late evenings and weekends. Pilot walk-in centres have been established across the UK, with support from PCGs PCTs and GP services (NHS Executive, 1999). Greater accessibility in terms of GP services is also being considered, with a review of GPs' out-of-hours services being undertaken (Carson, 2000). NHS Direct Online gives access to options for health information via the computer and Internet. All the above options are now in pilot stages at different levels, across the UK. The evaluation of these services should provide information which will shape the future of health care delivery in the new century.

Primary care groups (PCGs) and primary care trusts (PCTs)

The process of reforming the NHS was aimed at ensuring that the services being offered would contribute to a modern and improved NHS with primary care as the new focus, at the heart of the proposals.

As a key requirement, the White Paper *The New NHS: Modern, Dependable* (DoH, 1997) recommends closer working partnerships within and across organisations in order to enhance positive health outcomes for individuals in the community. A PCG is a committee of the local health authority/Trust, and consists of representatives of nurses, GPs, social services, health trusts, the public and a general manager. The main function of the PCG is to ensure that the health needs of the locality are appropriately identified, so that programmes to improve health outcomes for the community can be implemented. Key factors in the setting up of PCGs include the following:

- In April 1999, the groups eventually replaced the wide range of commissioning models that have been used over the years, including GP fundholding.

- The establishment of health action zones (HAZs) would immediately follow the setting up of PCGs, and health improvement programmes would be the natural follow on.

- PCGs will reflect locality circumstances; hence they will remain flexible rather than prescriptive.

- Development of PCGs was able to take place at rates appropriate within specific local environments, so that eventually they could assume full functional responsibilities.

Student Activity 15.5

◆ Talk to your assessor to find out whether he or she is a member of a local PCG/PCT.

◆ If not, find out whether there is a nurse member (DN) in your locality.

◆ Negotiate some time with your assessor to plan an interview with this person.

◆ Find out what the composition in terms of ratio is, of members on the team, and what the DN considers his or her role to be as part of the team.

◆ If possible attend a public meeting of a PCG/PCT, to find out how well they are attended and how this might affect their effectiveness.

◆ Make notes in your portfolio.

- They should be representative of all GPs in the locality, as well as have a governing body, consisting of community nursing, social services, and local lay members.

- The recognition of boundaries for social services and health authorities and trusts needs to be taken into consideration to ensure that service planning and provision will be integrated.

- Typical numbers of patients per PCG should average around 100,000, although this can be flexible to reflect not only local issues, but eventual evidence in terms of the effectiveness of groups of different sizes.

- The establishment of independent PCTs was a clear expectation of progression of PCGs.

To summarise, PCGs were established as freestanding and accountable to local health authorities. They have the responsibility of providing community services for their locality.

Responsibility for managing the budget was devolved to them, and they are expected to act in an advisory capacity to the health authority regarding the commissioning of care to its local population. The role of the community nurse is seen as an important part of the PCG, with greater partnerships encouraged across all professions.

Student Activity 15.6

◆ Talk to your DN about the development of PCTs in your locality, and find out whether one has already been set up, and if not whether a timetable has been set.

◆ Discuss the possible role of the community nurse (DN) in these developments.

◆ Talk to some of your peers in different localities to see if information about developments is similar.

◆ Make notes in your portfolio.

Primary care trusts (PCTs)

Configuring and establishing PCTs was left to the discretion of local PCGs, with the health authorities/Trusts expected to act as organiser in terms of strategic planning and service configuration. By the time this text is published, most local health authorities and Trusts would have held discussions with PCGs, and come to an agreement regarding configuring and launching their PCTs. PCTs are independent PCGs that are able to sustain their independence with a devolved budget, including resourcing for general medical services, hospital and community health services and prescribing. It is envisaged that community health services will be eventually provided by PCTs, thus employing all the staff, community hospitals, and other facilities in the community, to ensure that services are integrated. Mental health and learning disability services were not seen as being part of the remit of the PCT.

PCTs will be accountable to local health authorities and the government intends to evaluate them, once they have been set up, to ensure that they are meeting required operational standards. Some areas have already set up PCTs and more are in the process of doing so.

The evaluation of these new developments will form the basis of planning for future health services delivery, and the role of the community nurse within these developments will also need to be monitored to ensure effective participation in policy and planning for local health outcomes.

Conclusion

The future of community nursing is being influenced by present changes in policy and practice, which place primary care at the leading edge of health care delivery. There are a number of significant factors, which have influenced these changes, and these include, among others, global and national economic, political demographic and epidemiological issues. The increasing technological advances contribute to a better informed public, who are able to demand a more flexible and responsive service, due to availability of an 'information superhighway'. The political response for change is based within the concept of modernising services and encouraging greater partnerships to provide for truly integrated services to patients. Community nurses have a key role to play in these developments, as identified in the White Paper *The New NHS: Modern, Dependable* (DoH, 1997) and The Health Act (DoH, 1999). The Information for Health Strategy (NHS Executive, 1998), aims to ensure that members of the public are more involved in decisions about their health by providing accurate and reliable information which they can use to help them remain well. The benefits for nurses and health care workers include access to latest medical research and up to the minute details about medical histories. This national electronic library for health is designed to keep pace with advances in technological developments, to ensure that the NHS is not left behind.

The extent to which community nurses are able to participate effectively will depend on their ability to place themselves in a position which is firmly based within the evidence from their practice, and to generate further evidence through contribution to research and dissemination of good practice. For example, evaluation of the newly configured PCTs should provide many opportunities for active participation, which should be effective in contributing to strengthening the literature base for nursing interventions relevant to clinical practice and the management functions related to PCTs. Clinical effectiveness must be measurable, and community nurses will need to find new ways of engaging with the current requirements to ensure a quality provision through effective leadership. The National Institute for Clinical Excellence (NICE) contributes to this process, and one could argue, is directly answerable to the public for decisions made about effectiveness and reliability of NHS interventions. DeBell (1998) argues that the challenge for all nurses depends on a sound research base. Clinical governance now provides the framework within which all nurses, and specifically community nurses, can confidently participate in shaping the new face of the NHS by positive and responsive actions. This will ensure that their voices are effective in being heard as part of the current changes, and their role as key contributors to future developments will be secured.

Further reading

Gallen, D. and Buckle, G. (1997) *Top Tips in Primary Care Management.* London, Blackwell Science. Chapter 10.
Royce, R. (2000) *Primary Care and the NHS Reforms. A Manager's View.* London, Office of Health Economics.
Warner, M., Longley, M., Gould E. and Picek, A. (1998) *Health Care Futures 2010.* Cardiff, Welsh Institute for Health and Social Care.

USEFUL WEB SITES

Department of Health www.doh.gov.uk

NHS Exectutive hwww.open.gov.uk/doh/nhs.htm

NHS Direct Online www.nhsdirect.nhs.uk/

References

Acheson, D. (1998) *Independent Inquiry into Inequalities in Health.* London, HMSO.
Audit Commission (2000) *Forget-me-not: Mental Health Services for Older People.* London, Audit Commission.
Butler, R. (1997) *Ageing beyond the Millennium.* London, Nuffield Trust and Age Concern Cymru Wales.
Calman, K. (1995) On the state of the public health. *Health Trends,* **26**(2): 35–7.
Carson, D. (2000) *The GP Out of Hours Review.* London, Royal College of Surgeons.
DeBell, D. (1998) The challenge of leadership in community health care nursing. *British Journal of Community Nursing,* **3**(2): 62–3.
Department of Health (1990) *NHS and Community Care Act.* London, HMSO.
Department of Health (1994) *The Challenges for Nursing and Midwifery in the 21st Century* (The Heathrow Debate). London, HMSO.

Department of Health (1997) *The New NHS: Modern, Dependable.* London, HMSO.
Department of Health (1998) *Our Healthier Nation.* London, DoH.
Department of Health (1999) *The Health Act.* London, HMSO
Department of Health (2000) *The NHS Plan.* London, HMSO.
Department of Health and Social Security (1980) *Inequalities in Health* (Black Report). London, DHSS.
Donnellan, C. (1995) *Our Ageing Generation: Issues for the Nineties.* Cambridge, Independence Educational Publishers.
Gallen, D. and Buckle, G. (1997) *Top Tips in Primary Care Management.* Oxford, Blackwell Science.
Hunt, R. and Zurek, E.L. (1997) *Introduction to Community Nursing.* Philadelphia and New York, Lippincott.
Jellinek, D. (1998) *Official UK: The Essential Guide to Government Websites.* London, HMSO.
Jennings, K., Miller, K. and Materna, S. (1997) *Changing Health Care.* Santa Monica, Knowledge Exchange.
NHS Executive (1998) *Investment to put Information to Work for NHS Patients and Staff.* London, HMSO.
NHS Executive (1999) *NHS Primary Care Walk-in Centres.* London, HMSO.
Nursing Times (NT) and NHS Executive (1998) *Clinical Effectiveness for Nurses, Midwives and Health Visitors.* London, *NT Books* and NHS Executive.
Office of Economic and Cultural Development (1997) *The World in 2020: Towards a Global Age.* Paris, OECD.
Rogers, A., Hassell, K. and Nicolaas, G. (1999) *Demanding Patients? Analysing the Use of Primary Care.* Buckingham, Open University Press.
Royce, R. (2000) *Primary Care and the NHS Reforms: A Manager's View.* London, Office of Health Economics.
Townsend, P., Davidson, N. and Whitehead, M. (1990) *Inequalities in Health – The Black Report, the Health Divide.* London, Penguin.
Trent Health (1993) *Every Nurses' Business: The Nursing, Midwifery and Health Visiting Contribution to the Achievement of the Trent Strategy for Health and the Health of the Nation.* Leicester, Trent Health.
United Kingdom Central Council for Nursing, Midwifery and Health Visiting (1992) *The Scope of Professional Practice.* London, UKCC.
Warner, M. (1997) *Health Systems and Primary Care for the 21st Century.* Geneva, WHO.
Warner, M., Longley, M., Gould, E. and Picek, A. (1998) *Health Care Futures 2010.* Cardiff, Welsh Institute for Health and Social Science.
Whitehead, M. (1987) *The Health Divide. Inequalities in Health in the 1980s.* London, HEA.
World Health Organization, Regional Office for Europe (WHO) (1996) Third Consultation on Future Trends and the European HFA Strategy. Copenhagen, WHO.

Index

Page numbers in **bold** refer to figures; those in *italic* to tables